ROLE
DEVELOPMENT

in Professional Nursing Practice

The Pedagogy

Role Development in Professional Nursing Practice, Third Edition drives comprehension through various strategies that meet the learning needs of students, while also generating enthusiasm about the topic. This interactive approach addresses different learning styles, making this the ideal text to ensure mastery of key concepts. The pedagogical aids that appear in most chapters include the following:

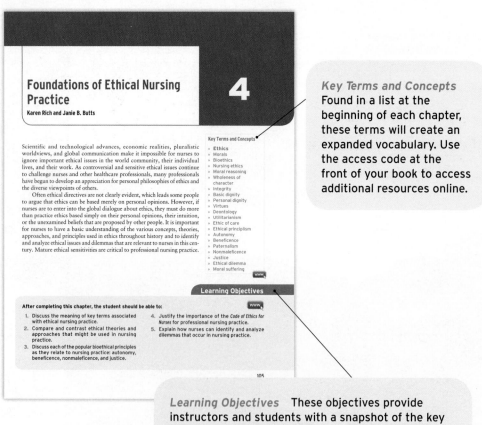

Key Terms and Concepts Found in a list at the beginning of each chapter, these terms will create an expanded vocabulary. Use the access code at the front of your book to access additional resources online.

Learning Objectives These objectives provide instructors and students with a snapshot of the key information they will encounter in each chapter. They serve as a checklist to help guide and focus study. Objectives can also be found within the text's online resources.

Case Studies Case studies encourage active learning and promote critical thinking skills in learners. Students can read about real-life scenarios, and then analyze the situation they are presented with. Complete questions online using the access code in the front of your book.

Critical Thinking Questions Review key concepts with these questions in each chapter. Review these questions online and submit your answers directly to your professor.

Classroom Activities Each chapter includes classroom activities that focus on how the information in the text applies to everyday practice. Students can answer questions in a group or as individuals. Activities can also be found within the text's online resources.

indications, patient preferences, quality of life, and contextual features (Jonsen et al., 2006). Nurses and other healthcare professionals on the team gather information in an attempt to answer the questions in each of the four boxes.

The Four Topics Method promotes a dialogue among the patient, family, and members of the healthcare ethics team. Each patient's case is unique and should be considered as such, but the subject matter concerning the dilemma involves common threads among cases, such as withdrawing or withholding treatment and right to life. Applicability of the four fundamental bioethical principles—autonomy, beneficence, nonmaleficence, and justice—is considered along with data generated by using the Four Topics Method in analyzing a patient's case. In Table 4-1, each box includes principles appropriate for each of the four topics. The additional principles of fairness and loyalty are included in the contextual features section.

CASE STUDY ▪ MS. CRANFORD

You are a student nurse who is caring for Ms. Cranford. She is an 87-year-old mentally competent woman who has lived alone since her husband died 10 years ago. She was admitted to the hospital with chest pain, feeling faint, a pulse of 48, and a blood pressure of 98/56. The physician and nurses stabilized Ms. Cranford with medications and intravenous fluids but later informed Ms. Cranford and her only son that she would need a heart pacemaker to regulate her heartbeat. After the physician explained the procedure for a long while before discussing it with her son and the physician. Her medical history includes long-term adult-onset diabetes, chronic renal failure, and arterial insufficiency. She feels very tired. She decides that she does not want a pacemaker. Once Ms. Cranford tells her son her wishes, he is quite upset, and thus, he meets with the physician to discuss the options. The physician and Ms. Cranford's son revisited this issue with her in an attempt to persuade her to change her mind, but she continues to refuse the recommended treatment. She and her son argue. The physician tries to explain to

She feels as if they are "ganging up" on her. Once the registered nurse becomes aware of the problem, you and the nurse visit with Ms. Cranford and son to assess and evaluate the ethical issues involved with her case.

Case Study Questions
Imagine that you are a nurse on the ethics committee consulted about Ms. Cranford's case. Answer the following questions:

1. What are the central ethical issues and questions in this case?
2. Which principles are in conflict in this case?
3. What did the physician mean by "best interest" for Ms. Cranford?
4. Use the Four Topics Method to discuss issues, to identify additional information that might be needed, and to analyze this case. What are your recommendations on behalf of the ethics committee?
5. What is the role of the nurses caring for Ms. Cranford in resolving this situation with other healthcare providers, her son?

merely on subjective preferences or judgments of happiness. Commonsense ethical directives agreed upon by groups of people are usually applied.

▪ **Ethic of Care**

The ethic of care has a history in feminist ethics, which has a focus in the moral experiences of women. In the ethic of care approach, personal relationships and relationship responsibilities are emphasized. Important concepts in this approach are compassion, empathy, sympathy, concern for others, and caring for others. Carol Gilligan with her study on gender differences in moral development (see the Moral Reasoning section earlier in this chapter) has had an influence on the ethic of care approach.

People who uphold the ethic of care think in terms of particular situations and individual contexts, not in terms of impersonal universal rules and principles. In resolving moral conflicts and understanding a complex situation, a person must use critical thinking to inquire about relationships, circumstances, and the problem at hand. The situation must be brought to light with "caring, consideration, understanding, generosity, sympathy, helpfulness, and a willingness to assume responsibility" (Munson, 2004, p. 788).

▪ **Ethical Principlism**

Ethical principlism, a popular approach to ethics in health care, involves using a set of ethical principles that is drawn from the common or widely shared conception of morality. The four principles that are most commonly used in bioethics are autonomy, beneficence, nonmaleficence, and justice. In 1979, Tom Beauchamp and James Childress published the first edition of *Principles of Biomedical Ethics*, which featured these four principles. Currently, the book is in its sixth edition, and the four principles have become an essential foundation for analyzing and resolving bioethical problems.

These principles, which are closely associated with rule-based ethics, provide a framework to support moral behavior and decision making. However, the principles neither form a theory nor provide a well-defined decision-making model. The framework of principlism provides a prima facie model. As a prima facie model, principles are applied based on rules and justifications for moral behavior. Often, more than one principle is relevant in ethical situations, and no conflict occurs. However, if relevant principles conflict in any situation, judgment must be used in weighing which principle should take precedence in guiding actions.

CRITICAL THINKING QUESTIONS ▪
Think about the ethical theories and approaches discussed in this section and think about moral conflicts you have experienced in the past. Have you used one of these approaches to resolve a conflict? Which approach or approaches have you used?

The four principles that are most commonly used in bioethics are autonomy, beneficence, nonmaleficence, and justice.

Classroom Activity: Nursing School Survival Game

Before class the instructor will prepare the board game. Spaces on the board will reflect self-care activities and give instructions for moving forward or backward depending on whether the activity reflected in the space promotes self-care or is detrimental. Divide students into small groups to play the Nursing School Survival Game. Students roll the dice to determine how many spaces to move. As they move around the board, they will progress from nursing school admission to second semester, third semester, fourth semester, and then graduation.

As the groups land on different spaces, take time to discuss the self-care activity and why it will help them to be successful in nursing school. Activities might include things such as buying a planner to get organized, reading assignments before class, finding a study group, getting regular exercise, eating nutritious meals,

and employing specific stress management techniques. This game is a good one to use at the beginning of the first semester to help students get to know one another as well as discuss ways in which students can begin using self-care strategies from the very beginning of their nursing school career.

Spaces on the board may alternately reflect categories if verbal questions will be asked during the game. If this approach is used, the group will answer questions about self-care categories to progress around the board. Another approach to this game that is fun is to have different colored pieces of paper labeled as categories of self-care questions on the floor, creating a game board effect and letting the students (either alone or in groups) move around the "game board" as they answer questions related to self-care.

References

American Association of Colleges of Nursing. (2002). *White paper on the professional practice setting*. Retrieved from http://www.aacn.nche.edu/Publications/positions/hallmarks.htm

Covey, S. R. (1989). *The 7 habits of highly effective people*. New York, NY: Simon & Schuster.

Joel, L. A. (2003). Career management. In L. A. Joel (Ed.), *Kelly's dimensions of professional nursing* (9th ed.). New York, NY: McGraw-Hill.

Massachusetts Department of Higher Education. (2010). *Nurse of the future: Nursing core competencies*. Retrieved from http://www.mass.edu/currentinit/documents/NursingCoreCompetencies.pdf

Miller, T. W. (2003). Work versus career. In T. W. Miller (Ed.), *Building and managing a career in nursing*. Indianapolis, IN: Sigma Theta Tau International.

Oxford University Press. (1996). *The Oxford English dictionary*. New York, NY: Oxford University Press.

Riley, J. B. (2004). Feedback. In J. B. Riley (Ed.), *Communication in nursing* (5th ed.). St. Louis, MO: Mosby.

THE INTEGRATED TEACHING AND LEARNING PACKAGE

Welcome to *Role Development in Professional Nursing Practice, Third Edition*. To help meet the changing needs of today's faculty and students, this text has been fully integrated with a suite of instructor and student ancillaries, helping instructors teach more efficiently and students learn more effectively.

STUDENT RESOURCES

The access code at the front of your book, specifically designed to accompany *Role Development in Professional Nursing Practice, Third Edition*, offers students a valuable integration of the text and online study tools, including:

- Interactive Glossary
- Flashcards
- Crossword
- Learning Objectives
- Critical Thinking Questions
- Case Studies
- Classroom Activities
- Web Links

Learn More About Student Resources Online:
http://www.jblearning.com

INSTRUCTOR RESOURCES

- **Test Bank**–Customize quizzes and tests that can be printed or administered online.

- **PowerPoint Presentations**–Modify pre-made classroom presentations and use them in your course.

- **Sample Syllabus**–Save time preparing course plans with this helpful guide.

- **Sample Professional Development Assignments**–Implement these assignments in your course to develop critical thinking skills in students.

Third Edition

ROLE DEVELOPMENT

in Professional Nursing Practice

Edited by

KATHLEEN MASTERS, DNS, RN

Associate Professor
University of Southern Mississippi
College of Nursing
Hattiesburg, Mississippi

JONES & BARTLETT
LEARNING

World Headquarters
5 Wall Street
Burlington, MA 01803
978-443-5000
info@jblearning.com
www.jblearning.com

Jones & Bartlett Learning books and products are available through most bookstores and online booksellers. To contact Jones & Bartlett Learning directly, call 800-832-0034, fax 978-443-8000, or visit our website, www.jblearning.com.

Substantial discounts on bulk quantities of Jones & Bartlett Learning publications are available to corporations, professional associations, and other qualified organizations. For details and specific discount information, contact the special sales department at Jones & Bartlett Learning via the above contact information or send an email to specialsales@jblearning.com.

Role Development in Professional Nursing Practice, Third Edition is an independent publication and has not been authorized, sponsored, or otherwise approved by the owners of the trademarks or service marks referenced in this product.

Some images in this book feature models. These models do not necessarily endorse, represent, or participate in the activities represented in the images.

The authors, editor, and publisher have made every effort to provide accurate information. However, they are not responsible for errors, omissions, or for any outcomes related to the use of the contents of this book and take no responsibility for the use of the products and procedures described. Treatments and side effects described in this book may not be applicable to all people; likewise, some people may require a dose or experience a side effect that is not described herein. Drugs and medical devices are discussed that may have limited availability controlled by the Food and Drug Administration (FDA) for use only in a research study or clinical trial. Research, clinical practice, and government regulations often change the accepted standard in this field. When consideration is being given to use of any drug in the clinical setting, the health care provider or reader is responsible for determining FDA status of the drug, reading the package insert, and reviewing prescribing information for the most up-to-date recommendations on dose, precautions, and contraindications, and determining the appropriate usage for the product. This is especially important in the case of drugs that are new or seldom used.

Production Credits

Executive Publisher: Kevin Sullivan
Acquisitions Editor: Amanda Harvey
Editorial Assistant: Sara Bempkins
Associate Production Editor: Sara Fowles
Marketing Communications Manager: Katie Hennessy
V.P., Manufacturing and Inventory Control: Therese Connell

Composition: diacriTech
Cover Design: Kristin E. Parker
Cover Image: © Anton Petrus/ShutterStock; Inc.
Printing and Binding: Courier Companies
Cover Printing: Courier Companies

To order this product, use ISBN: 978-1-4496-9150-9

Library of Congress Cataloging-in-Publication Data
Role development in professional nursing practice / [edited by] Kathleen Masters. — 3rd ed.
p. ; cm.
Includes bibliographical references and index.
ISBN 978-1-4496-8198-2 (pbk.)
I. Masters, Kathleen.
[DNLM: 1. Nursing—standards. 2. Nursing—trends. 3. Nurse's Role. 4. Philosophy, Nursing. 5. Professional Practice. WY 16]
610.73—dc23
                            2012031815
6048

Printed in the United States of America
17 16 15 14   10 9 8 7 6 5

Dedication

*This book is dedicated to my Heavenly Father
and to my loving family: my husband, Eddie, and
my two daughters, Rebecca and Rachel. Words
cannot express my appreciation for their ongoing
encouragement and support throughout my career.*

Contents

7 Career Management and Care of the Professional Self   167
Luann M. Daggett

UNIT II: PROFESSIONAL NURSING PRACTICE AND THE MANAGEMENT OF PATIENT CARE   194

8 The Healthcare Delivery System and the Role of the Professional Nurse   195
Sharon Vincent

9 Critical Thinking and Clinical Judgment in Professional Nursing   217
Jill Rushing

14 Informatics and Technology in Professional Nursing Practice 325
Cathy K. Hughes

15 Future Directions in Professional Nursing Practice 349
Katherine Elizabeth Nugent

Preface

Although the process of professional development is a lifelong journey, it is a journey that begins in earnest during the time of academic preparation. The goal of this book is to provide nursing students with a road map to help guide them along their journey as a professional nurse.

This book is organized into two units. The chapters in the first unit focus on the foundational concepts that are essential to the development of the individual professional nurse. The chapters in Unit II address issues related to professional nursing practice and the management of patient care.

The chapters included in Unit I provide the student nurse with a basic foundation in areas such as nursing history, theory, philosophy, ethics, socialization into the nursing role, and the social context of nursing. Also included in Unit I is content related to the care of the professional self and career development in nursing.

The chapters in Unit II are more directly related to patient care issues. Included are topics such as patient education, ethical issues in nursing practice, the law as it relates to patient care and nursing, clinical judgment, informatics and technology, and evidence-based nursing practice. Unit II concludes with a chapter addressing future directions in professional nursing practice.

New to the third edition is the incorporation of the *Nurse of the Future: Nursing Core Competencies* throughout each chapter. The *Nurse of the Future: Nursing Core Competencies* "emanate from the foundation of nursing knowledge" (Massachusetts Department of Higher Education, 2010, p. 4) and are based on the American Association of Colleges of Nursing *Essentials of Baccalaureate Education for Professional Nursing Practice*, National League for Nursing Council of Associate Degree Nursing competencies, Institute of Medicine recommendations, Quality and Safety Education for Nursing competencies, and American Nurses Association standards, as well as other professional organization standards and recommendations. The 10 competencies included in the model include patient-centered care, professionalism, informatics and technology, evidence-based practice, leadership, systems-based practice, safety, communication, teamwork and collaboration, and quality improvement. Essential knowledge, skills, and attitudes (KSA), reflecting cognitive, affective, and psychomotor learning domains, are specified for each competency. The KSA identified in the model reflect the expectations for initial nursing practice following the completion of a prelicensure professional nursing education program (Massachusetts Department of Higher Education, 2010, p. 4).

The *Nurse of the Future: Nursing Core Competencies* graphic illustrates through the use of broken lines the reciprocal and continuous relationship between each of the competencies and nursing knowledge, that the competencies can overlap and are not mutually exclusive, and that all competencies are of equal importance. In addition, nursing knowledge is placed as the core in the graphic to illustrate that nursing knowledge reflects the overarching art and science of professional nursing practice (Massachusetts Department of Higher Education, 2010, p. 4).

This new edition has competency boxes throughout the chapters that link examples of the knowledge, skills, and attitudes (KSA) appropriate to the chapter content to *Nurse of the Future: Nursing Core Competencies* required of entry-level professional nurses. The competency model in its entirety is available online at www.mass.edu/currentinit/documents/NursingCoreCompetencies.pdf.

This new edition also contains more case studies with questions, which is congruent with Benner, Sutphen, Leonard, and Day's (2010) Carnegie Report recommendations that nursing educators teach for "situated cognition" using narrative strategies to lead to "situated action," thus increasing the clinical connection in our teaching or that we teach for "clinical salience." Although the topics included in this textbook are not inclusive of all that could be discussed in relationship to the broad theme of role development in professional nursing practice, it is my prayer that the subjects herein make a contribution to the profession of nursing by providing the student with a solid foundation and a desire to grow as a professional nurse throughout the journey that we call a professional nursing career. Let the journey begin.

Kathleen Masters

References

Benner, P., Sutphen, M., Leonard, V., & Day, L. (2010). *Educating nurses: A call for radical transformation.* San Francisco, CA: Jossey-Bass.

Massachusetts Department of Higher Education. (2010). *Nurse of the future: Nursing core competencies.* Retrieved from http://www.mass.edu/currentinit/documents/NursingCoreCompetencies.pdf

Contributors

Janie B. Butts, DSN, RN
University of Southern Mississippi
College of Nursing
Hattiesburg, Mississippi

Luann M. Daggett, DSN, RN
Brentwood, Tennessee

Kathleen Driscoll, JD, MS, RN
University of Cincinnati
College of Nursing
Cincinnati, Ohio

Rowena W. Elliott, PhD, RN, FAAN
University of Southern Mississippi
College of Nursing
Hattiesburg, Mississippi

Melanie Gilmore, PhD, RN
University of Southern Mississippi
College of Nursing
Meridian, Mississippi

Cathy K. Hughes, DNP, RN
University of Southern Mississippi
College of Nursing
Hattiesburg, Mississippi

Karen Saucier Lundy, PhD, RN, FAAN
Professor Emeritus
University of Southern Mississippi
College of Nursing
Hattiesburg, Mississippi

Evadna Lyons, PhD, RN
East Central Community College
School of Nursing
Decatur, Mississippi

Katherine Elizabeth Nugent, PhD, RN
Dean, College of Nursing
University of Southern Mississippi
Hattiesburg, Mississippi

Karen Rich, PhD, RN
University of Southern Mississippi
College of Nursing
Long Beach, Mississippi

Jill Rushing, MSN, RN
University of Southern Mississippi
College of Nursing
Hattiesburg, Mississippi

Mary W. Stewart, PhD, RN
Director of PhD Program
University of Mississippi Medical Center
School of Nursing
Jackson, Mississippi

Sharon Vincent, DNP, RN, CNOR
University of Southern Mississippi
College of Nursing
Hattiesburg, Mississippi

UNIT I

Foundations of Professional Nursing Practice

A History of Health Care and Nursing

Karen Saucier Lundy

1

Although no specialized nurse role per se developed in early civilizations, human cultures recognized the need for nursing care. The truly sick person was weak and helpless and could not fulfill the duties that were normally expected of a member of the community. In such cases, someone had to watch over the patient, nurse him or her, and provide care. In most societies, this nurse role was filled by a family member, usually female. As in most cultures, the childbearing woman had special needs that often resulted in a specialized role for the caregiver. Every society since the dawn of time had someone to nurse and take care of the mother and infant around the childbearing events. In whatever form the nurse took, the role was associated with compassion, health promotion, and kindness (Bullough & Bullough, 1978).

Learning Objectives

After completing this chapter, the student should be able to:

1. Identify social, political, and economic influences on the development of professional nursing practice.

2. Identify important leaders and events that have significantly affected the development of professional nursing practice.

Classical Era

More than 4,000 years ago, Egyptian physicians and nurses used an abundant pharmacological repertoire to cure the ill and injured. The Ebers Papyrus lists more than 700 remedies for ailments ranging from snakebites to puerperal fever. The Kahun Papyrus (circa 1850 B.C.) identified suppositories (e.g., crocodile feces) that could be used for contraception (Kalisch & Kalisch, 1986). Healing appeared in the Egyptian culture as the successful result of

Key Terms and Concepts

» **Greek era**
» Roman era
» Deaconesses
» Florence Nightingale
» Black Death
» Edward Jenner
» Louis Pasteur

Note: This chapter is adapted from Lundy, K. S., & Bender, K. W. (2009). History of community health and public health nursing. In K. S. Lundy & S. Janes (Eds.), *Community health nursing: Caring for the public's health* (2nd ed.). Sudbury, MA: Jones and Bartlett.

a contest between invisible beings of good and evil (Shryock, 1959). The physician was not a shaman; instead there was specialization and separation of function, with physicians, priests, and sorcerers all practicing separately and independently. Some clients would consult the physician, some the shaman, and others sought healing from magical formulas. Many tried all three approaches. The Egyptians, quite notably, did not accept illness and death as inevitable but believed that life could be prolonged indefinitely. Because Egyptians blended medicine and magic, the concoctions believed to be the most effective were often bizarre and repulsive by today's standards. For example, lizard's blood, swine's ears and teeth, putrid meat and fat, tortoise brains, the milk of a lactating woman, the urine of a chaste woman, and excreta of donkeys and lions were frequently used ingredients. At least some explanation for these odd ingredients can be found in the following: "These pharmacological mixtures were intended to sicken and drive out the intruding demon which was thought to cause the disease. Drugs containing fecal matter were in fact used until the end of the 1700s in Europe as common practice" (Kalisch & Kalisch, 1986).

As early as 3000 to 1400 B.C., the Minoans created ways to flush water and construct drainage systems. Around 1000 B.C., the Egyptians constructed elaborate drainage systems, developed pharmaceutical herbs and preparations, and embalmed the dead. The Hebrews formulated an elaborate hygiene code that dealt with laws governing both personal and community hygiene, such as contagion, disinfection, and sanitation through the preparation of food and water. Hebrews, although few in number, exercised great influence in the development of religious and health doctrine. According to Bullough and Bullough (1978), most of their genius was religious, giving birth to both Christianity and Islam. The Jewish contribution to public health is greater in sanitation than in their concept of disease. Garbage and excreta were disposed of outside the city or camp, infectious diseases were quarantined, spitting was outlawed as unhygienic, and bodily cleanliness became a prerequisite for moral purity. Although many of the Hebrew ideas about hygiene were Egyptian in origin, Moses and the Hebrews were the first to codify them and link them with spiritual godliness. Their notion of disease was rooted in the "disease as God's punishment for sin" idea.

The civilization that grew up between the Tigris and Euphrates Rivers is known geographically as Mesopotamia (modern Iraq) and includes the Sumerians. Disease and disability in the Mesopotamian area, at least in the earlier period, were considered a great curse, a divine punishment for grievous acts against the gods. Having such a curse of illness resulting from sin did not exactly put the sick person in a valued status in the society. Experiencing illness as punishment for a sin linked the sick person to anything even remotely deviant; such acts as murder, perjury, adultery, and drunkenness could be the identified sins. Not only was the person suffering from the illness, but he or she also was branded by all of society as having deserved it. The illness made the sin apparent to all; the sick person was isolated and disgraced. Those who obeyed God's law lived in health and happiness. Those who transgressed the law were punished, with illness and suffering thought to be consequences. The sick person then had to make atonement for the sins, enlist a priest or other spiritual healer to lift the spell or curse, or live with the illness to its ultimate outcome. In simple terms, the person had to get right with the gods or live with the consequences (Bullough & Bullough, 1978). Nursing care by a family member or relative would be needed in any case, regardless of the outcome of the sin, curse, disease-atonement-recovery, or death cycle. This logic became the basis for explanation of why some people "get sick and some don't" for many centuries and still persists to some degree in most cultures today.

■ The Greeks and Health

In Greek mythology, the god of medicine, Asclepias, cured disease. One of his daughters, Hygeia, from whom we derive the word *hygiene*, was the goddess of preventive health and protected humans from disease. Panacea, Asclepias' other daughter, was known as the all-healing "universal remedy," and today her name is used to describe any ultimate cure-all in medicine. She was known as the "light" of the day, and her name was invoked and shrines built to her during times of epidemics (Brooke, 1997).

During the **Greek era**, Hippocrates of Cos emphasized the rational treatment of sickness as a natural rather than god-inflicted phenomenon. Hippocrates (460–370 B.C.) is considered the father of medicine because of his arrangements of the oral and written remedies and diseases, which had long been secrets held by priests and religious healers, into a textbook of medicine that was used for centuries (Bullough & Bullough, 1978). Hippocrates' contribution to the science of public health was his recognition that making accurate observations of and drawing general conclusions from actual phenomena formed the basis of sound medical reasoning (Shryock, 1959).

In Greek society, health was considered to result from a balance between mind and body. Hippocrates wrote a most important book, *Air, Water and Places*, which detailed the relationship between humans and the environment. This is considered a milestone in the eventual development of the science of epidemiology as the first such treatise on the connectedness of the web of life. This topic of the relationship between humans and their environment did not reoccur until the development of bacteriology in the late 1800s (Rosen, 1958).

Perhaps the idea that most damaged the practice and scientific theory of medicine and health for centuries was the doctrine of the four humors, first spoken of by Empedodes

> Hippocrates wrote a most important book, *Air, Water and Places*, which detailed the relationship between humans and the environment. This is considered a milestone in the eventual development of the science of epidemiology as the first such treatise on the connectedness of the web of life.

of Acragas (493–433 B.C.). Empedodes was a philosopher and a physician, and as a result, he synthesized his cosmological ideas with his medical theory. He believed that the same four elements (or "roots of things") that made up the universe were found in humans and in all animate beings (Bullough & Bullough, 1978). Empedodes believed that man was a microcosm, a small world within the macrocosm, or external environment. The four humors of the body (blood, bile, phlegm, and black bile) corresponded to the four elements of the larger world (fire, air, water, and earth) (Kalisch & Kalisch, 1986). Depending on the prevailing humor, a person was sanguine, choleric, phlegmatic, or melancholic. Because of this strongly held and persistent belief in the connection between the balance of the four humors and health status, treatment was aimed at restoring the appropriate balance of the four humors through the control of their corresponding elements. Through manipulating the two sets of opposite qualities—hot and cold, wet and dry—balance was the goal of the intervention. Fire was hot and dry, air was hot and wet, water was cold and wet, and earth was cold and dry. For example, if a person had a fever, cold compresses would be prescribed for a chill and the person would be warmed. Such doctrine gave rise to faulty and ineffective treatment of disease that influenced medical education for many years (Taylor, 1922).

Plato, in *The Republic*, details the importance of recreation, a balanced mind and body, nutrition, and exercise. A distinction was made among sex, class, and health as early as the Greek era; only males of the aristocracy could afford the luxury of maintaining a healthful lifestyle (Rosen, 1958).

In *The Iliad*, a poem about the attempts to capture Troy and rescue Helen from her lover Paris, 140 different wounds are described. The mortality rate averaged 77.6%, the highest as a result of sword and spear thrusts and the lowest from superficial arrow wounds. There was considerable need for nursing care, and Achilles, Patroclus, and other princes often acted as nurses to the injured. The early stages of Greek medicine reflected the influences of Egyptian, Babylonian, and Hebrew medicine. Therefore, good medical and nursing techniques were used to treat these war wounds: The arrow was drawn or cut out, the wound washed, soothing herbs applied, and the wound bandaged. However, in sickness in which no wound occurred, an evil spirit was considered the cause. For example, the cause of the plague was unknown, so the question became how and why affected soldiers had angered the gods. According to *The Iliad*, the true healer of the plague was the prophet who prayed for Apollo to stop shooting the "plague arrows." The Greeks applied rational causes and cures to external injuries, while internal ailments continued to be linked to spiritual maladies (Bullough & Bullough, 1978).

▪ Roman Era

During the rise and the fall of the **Roman era** (31 B.C.–A.D. 476), Greek culture continued to be a strong influence. The Romans easily adopted Greek culture and expanded the Greeks' accomplishments, especially in the fields of engineering, law, and government. The development of policy, law, and protection of the public's health was an important precursor to our modern public health systems. For Romans, the government had an obligation to protect its citizens, not only from outside aggression such as warring neighbors, but from inside the civilization, in the form of health laws. According to Bullough and Bullough (1978), Rome was essentially a "Greek cultural colony" (p. 20).

During the third century B.C., Rome began to dominate the Mediterranean, Egypt, the Tigris-Euphrates Valley, the Hebrews, and the Greeks (Boorstin, 1985). Greek science and Roman engineering then spread throughout the ancient world, providing a synthesized Greco-Roman foundation for eventual public health policies (Bullough & Bullough, 1978).

Galen of Pergamum (A.D. 129–199), often known as the greatest Greek physician after Hippocrates, left for Rome after studying medicine in Greece and Egypt and gained great fame as a medical practitioner, lecturer, and experimenter. In his lifetime, medicine evolved into a science; he submitted traditional healing practices to experimentation and was possibly the greatest medical researcher before the 1600s (Bullough & Bullough, 1978). He was considered the last of the great physicians of antiquity (Kalisch & Kalisch, 1986).

The Greek physicians and healers certainly made the most contributions to medicine, but the Romans surpassed the Greeks in promoting the evolution of nursing. Roman armies developed the notion of a mobile war nursing unit because their battles took them far from home where they could be cared for by wives and family. This portable hospital was a series of tents arranged in corridors; as battles wore on, these tents gave way to buildings that became permanent convalescent camps at the battle sites (Rosen, 1958). Many of these early military hospitals have been excavated by archaeologists along the banks of the Rhine and Danube Rivers. They had wards, recreation areas, baths, pharmacies, and even rooms for officers who needed a "rest cure" (Bullough & Bullough, 1978). Coexisting were the Greek dispensary forms of temples, or the *iatreia*, which started out as a type of physician waiting room. These eventually developed into a primitive type of hospital, places for surgical clients to stay until they could be taken home by their families. Although nurses during the Roman era were usually family members, servants, or slaves, nursing had strengthened its position in medical care and emerged during the Roman era as a separate and distinct specialty.

The Romans developed massive aqueducts, bathhouses, and sewer systems during this era. At the height of the Roman Empire, Rome provided 40 gallons of water per person per day to its 1 million inhabitants, which is comparable to our rates of consumption today (Rosen, 1958). Even though these engineering feats were remarkable at the

> **The Greek physicians and healers certainly made the most contributions to medicine, but the Romans surpassed the Greeks in promoting the evolution of nursing.**

time, poorer and less fortunate residents often did not benefit from the same level of public health amenities, such as sewer systems and latrines (Bullough & Bullough, 1978). However, the Romans did provide many of their citizens with what we would consider public health services.

Middle Ages

Many of the advancements of the Greco-Roman era were reversed during the Middle Ages (A.D. 476–1453) after the decline of the Roman Empire. The Middle Ages, or the medieval era, served as a transition between ancient and modern civilizations. Once again, myth, magic, and religion were explanations and cures for illness and health problems. The medieval world was the result of a fusion of three streams of thought, actions, and ways of life— Greco-Roman, Germanic, and Christian—into one (Donahue, 1985). Nursing was most influenced by Christianity with the beginning of **deaconesses**, or female servants, doing the work of God by ministering to the needs of others. Deacons in the early Christian churches were apparently available only to care for men, while deaconesses cared for the needs of women. The role of deaconesses in the church was considered a forward step in the development of nursing and in the 1800s would strongly influence the young **Florence Nightingale**. During this era, Roman military hospitals were replaced by civilian ones. In early Christianity, the *Diakonia*, a kind of combination outpatient and welfare office, was managed by deacons and deaconesses and served as the equivalent of a hospital. Jesus served as the example of charity and compassion for the poor and marginal of society.

Communicable diseases were rampant during the Middle Ages, primarily because of the walled cities that emerged in response to the paranoia and isolation of the populations. Infection was next to impossible to control. Physicians had little to offer, deferring to the Church for management of disease. Nursing roles were carried out primarily by religious orders.

The oldest hospital (other than military hospitals in the Roman era) in Europe was most likely the Hôtel-Dieu in Lyons, France, founded about 542 by Childebert I, king of France. The Hôtel-Dieu in Paris was founded around 652 by Saint Landry, bishop of Paris. During the Middle Ages, charitable institutions, hospitals, and medical schools increased in number, with the religious leaders as caregivers. The word *hospital*, which is derived from the Latin word *hospitalis*, meaning service of guests, was most likely more of a shelter for travelers and other pilgrims as well as the occasional person who needed extra care (Kalisch & Kalisch, 1986). Early European hospitals were more like hospices or homes for the aged, sick pilgrims, or orphans. Nurses in these early hospitals were religious deaconesses who chose to care for others in a life of servitude and spiritual sacrifice.

■ Black Death

During the Middle Ages, a series of horrible epidemics, including the **Black Death** or bubonic plague, ravaged the civilized world (Diamond, 1997). In the 1300s, Europe, Asia, and Africa saw nearly half their populations lost to the bubonic plague. According to Bullough and Bullough (1978), an interesting account of the arrival of the bubonic plague in 1347 claims that the disease started in the Genoese colony of Kaffa in the Crimea. The story passed down through the ages is that the city was besieged by a Mongol khan. When the disease broke out among the khan's men, he catapulted the bodies of its victims into Kaffa to infect and weaken his enemies. The soldiers and colonists of Kaffa carried the disease back to Genoa. Worldwide, more than 60 million deaths were eventually attributed to this horrible plague. In some parts of Europe, only one-fourth of the population survived, with some places having too few survivors alive to bury the dead. Families abandoned sick children, and the sick were often left to die alone (Cartwright, 1972).

Nurses and physicians were powerless to avert the disease. Black spots and tumors on the skin appeared, and petechiae and hemorrhages gave the skin a darkened appearance. There was also acute inflammation of the lungs, burning sensations, unquenchable thirst, and inflammation of the entire body. Hardly anyone afflicted survived the third day of the attack. So great was the fear of contagion that ships carrying bodies of infected persons were set to sail without a crew to drift from port to port through the North, Black, and Mediterranean Seas with their dead passengers (Cohen, 1989).

Bubonic plague is caused by the bacillus *Yersinia pestis* (formerly *Pasteurella pestis*), which is usually transmitted by the bite of a flea carried by an animal vector, typically a rat. After the initial flea bite, the infection spreads through the lymph nodes and the nodes swell to enormous size; the inflamed nodes are called bubos, from which the bubonic plague derives its name. Medieval people knew that this disease was in some way communicable, but they were unsure of the mode of transmission (Diamond, 1997); hence the avoidance of victims and a reliance on isolation techniques. The practice of quarantine in city ports was developed as a preventive measure and is still used today (Bullough & Bullough, 1978; Kalisch & Kalisch, 1986).

The Renaissance

During the rebirth of Europe, great political, social, and economic advances occurred along with a tremendous revival of learning. Donahue (1985) contends that the Renaissance has been "viewed as both a blessing and a curse" (p. 188). There was a renewed interest in the arts and sciences, which helped advance medical science (Boorstin, 1985; Bullough & Bullough, 1978). Columbus and other explorers discovered new worlds, and belief in a sun-centered rather than earth-centered universe was promoted by Copernicus (1473–1543). Sir Isaac Newton's (1642–1727) theory of gravity changed the world forever. Gunpowder was introduced, and social and religious upheavals resulted in the American and French Revolutions at the end of the 1700s. In the arts and sciences, Leonardo da Vinci, known as one of "the greatest geniuses of all time," made a number of anatomic drawings based on dissection experiences. These drawings have become classics in the progression of knowledge about the human anatomy. Many artists of this time left an indelible mark and continue to exert influence today, including Michelangelo, Raphael, and Titian (Donahue, 1985).

The Advancement of Science and Health of the Public

> **It took the first 50 years of the 1700s for the new knowledge from the Enlightenment to be organized and digested.**

It took the first 50 years of the 1700s for the new knowledge from the Enlightenment to be organized and digested, according to Donahue (1985). In Britain, **Edward Jenner** discovered an effective method of vaccination against the dreaded smallpox virus in 1798. Psychiatry developed as a separate branch of medicine, and instruments that measured and allowed for assessment of the body such as the pulse watch and the stethoscope were invented.

One of the greatest scientists of this period was **Louis Pasteur** (1822–1895). A French chemist, Pasteur first became interested in pathogenic organisms through his studies of the diseases of wine. He discovered that if wine was heated to a temperature of 55°C to 60°C, the process killed the microorganisms that spoiled wine. This discovery of pasteurization was critical to the wine industry's success in France. Pasteur investigated many fields and saved many lives from the consequences of contaminated milk and food.

Joseph Lister (1827–1912) was a physician who set out to decrease the mortality resulting from infection after surgery. He used Pasteur's research to eventually arrive at a chemical antiseptic solution of carbolic acid for use in surgery. Widely regarded as the father of modern surgery, he practiced his antiseptic surgery with great results, and the Listerian principles of asepsis changed the way physicians and nurses practice to this day (Dietz & Lehozky, 1963). **Robert Koch** (1843–1910), a physician known for his research on anthrax, is regarded as the father of microbiology. After identifying the organism that caused cholera, *Vibrio cholerae*, he also demonstrated its transmission by water, food, and clothing. **Edwin Klebs** (1834–1913) proved the germ theory, that is, that germs are the causes of infectious diseases. This discovery of the bacterial origin of diseases can be considered the greatest achievement of the 1800s. Although the microscope had been around for two centuries, it remained for Lister, Pasteur, and Koch—and ultimately Klebs—to provide the missing link (Dietz & Lehozky, 1963; Rosen, 1958).

The Emergence of Home Visiting

In 1633, **Saint Vincent de Paul** founded the Sisters of Charity in France, an order of nuns who traveled from home to home visiting the sick. As the services of the sisters grew, de Paul appointed Mademoiselle Le Gras as supervisor of these visitors. These nurses functioned as the first organized visiting nurse service, making home visits and caring for the sick in their homes. De Paul believed that for family members to go to the hospital was disruptive to family life and that taking nursing services to the home enabled health to be restored more effectively and more efficiently.

The Reformation

Religious changes during the Renaissance influenced nursing perhaps more than any other aspect of society. Particularly important was the rise of Protestantism as a result of the reform movements of Martin Luther (1483–1546) in Germany and John Calvin (1509–1564) in France and Geneva. Although the various sects were numerous in the Protestant movement, the agreement among the leaders was almost unanimous on the abolition of the monastic or cloistered career. The effects on nursing were drastic: Monastic-affiliated institutions, including hospitals and schools, were closed, and orders of nuns, including nurses, were dissolved. Even in countries where Catholicism flourished, royal leaders seized monasteries frequently.

> **Religious changes during the Renaissance influenced nursing perhaps more than any other aspect of society.**

Religious leaders, such as Martin Luther, who led the **Reformation** in 1517, were well aware of the lack of adequate nursing care as a result of these sweeping changes. Luther advocated that each town establish something akin to a "community chest" to raise funds for hospitals and nurse visitors for the poor (Dietz & Lehozky, 1963). For example, in England, where there had been at least 450 charitable foundations before the Reformation, only a few survived the reign of Henry VIII, who closed most of the monastic hospitals (Donahue, 1985). Eventually, Henry VIII's son Edward VI, who reigned from 1547 to 1553, was convinced and did endow some hospitals, namely, St. Bartholomew's Hospital and St. Thomas' Hospital, which would eventually house the Nightingale School of Nursing later in the 1800s (Bullough & Bullough, 1978).

The Dark Period of Nursing

The last half of the period between 1500 and 1860 is widely regarded as the "dark period of nursing" because nursing conditions were at their worst (Donahue, 1985). Education for girls, which had been provided by the nuns in religious schools, was lost. Because of the elimination of hospitals and schools, there was no one to pass on knowledge about caring for the sick. As a result, the hospitals were managed and staffed by municipal authorities; women entering nursing service often came from illiterate classes, and even then there were too few to serve (Dietz & Lehozky, 1963). The lay attendants who filled the nursing role were illiterate, rough, inconsiderate, and often immoral and alcoholic. Intelligent women and men could not be persuaded to accept such a degraded and low-status position in the offensive municipal hospitals of London. Nursing slipped back into a role of servitude as menial, low-status work. According to Donahue (1985), when a woman could no longer make it as a gambler, prostitute, or thief, she might become a nurse. Eventually, women serving jail sentences for crimes such as prostitution and stealing were ordered to care for the sick in the hospitals instead of serving their sentences in the city jail (Dietz & Lehozky, 1963). The nurses of this era took bribes from clients, became inappropriately involved with them, and survived the best way they could, often at the expense of their assigned clients.

Nursing had, during this era, virtually no social standing or organization. Even Catholic sisters of the religious orders throughout Europe "came to a complete standstill" professionally because of the intolerance of society (Donahue, 1985, p. 231). Charles Dickens, in *Martin Chuzzlewit* (1844), created the enduring characters of Sairey Gamp and Betsy Prig. Sairey Gamp was a visiting nurse based on an actual hired attendant whom Dickens had met in a friend's home. Sairey Gamp was hired to care for sick family members but was instead cruel to her clients, stole from them, and ate their rations; she was an alcoholic and has been immortalized forever as a reminder of the world in which Florence Nightingale came of age (Donahue, 1985):

> She was a fat old woman, this Mrs. Gamp, with a husky voice and a moist eye, which she had a remarkable power of turning up and showing the white of it. Having very little neck, it cost her some trouble to look over herself, if one may say so, to those to whom she talked. She wore a very rusty black gown, rather the worse for snuff, and a shawl and bonnet to correspond…. The face of Mrs. Gamp—the nose in particular—was somewhat red and swollen, and it was difficult to enjoy her society without becoming conscious of the smell of spirits. Like most persons who have attained to great eminence in their profession, she took to hers very kindly; insomuch, that setting aside her natural predilections as a woman, she went to a lying-in [birth] or a laying-out [death] with equal zest and relish.
>
> —Charles Dickens, 1844

Early Organized Health Care in the Americas: A Brave New World

In the New World, the first hospital in the Americas, the Hospital de la Purisima Concepcion, was founded some time before 1524 by Hernando Cortez, the conqueror of Mexico. The first hospital in the continental United States was erected in Manhattan in 1658 for the care of sick soldiers and slaves. In 1717, a hospital for infectious diseases was built in Boston; the first hospital established by a private gift was the Charity Hospital in New Orleans. A sailor, Jean Louis, donated the endowment for the hospital's founding (Bullough & Bullough, 1978).

During the 1600s and 1700s, colonial hospitals with little resemblance to modern hospitals were often used to house the poor and downtrodden. Hospitals called "pesthouses" were created to care for clients with contagious diseases; their primary purpose was to protect the public at large, rather than to treat and care for the clients. Contagious diseases were rampant during the early years of the American colonies, often being spread by the large number of immigrants who brought these diseases with them on their long journey to America. Medicine was not as developed as in Europe, and nursing remained in the hands of the uneducated. By 1720, average life expectancy at birth was only around 35 years. Plagues were a constant nightmare, with outbreaks of smallpox and yellow fever. In 1751, the first true hospital in the new colonies, Pennsylvania Hospital, was erected in Philadelphia on the recommendation of Benjamin Franklin (Kalisch & Kalisch, 1986).

By today's standards, hospitals in the 1800s were disgraceful, dirty, unventilated, and contaminated by infections; to be a client in a hospital actually increased one's risk of dying. As in England, nursing was considered an inferior occupation. After the sweeping changes of the Reformation, educated religious health workers were replaced with lay people who were "down and outers," in prison, or had no option left but to work with the sick (Kalisch & Kalisch, 1986).

The Chadwick Report and the Shattuck Report

Edwin Chadwick became a major figure in the development of the field of public health in Great Britain by drawing attention to the cost of the unsanitary conditions that shortened the life span of the laboring class and threatened the wealth of Britain. Although the first sanitation legislation, which established a National Vaccination Board, was passed in 1837, Chadwick found in his classic study, *Report on an Inquiry into the Sanitary Conditions of the Laboring Population of Great Britain*, that death rates were high in large industrial cities such as Liverpool. A more startling finding, from what is often referred to simply as the **Chadwick Report**, was that more than half the children of labor-class workers died by age 5, indicating poor living conditions that affected the health of the most vulnerable. Laborers lived only half as long as the upper classes.

One consequence of the report was the establishment in 1848 of the first board of health, the General Board of Health for England (Richardson, 1887). More legislation followed that initiated social reform in the areas of child welfare, elder care, the sick, the mentally ill, factory health, and education. Soon sewers and fire plugs, based on an available water supply, appeared as indicators that the public health linkages from the Chadwick Report had an impact.

In the United States during the 1800s, waves of epidemics of yellow fever, smallpox, cholera, typhoid fever, and typhus continued to plague the population as in England and the rest of the world. As cities continued to grow in the industrialized young nation, poor workers crowded into larger cities and suffered from illnesses caused by the unsanitary living conditions (Hanlon & Pickett, 1984). Similar to Chadwick's classic study in England, Lemuel Shattuck, a Boston bookseller and publisher who had an interest in public health, organized the American Statistical Society in 1839 and issued a census of Boston in 1845. Shattuck's census revealed high infant mortality rates and high overall population mortality rates. In 1850, in his *Report of the Massachusetts Sanitary Commission*, Shattuck not only outlined his findings on the unsanitary conditions but made recommendations for public health reform that included the bookkeeping of population statistics and development of a monitoring system that would provide information to the public about environmental, food, and drug safety and infectious disease control (Rosen, 1958). He also called for services for well-child care, school-age children's health, immunizations, mental health, health education for all, and health planning. The **Shattuck Report** was revolutionary in its scope and vision for public health, but it was virtually ignored during Shattuck's lifetime. Nineteen years later, in 1869, the first state board of health was formed (Kalisch & Kalisch, 1986).

The Industrial Revolution

During the mid-1700s in England, capitalism emerged as an economic system based on profit. This emerging system resulted in mass production, as contrasted with the previous system of individual workers and craftsmen. In the simplest terms, the Industrial Revolution was the application of machine power to processes formerly done by hand. Machinery was invented during this era and ultimately standardized quality; individual craftsmen were forced to give up their crafts and lands and become factory laborers for the capitalist owners. All types of industries were affected; this new-found efficiency produced profit for owners of the means of production. Because of this, the era of invention flourished, factories grew, and people moved in record numbers to the work in the cities. Urban areas grew, tenement housing projects emerged, and overcrowding in cities seriously threatened individuals' well-being (Donahue, 1985).

Workers were forced to go to the machines, rather than the other way around. Such relocations meant giving up not only farming, but a way of life that had existed for centuries. The emphasis on profit over people led to child labor, frequent layoffs, and long work days filled with stressful, tedious, unfamiliar work. Labor unions did not exist, and neither was there any legal protection against exploitation of workers, including children (Donahue, 1985). All these rapid changes and often threatening conditions created the world of Charles Dickens, where, as in his book *Oliver Twist*, children worked as adults without question.

According to Donahue (1985), urban life, trade, and industrialization contributed to these overwhelming health hazards, and the situation was confounded by the lack of an adequate means of social control. Reforms were desperately needed, and the social reform movement emerged in response to the unhealthy by-products of the Industrial Revolution. It was in this world of the 1800s that reformers such as John Stuart Mill (1806–1873) emerged. Although the Industrial Revolution began in England, it quickly spread to the rest of Europe and to the United States (Bullough & Bullough, 1978). The reform movement is critical to understanding the emerging health concerns that were later addressed by Florence Nightingale. Mill championed popular education, the emancipation of women, trade unions, and religious toleration. Other reform issues of the era included the abolition of slavery and, most important for nursing, more humane care of the sick, the poor, and the wounded (Bullough & Bullough, 1978). There was a renewed energy in the religious community with the reemergence of new religious orders in the Catholic Church that provided service to the sick and disenfranchised.

Epidemics had ravaged Europe for centuries, but they became even more serious with urbanization. Industrialization brought people to cities, where they worked in close quarters (as compared with the isolation of the farm), and contributed to the social decay of the second half of the 1800s. Sanitation was poor or nonexistent, sewage disposal from the growing population was lacking, cities were filthy, public laws were weak or nonexistent, and congestion of the cities inevitably brought pests in the form of rats, lice, and bedbugs, which transmitted many pathogens. Communicable diseases continued to plague the population, especially those who lived in these unsanitary environments. For example, during the mid-1700s typhus and typhoid fever claimed twice as many lives each year as did the Battle of Waterloo (Hanlon & Pickett, 1984). Through

> **Epidemics had ravaged Europe for centuries, but they became even more serious with urbanization.**

foreign trade and immigration, infectious diseases were spread to all of Europe and eventually to the growing United States.

John Snow and the Science of Epidemiology

John Snow, a prominent physician, is credited with being the first epidemiologist. In 1854, Snow demonstrated that cholera rates were linked with water pump use in London (Cartwright, 1972). Snow investigated the area around Golden Square in London and arrived at the conclusion that cholera was not carried by bad air or necessarily by direct contact. He formed the opinion that diarrhea, unwashed hands, and shared food somehow played a large part in spreading the disease.

People around Golden Square in London were not supplied with water by pipes but drew their water from surface wells by means of hand-operated pumps. A severe outbreak of cholera occurred at the end of August 1853, resulting in at least 500 deaths in just 10 days in Golden Square. By mapping rates of cholera, Snow for the first time linked the sources of the drinking water at the Broad Street pump to the outbreaks of cholera. This proved that cholera was a waterborne disease. Dr. Snow's epidemiological investigation started a train of events that eventually would end the great epidemics of cholera, dysentery, and typhoid.

When Snow attended the now-famous community meeting of Golden Square and gave his evidence, government officials asked him what measures were necessary. His reply was, "Take the handle off the Broad Street pump." The handle was removed the next day, and no more cholera cases occurred (Snow, 1855). Although he did not discover the true cause of the cholera—the identification of the organism—he came very close to the truth (Rosen, 1958).

And Then There Was Nightingale ...

Florence Nightingale was named one of the 100 most influential persons of the last millennium by *Life* magazine (The 100 people who made the millennium, 1997). She was one of only eight women identified as such. Of those eight women, including Joan of Arc, Helen Keller, and Elizabeth I, Nightingale was identified as a true "angel of mercy," having reformed military health care in the Crimean War and used her political savvy to forever change the way society views the health of the vulnerable, the poor, and the forgotten. She is probably one of the most written about women in history (Bullough & Bullough, 1978). *Florence Nightingale* has become synonymous with modern nursing.

Florence Nightingale was the second child born on May 12, 1820, to the wealthy English family of William and Frances Nightingale in her namesake city, Florence, Italy. As a young child, Florence displayed incredible curiosity and intellectual abilities not common to female children of the Victorian age. She mastered the fundamentals of Greek and Latin, and she studied history, art, mathematics, and

> **Florence Nightingale has become synonymous with modern nursing.**

philosophy. To her family's dismay, she believed that God had called her to be a nurse. Nightingale was keenly aware of the suffering that industrialization created; she became obsessed with the plight of the miserable and suffering people: Conditions of general starvation accompanied the Industrial Revolution, prisons and workhouses overflowed, and persons in all sections of British life were displaced. She wrote in the spring of 1842, "My mind is absorbed with the sufferings of man; it besets me behind and before.... All that the poets sing of the glories of this world seem to me untrue. All the people that I see are eaten up with care or poverty or disease" (Woodham-Smith, 1951, p. 31).

For Nightingale, her entire life would be haunted by this conflict between the opulent life of gaiety that she enjoyed and the plight and misery of the world, which she was unable to alleviate. She was, in essence, an "alien spirit in the rich and aristocratic social sphere of Victorian England" (Palmer, 1977, p. 14). Nightingale remained unmarried, and at the age of 25, she expressed a desire to be trained as a nurse in an English hospital. Her parents emphatically denied her request, and for the next 7 years, she made repeated attempts to change their minds and allow her to enter nurse training. She wrote, "I crave for some regular occupation, for something worth doing instead of frittering my time away on useless trifles" (Woodham-Smith, 1951, p. 162). During this time, she continued her education through the study of math and science and spent 5 years collecting data about public health and hospitals (Dietz & Lehozky, 1963). During a tour of Egypt in 1849 with family and friends, Nightingale spent her 30th year in Alexandria with the Sisters of Charity of St. Vincent de Paul, where her conviction to study nursing was only reinforced (Tooley, 1910). While in Egypt, Nightingale studied Egyptian, Platonic, and Hermetic philosophy; Christian scripture; and the works of poets, mystics, and missionaries in her efforts to understand the nature of God and her "calling" as it fit into the divine plan (Calabria, 1996; Dossey, 1999).

The next spring, Nightingale traveled unaccompanied to the Kaiserwerth Institute in Germany and stayed there for 2 weeks, vowing to return to train as a nurse. In June 1851, Nightingale took her future into her own hands and announced to her family that she planned to return to Kaiserwerth and study nursing. According to Dietz and Lehozky (1963, p. 42), her mother had "hysterics" and scene followed scene. Her father "retreated into the shadows," and her sister, Parthe, expressed that the family name was forever disgraced (Cook, 1913).

In 1851, at the age of 31, Nightingale was finally permitted to go to Kaiserwerth, and she studied there for 3 months with Pastor Fliedner. Her family insisted that she tell no one outside the family of her whereabouts, and her mother forbade her to write any letters from Kaiserwerth. While there, Nightingale learned about the care of the sick and the importance of discipline and commitment of oneself to God (Donahue, 1985). She returned to England and cared for her then ailing father, from whom she finally gained some support for her intent to become a nurse—her lifelong dream.

In 1852, Nightingale wrote the essay "Cassandra," which stands today as a classic feminist treatise against the idleness of Victorian women. Through her voluminous journal writings, Nightingale reveals her inner struggle throughout her adulthood with what was expected of a woman and what she could accomplish with her life. The life expected of an aristocratic woman in her day was one she grew to loathe; throughout her writings, she poured out her detestation of the life of an idle woman (Nightingale, 1979, p. 5). In "Cassandra," Nightingale put her thoughts to paper, and many scholars believe that her eventual intent was to extend the essay to a novel. She wrote in "Cassandra," "Why have women passion, intellect, moral activity—these three—in a place in society where no one of the three can be exercised?" (Nightingale, 1979, p. 37). Although uncertain about the meaning of the name Cassandra, many scholars believe that it came from the Greek goddess Cassandra, who was cursed by Apollo and doomed to see and speak the truth but never to be believed. Nightingale saw the conventional life of women as a waste of time and abilities. After receiving a generous yearly endowment from her father, Nightingale moved to London and worked briefly as the superintendent of the Establishment for Gentlewomen During Illness hospital, finally realizing her dream of working as a nurse (Cook, 1913).

■ The Crimean Experience: "I Can Stand Out the War with Any Man"

Nightingale's opportunity for greatness came when she was offered the position of female nursing establishment of the English General Hospitals in Turkey by the secretary of war, Sir Sidney Herbert. Soon after the outbreak of the Crimean War, stories of the inadequate care and lack of medical resources for the soldiers became widely known throughout England (Woodham-Smith, 1951). The country was appalled at the conditions so vividly portrayed in the *London Times*. Pressure increased on Sir Herbert to react. He knew of one woman who was capable of bringing order out of the chaos and wrote the following now-famous letter to Nightingale on October 15, 1854, as a plea for her service:

> There is but one person in England that I know of who would be capable of organising and superintending such a scheme.... The difficulty of finding women equal to a task after all, full of horrors,

and requiring besides knowledge and good will, great energy and great courage, will be great. Your own personal qualities, your knowledge and your power of administration and among greater things your rank and position in Society give you advantages in such a work which no other person possesses. (Woodham-Smith, 1951, pp. 87–89)

Nightingale took the challenge from Sir Herbert and set sail with 38 self-proclaimed nurses with varied training and experiences, of whom 24 were Catholic and Anglican nuns. Their journey to the Crimea took a month, and on November 4, 1854, the brave nurses arrived at Istanbul and were taken to Scutari the same day. Faced with 3,000 to 4,000 wounded men in a hospital designed to accommodate 1,700, the nurses went to work (Kalisch & Kalisch, 1986). The nurses were faced with 4 miles of beds 18 inches apart. Most soldiers were lying naked with no bedding or blanket. There were no kitchen or laundry facilities. The little light present took the form of candles in beer bottles. The hospital was literally floating on an open sewage lagoon filled with rats and other vermin (Donahue, 1985).

The barrack "hospital" was more of a death trap than a place for healing before Nightingale's arrival. In a letter to Sir Herbert, Nightingale, demonstrating her sense of humor, wrote, with tongue in cheek, that "the vermin might, if they had but unity of purpose, carry off the four miles of beds on their backs and march them into the War Office" (Stanmore, 1906, pp. 393–394).

By taking the newly arrived medical equipment and setting up kitchens, laundries, recreation rooms, reading rooms, and a canteen, Nightingale and her team of nurses proceeded to clean the barracks of lice and filth. Nightingale was in her element. She set out not only to provide humane health care for the soldiers but to essentially overhaul the administrative structure of the military health services (Williams, 1961). Nightingale and her nurses were faced with overwhelming odds and deplorable conditions. No accommodations had been made for their quarters, so they ended up in one of the hospital towers, 39 women crowded into six small rooms. In addition to having no furniture, one of the rooms even had a long-neglected, forgotten corpse swarming with vermin! Ever the disciplinarian, Nightingale insisted on strict adherence to a standard nurse uniform: gray tweed dresses, gray worsted jackets, plain white caps, short woolen cloaks, and brown scarves embroidered in red with the words "Scutari Hospital" (Bullough & Bullough, 1978).

■ Florence Nightingale and Sanitation

Although Nightingale never accepted the germ theory, she demanded clean dressings; clean bedding; well-cooked, edible, and appealing food; proper sanitation; and fresh air. After the other nurses were asleep, Nightingale made her famous solitary rounds with a lamp or lantern to check on the soldiers. Nightingale had a lifelong pattern of sleeping few hours, spending many nights writing, developing elaborate plans, and evaluating implemented changes. She seldom believed in the "hopeless" soldier, only one who needed extra attention. Nightingale was convinced that most of the maladies that the soldiers suffered and died from were preventable (Williams, 1961).

Many soldiers wrote about their experiences of the Angel of Mercy, Florence Nightingale. One soldier wrote perhaps one of the most revealing tributes to this "Lady with the Lamp":

> What a comfort it was to see her pass even. She would speak to one and nod and smile to as many more, but she could not do it all, you know. We lay there by hundreds, but we could kiss her shadow as it fell, and lay our heads on the pillow again content. (Tyrell, 1856, p. 310)

Before Nightingale's arrival and her radical and well-documented interventions based on sound public health principles, the mortality rate from the Crimean War was estimated to be from 42% to 73%. Nightingale is credited with reducing that rate to 2% within 6 months of her arrival at Scutari. She did this through careful, scientific epidemiological research (Dietz & Lehozky, 1963). Upon arriving at Scutari, Nightingale's first act was to order 200 scrubbing brushes. The death rate fell dramatically once Nightingale discovered that the hospital was built literally over an open, sewage lagoon. A dead horse was even retrieved from the sewer system under Scutari (Andrews, 2003).

According to Palmer (1982), Nightingale possessed the qualities of a good researcher: insatiable curiosity, command of her subject, familiarity with methods of inquiry, a good background of statistics, and the ability to discriminate and abstract. She used these skills to maintain detailed and copious notes and to codify observations. Nightingale relied on statistics and attention to detail to back up her conclusions about sanitation, management of care, and disease causation. Her now-famous "cox combs" are a hallmark of military health services management by which she diagrammed deaths in the Army from wounds and from other diseases and compared them with deaths that occurred in similar populations in England (Palmer, 1977).

Nightingale was first and foremost an administrator: She believed in a hierarchical administrative structure with ultimate control lodged in one person to whom all subordinates and offices reported. Within a matter of weeks of her arrival in the Crimea, Nightingale was the acknowledged administrator and organizer of a mammoth humanitarian effort. From her Crimean experience on, Nightingale involved herself primarily in organizational activities and health planning administration. Palmer contends that Nightingale "perceived the Crimean venture, which was set up as an experiment, as a golden opportunity to demonstrate the efficacy of female nursing" (Palmer, 1982, p. 4). Although Nightingale faced initial resistance from the unconvinced and oppositional medical officers and surgeons, she boldly defied convention and remained steadfastly focused on her mission to create a sanitary and highly structured environment for her "children"—the British soldiers who dedicated their lives to the defense of Great Britain. Through her resilience and insistence on absolute authority regarding nursing and the hospital environment, Nightingale was known to send nurses home to England from the Crimea for suspicious alcohol use and character weakness.

It was through this success at Scutari that she began a long career of influence on the public's health through social activism and reform, health policy, and the reformation of career nursing. Using her well-publicized successful "experiment" and supportive evidence from the Crimea, Nightingale effectively argued the case for the reform and creation of military health care that would serve as the model for people in uniform to the present (D'Antonio, 2002). Nightingale's ideas about proper hospital architecture and administration influenced a generation of medical doctors and the entire world, in both military and civilian service. Her work in *Notes on Hospitals*, published in 1860, provided the template for the organization of military health care in the Union Army when the U.S. Civil War erupted in 1861. Her vision for health care of soldiers and the responsibility of the governments that send them to war continues today; her influence can be seen throughout the previous century and into this century as health care for the women and men who serve their country is a vital part of the well-being of not only the soldiers but for society in general (D'Antonio, 2002).

Mary Grant Seacole, an African nurse from Jamaica, offered her services to Nightingale after hearing of the need in Scutari. Although Nightingale was unwilling to hire Seacole as part of the nursing staff, Seacole volunteered her services without pay. Seacole was so committed to providing care to the British military that she set up an inn with her own money that provided food and lodging for soldiers and their families near Scutari (Hine, 1989). Although Seacole is less well known than Nightingale, her contributions to nursing in wartime were significant in the history of minority nursing. The School of Nursing in Kingston, Jamaica, is today named in her honor.

Scores have been written about Nightingale—an almost mythic figure in history. She truly was a beloved legend throughout Great Britain by the time she left the Crimea in July 1856, 4 months after the war. Longfellow immortalized this "Lady with the Lamp" in his poem "Santa Filomena" (Longfellow, 1857).

■ Returning Home a Heroine: The Political Reformer

When Nightingale returned to London, she found that her efforts to provide comfort and health to the British soldier succeeded in making heroes of both herself and the soldiers (Woodham-Smith, 1951). Both had suffered from negative stereotypes: The soldier was often portrayed as a drunken oaf with little ambition or honor, the nurse as a tipsy, self-serving, illiterate, promiscuous loser. After the Crimean War and the efforts of Nightingale and her nurses, both returned with honor and dignity, nevermore the downtrodden and disrespected.

After her return from the Crimea, Florence Nightingale never made a public appearance, never attended a public function, and never issued a public statement (Bullough & Bullough, 1978). She single-handedly raised nursing from, as she put it, "the sink it was" into a respected and noble profession (Palmer, 1977). As an avid scholar and student of the Greek writer Plato, Nightingale believed that she had a moral obligation to work primarily for the good of the community. Because she believed that education formed character, she insisted that nursing must go beyond care for the sick; the mission of the trained nurse must include social reform to promote the good. This dual mission of nursing—caregiver and political reformer—has shaped the profession as we know it today. LeVasseur (1998) contends that Nightingale's insistence on nursing's involvement in a larger political ideal is the historical foundation of the field and distinguishes us from other scientific disciplines, such as medicine.

How did Nightingale accomplish this? You will learn throughout this text how nurses effect change through others. Florence Nightingale is the standard by which we measure our effectiveness. She effected change through her wide command of acquaintances: Queen Victoria was a significant admirer of her intellect and ability to effect change, and Nightingale used her position as national heroine to get the attention of elected officials in Parliament. She was tireless and had an amazing capacity for work. She used people. Her brother-in-law, Sir Harry Verney, was a member of Parliament and often delivered her "messages" in the form of legislation. When she wanted the public incited, she turned to the press, writing letters to the *London Times* and having others of influence write articles. She was not above threats to "go public" by certain dates if an elected official refused to establish a commission or appoint a committee. And when those commissions were formed, Nightingale was ready with her list of selected people for appointment (Palmer, 1982).

■ Nightingale and Military Reforms

The first real test of Nightingale's military reforms came in the United States during the Civil War. Nightingale was asked by the Union to advise on the organization of hospitals and care of the sick and wounded. She sent recommendations back to the United States based on her experiences and analysis in the Crimea, and her advisement and influence gained wide publicity. Following her recommendations, the Union set up a sanitary commission and provided for regular inspection of camps. She expressed a desire to help with the Confederate military also but, unfortunately, had no channel of communication with them (Bullough & Bullough, 1978).

■ The Nightingale School of Nursing at St. Thomas: The Birth of Professional Nursing

The British public honored Nightingale by endowing 50,000 pounds sterling in her name upon her return to England from the Crimea. The money had been raised from the soldiers under her care and donations from the public. This Nightingale Fund eventually was used to create the Nightingale School of Nursing at St. Thomas, which was to be the beginning of professional nursing (Donahue, 1985). Nightingale, at the age of 40, decided that St. Thomas' Hospital was the place for her training school for nurses. While the negotiations for the school went forward, she spent her time writing *Notes on Nursing: What It Is and What It Is Not* (Nightingale, 1860). The small book of 77 pages, written for the British mother, was an instant success. An expanded library edition was written for nurses and used as the textbook for the students at St. Thomas. The book has since been translated into many languages, although it is believed that Nightingale refused all royalties earned from the publication of the book (Cook, 1913; Tooley, 1910). The nursing students chosen for the new training school were handpicked; they had to be of good moral character, sober, and honest. Nightingale believed that the strong emphasis on morals was critical to gaining respect for the new "Nightingale nurse," with no possible ties to the disgraceful association of past nurses. Nursing students were monitored throughout their 1-year program both on and off the hospital grounds; their activities were carefully watched for character weaknesses, and discipline was severe and swift for violators. Accounts from Nightingale's journals and notes reveal instant dismissal of nursing students for such behaviors as "flirtation, using the eyes unpleasantly, and being in the company of unsavory persons." Nightingale contended that "the future of nursing depends on how these young women behave themselves" (Smith, 1934, p. 234). She knew that the experiment at St. Thomas to educate nurses and raise nursing to a moral and professional calling was a drastic departure from the past images of nurses and would take extraordinary women of high moral character and intelligence. Nightingale knew every nursing student, or probationer, personally, often having the students at her house for weekend visits. She devised a system of daily journal keeping for the probationers; Nightingale herself read the journals monthly to evaluate their character and work habits. Every nursing student admitted to St. Thomas had to submit an acceptable "letter of good character" and Nightingale herself placed graduate nurses in approved nursing positions.

One of the most important features of the Nightingale School was its relative autonomy. Both the school and the hospital nursing service were organized under the head matron. This was especially significant because it meant that nursing service began independently of the medical staff in selecting, retaining, and disciplining students and nurses (Bullough & Bullough, 1978).

Nightingale was opposed to the use of a standardized government examination and the movement for licensure of trained nurses. She believed that schools of nursing would lose control of educational standards with the advent of national licensure, most notably those related to moral character. Nightingale led a staunch opposition to the movement by the British Nurses Association (BNA) for licensure of trained nurses, one the BNA believed critical to protecting the public's safety by ensuring the qualification of nurses by licensure exam. Nightingale was convinced that qualifying a nurse by examination tested only the acquisition of technical skills, not the equally important evaluation of character. She believed nursing involved "divergencies too great for a single standard to be applied" (Nutting & Dock, 1907; Woodham-Smith, 1951).

■ Taking Health Care to the Community: Nightingale and Wellness

Early efforts to distinguish hospital from community health nursing are evidence of Nightingale's views on "health nursing," which she distinguished from "sick nursing." She wrote two influential papers, one in 1893, "Sick-Nursing and Health-Nursing" (Nightingale, 1893), which was read in the United States at the Chicago Exposition, and the second, "Health Teaching in Towns and Villages" in 1894 (Monteiro, 1985). Both papers praised the success of prevention-based nursing practice. Winslow (1946) acknowledged Nightingale's influence in the United States by being one of the first in the field of public health to recognize the importance of taking responsibility for one's health. She wrote in 1891 that "There are more people to pick us up and help us stand on our own two feet" (Attewell, 1996). According to Palmer (1982), Nightingale was a leader in the wellness movement long before the concept was identified. Nightingale saw the nurse as the key figure in establishing a healthy society. She saw a logical extension of nursing in acute hospital settings to the broadest sense of community used in nursing today. Clearly, through her *Notes on Nursing*, she visualized the nurse as "the nation's first bulwark in health maintenance, the promotion of wellness, and the prevention of disease" (Palmer, 1982, p. 6).

William Rathbone, a wealthy ship owner and philanthropist, is credited with the establishment of the first visiting nurse service, which eventually evolved into district nursing in the community. He was so impressed with the private duty nursing care that his sick wife had received at home that he set out to develop a "district nursing service" in Liverpool, England. At his own expense, in 1859, he developed a corps of nurses trained to care for the sick poor in their homes (Bullough & Bullough, 1978). He divided the community into 16 districts; each was assigned a nurse and a social worker who provided nursing and health education. His experiment in district nursing was so successful that he was unable to find enough nurses to work in the districts. Rathbone contacted Nightingale for assistance. Her recommendation was to train more nurses, and she advised Rathbone to approach the Royal Liverpool Infirmary with a proposal for opening another training school for nurses (Rathbone, 1890; Tooley, 1910). The infirmary agreed to Rathbone's proposal, and district nursing soon spread throughout England as successful "health nursing" in the community for the sick poor through voluntary agencies (Rosen, 1958). Ever the visionary, Nightingale contended that "Hospitals are but an intermediate stage of civilization. The ultimate aim is to nurse the sick poor in their own homes (1893)" (Attewell, 1996). She also wrote in regard to visiting families at home: "We must not talk to them or at them but with them (1894)" (Attewell, 1996). A similar service, health visiting, began in Manchester, England, in 1862 by the Manchester and Salford Sanitary Association. The purpose of placing "health visitors" in the home was to provide health information and instruction to families. Eventually, health visitors evolved to provide preventive health education and district nurses to care for the sick at home (Bullough & Bullough, 1978).

Although Nightingale is best known for her reform of hospitals and the military, she was a great believer in the future of health care, which she anticipated should be preventive in nature and would more than likely take place in the home and community. Her accomplishments in the field of "sanitary nursing" extended beyond the walls of the hospital to include workhouse reform and community sanitation reform. In 1864, Nightingale and William Rathbone once again worked together to lead the reform of the Liverpool Workhouse Infirmary, where more than 1,200 sick paupers were crowded into unsanitary and unsafe conditions. Under the British Poor Laws, the most desperately poor of the large cities were gathered into large workhouses. When sick, they were sent to the Workhouse Infirmary. Trained nursing care was all but nonexistent. Through legislative pressure and a well-designed public campaign describing the horrors of the Workhouse Infirmary, reform of the workhouse system was accomplished by 1867. Although not as complete as Nightingale had wanted, nurses were in place and being paid a salary (Seymer, 1954).

■ The Legacy of Nightingale

When Nightingale returned to London after the Crimean War, she remained haunted by her experiences related to the soldiers dying of preventable diseases. She was troubled by nightmares and had difficulty sleeping in the years that followed. She wrote in her journal: "Oh my poor men; I am a bad mother to come home and leave you in your Crimean graves.... I can never forget.... I stand at the altar of the murdered men and while I live, I fight their cause" (Woodham-Smith, 1983, pp. 178, 193). Nightingale became a prolific writer and a staunch defender of the causes of the British soldier, sanitation in England and India, and trained nursing.

As a woman, she was not able to hold an official government post, nor could she vote. Historians have had varied opinions about the exact nature of the disability that kept her homebound for the remainder of her life. Recent scholars have speculated that she experienced post-traumatic stress disorder (PTSD) from her experiences in the Crimea; there is also considerable evidence that she suffered from the painful disease brucellosis (Barker, 1989; Young, 1995). She exerted incredible influence through friends and acquaintances, directing from her sick room sanitation and poor law reform. Her mission to "cleanse" spread from the military to the British Empire; her fight for improved sanitation both at home and in India consumed her energies for the remainder of her life (Vicinus & Nergaard, 1990).

According to Monteiro (1985), two recurrent themes are found throughout Nightingale's writings about disease prevention and wellness outside the hospital. The most persistent theme is that nurses must be trained differently and instructed specifically in district and instructive nursing. She consistently wrote that the "health nurse" must be trained in the nature of poverty and its influence on health, something she referred to as the "pauperization" of the poor. She also believed that above all, health nurses must be good teachers about hygiene and helping families learn to better care for themselves (Nightingale, 1893). She insisted that untrained, "good intended women" could not substitute for nursing care in the home. Nightingale pushed for an extensive orientation and additional training, including prior hospital experience, before one was hired as a district nurse. She outlined the qualifications in her paper "On Trained Nursing for the Sick Poor," in which she called for a month's "trial" in district nursing, a year's training in hospital nursing, and 3 to 6 months training in district nursing (Monteiro, 1985). She said, "There is no such thing as amateur nursing."

The second theme that emerged from her writings was the focus on the role of the nurse. She clearly distinguished the role of the health nurse in promoting what we today call self-care. In the past, philanthropic visitors in the form of Christian charity would visit the homes of the poor and offer them relief (Monteiro, 1985). Nightingale believed that such activities did little to teach the poor to care for themselves and further "pauperized" them—dependent and vulnerable—keeping them unhealthy, prone to disease, and reliant on others to keep them healthy. The nurse then must help the families at home manage a healthy environment for themselves, and Nightingale saw a trained nurse as being the only person who could pull off such a feat. She stated, "Never think that you have done anything effectual in nursing in London, till you nurse, not only the sick poor in workhouses, but those at home."

By 1901, Nightingale lived in a world without sight or sound, leaving her unable to write. Over the next 5 years,

> ...My view you know is that the ultimate destination of all nursing is the nursing of the sick in their own homes.... I look to the abolition of all hospitals and workhouse infirmaries. But no use to talk about the year 2000.
> —Nightingale, 1894

Nightingale lost her ability to communicate and most days existed in a state of unconsciousness. In November of 1907, Nightingale was honored with the Order of Merit by King Edward VII, the first time ever given to a woman. After 50 years, in May 1910, the Nightingale Training School of Nursing at St. Thomas celebrated its Jubilee. There were now more than a thousand training schools for nurses in the United States alone (Cook, 1913; Tooley, 1910).

Nightingale died in her sleep around noon on August 13, 1910, and was buried quietly and without pomp near the family's home at Embley, her coffin carried by six sergeants of the British Army. Only a small cross marks her grave at her request: "FN. Born 1820. Died 1910." (Brown, 1988). The family refused a national funeral and burial at Westminster Abbey out of respect for Nightingale's last wishes. She had lived for 90 years and 3 months.

www] **CRITICAL THINKING QUESTIONS** ✳

Some nurses believe that Florence Nightingale holds nursing back and represents the negative and backward elements of nursing. This view cites as evidence that Nightingale supported the subordination of nurses to physicians, opposed registration of nurses, and did not see mental health nurses as part of the profession. Wheeler has gone so far as to say, "The nursing profession needs to exorcise the myth of Nightingale, not necessarily because she was a bad person, but because the impact of her legacy has held the profession back too long." After reading this chapter, what do you think? Is Nightingale relevant in the 21st century to the nursing profession? Why or why not? ✳

Early Nursing Education and Organization in the United States

In the United States, the first training schools for nursing were modeled after the Nightingale School of Nursing at St. Thomas in London. The earliest programs for trained nurses in the United States were the Bellevue Training School for Nurses in New York City; Connecticut Training School for Nurses in New Haven, Connecticut; and the Boston Training School for Nurses at Massachusetts General Hospital (Christy, 1975; Nutting & Dock, 1907). Based on the Victorian belief in the natural abilities of women to be sensitive, possess high morals, and be caregivers, early nursing training required that applicants be female. Sensitivity, high moral character, purity of character, subservience, and "ladylike" behavior became the associated traits of a "good nurse," thus setting the "feminization of nursing" as the ideal standard for a good nurse. These historical roots of gender- and race-based caregiving continued to exclude males and minorities from the nursing profession for many years and still influence career choices for men and women today. These early training schools provided a stable, subservient, white female workforce because student nurses served as the primary nursing staff for these early hospitals.

A significant report, known simply as the **Goldmark Report**, *Nursing and Nursing Education in the United States*, was released in 1922 and advocated the establishment of university schools of nursing to train nursing leaders. The report, initiated by Nutting in 1918, was an exhaustive and comprehensive investigation into the state of nursing education and training resulting in a

500-page document. Josephine Goldmark, social worker and author of the pioneering research of nursing preparation in the United States, stated,

> From our field study of the nurse in public health nursing, in private duty, and as instructor and supervisor in hospitals, it is clear that there is need of a basic undergraduate training for all nurses alike, which should lead to a nursing diploma. (Goldmark, 1923, p. 35)

The first university school of nursing was developed at the University of Minnesota in 1909. Although the new nurse training school was under the college of medicine and offered only a 3-year diploma, the Minnesota program was nevertheless a significant leap forward in nursing education. *Nursing for the Future*, or the **Brown Report**, authored by Esther Lucille Brown in 1948 and sponsored by the Russell Sage Foundation, was critical of the quality and structure of nursing schools in the United States. The Brown Report became the catalyst for the implementation of educational nursing program accreditation through the National League for Nursing (Brown, 1936, 1948). As a result of the post–World War II nursing shortage, an Associate Degree in Nursing was established by Dr. Mildred Montag in 1952 as a 2-year program for registered nurses (RNs) (Montag, 1959). In 1950, nursing became the first profession for which the same licensure exam, the State Board Test Pool, was used throughout the nation to license registered nurses. This increased mobility for the registered nurse resulted in a significant advantage for the relatively new profession of nursing (State board test pool examination, 1952).

The Evolution of Nursing in the United States: The First Century of Professional Nursing

■ The Profession of Nursing Is Born in the United States

Early nurse leaders of the 20th century included **Isabel Hampton Robb**, who in 1896 founded the Nurses' Associated Alumnae, which in 1911 officially became known as the **American Nurses Association (ANA)**; and **Lavinia Lloyd Dock**, who became a militant suffragist linking women's roles as nurses to the emerging women's movement in the United States.

Mary Adelaide Nutting, Lavinia L. Dock, Sophia Palmer, and Mary E. Davis were instrumental in developing the first nursing journal, the *American Journal of Nursing (AJN)* in October 1900. Through the ANA and the *AJN*, nurses then had a professional organization and a national journal with which to communicate with each other (Kalisch & Kalisch, 1986).

State licensure of trained nurses began in 1903 with the enactment of North Carolina's licensure law for nursing. Shortly thereafter, New Jersey, New York, and Virginia passed similar licensure laws for nursing. Over the next several years, professional nursing was well on its way to public recognition of practice and educational standards as state after state passed similar legislation.

Margaret Sanger worked as a nurse on the Lower East Side of New York City in 1912 with immigrant families. She was astonished to find widespread ignorance among these families about conception, pregnancy, and childbirth. After a horrifying experience with the death of a woman from a failed self-induced abortion, Sanger devoted her life to teaching women about birth control. A staunch activist in the early family planning movement, Sanger is credited with founding Planned Parenthood of America (Sanger, 1928).

By 1917, the emerging new profession saw two significant events that propelled the need for additional trained nurses in the United States: World War I and the influenza epidemic. Nightingale and the devastation of the Civil War had well established the need for nursing care in wartime. Mary Adelaide Nutting, now Professor of Nursing and Health at Columbia University, chaired the newly established Committee on Nursing in response to the need for nurses as the United States entered the war in Europe. Nurses in the United States realized early that World War I was unlike previous wars. It was a global conflict that involved coalitions of nations against nations and vast amounts of supplies and demanded the organization of all the nations' resources for military purposes (Kalisch & Kalisch, 1986). Along with Lillian Wald and Jane A. Delano, Director of Nursing in the American Red Cross, Nutting initiated a national publicity campaign to recruit young women to enter nurses' training. The Army School of Nursing, headed by Annie Goodrich as dean, and the Vassar Training Camp for Nurses prepared nurses for the war as well as home nursing and hygiene nursing through the Red Cross (Dock & Stewart, 1931). The committee estimated that there were at the most about 200,000 active "nurses" in the United States, both trained and untrained, which was inadequate for the military effort abroad (Kalisch & Kalisch, 1986).

At home, the influenza epidemic of 1917 to 1919 led to increased public awareness of the need for public health nursing and public education about hygiene and disease prevention. The successful campaign to attract nursing students focused heavily on patriotism, which ushered in the new era for nursing as a profession. By 1918, nursing school enrollments were up by 25%. In 1920, Congress passed a bill that provided nurses with military rank (Dock & Stewart, 1931). Following close behind, the passage of the Nineteenth Amendment to the U.S. Constitution granted women the right to vote. According to Stewart:

KEY COMPETENCY 1-1

Examples of Applicable *Nurse of the Future: Nursing Core Competencies*

Professionalism:

Knowledge (K 8a) Understands the responsibilities inherent in being a member of the nursing profession

Skills (S 8a) Understands the history and philosophy of the nursing profession

Attitudes/Behaviors (A 8a) Recognizes the need for personal and professional behaviors that promote the profession of nursing

Source: Massachusetts Department of Higher Education (2010, p. 15).

The emerging new profession saw two significant events that propelled the need for additional trained nurses in the United States: World War I and the influenza epidemic.

Probably the greatest contribution of the war experience to nursing lies in the fact that the whole system of nursing education was shaken for a little while out of its well-worn ruts and brought out of its comparative seclusion into the light of public discussion and criticism. When so many lives hung on the supply of nurses, people were aroused to a new sense of their dependence on the products of nursing schools, and many of them learned for the first time of the hopelessly limited resources which nursing educators have had to work with in the training of these indispensable public servants. Whatever the future may bring, it is unlikely that nursing schools will willingly sink back again into their old isolation or that they will accept unquestionably the financial status which the older system imposed on them. (Stewart, 1921, p. 6)

■ The Emergence of Community and Public Health Nursing

The pattern for health visiting and district nursing practice outside the hospital was similar in the United States to that in England (Roberts, 1954). American cities were besieged by overcrowding and epidemics after the Civil War. The need for trained nurses evolved as in England, and schools throughout the United States developed along the Nightingale model. Visiting nurses were first sent to philanthropic organizations in New York City (1877), Boston (1886), Buffalo (1885), and Philadelphia (1886) to care for the sick at home. By the end of the century, most large cities had some form of visiting nursing program, and some headway was being made even in smaller towns (Heinrich, 1983). Industrial or occupational health nursing was first started in Vermont in 1895 by a marble company interested in the health and welfare of its workers and their families. Tuberculosis (TB) was a leading cause of death in the 1800s; nurses visited patients bedridden from TB and instructed persons in all settings about prevention of the disease (Abel, 1997).

■ Lillian Wald, Public Health Nursing, and Community Activism

Lillian Wald, a wealthy young woman with a great social conscience, graduated from the New York Hospital School of Nursing in 1891 and is credited with creating the title "public health nurse." After a year working in a mental institution, Wald entered medical school at Women's Medical College in New York. While in medical school, she was asked to visit immigrant mothers on New York's Lower East Side and instruct them on health matters. Wald was appalled by the conditions there. During one now famous home visit, a small child asked Wald to visit her sick mother. And the rest, as they say, is history (Box 1-1).

BOX 1-1 LILLIAN WALD TAKES A WALK

From the schoolroom where I had been giving a lesson in bed-making, a little girl led me one drizzling March morning. She had told me of her sick mother, and gathering from her incoherent account that a child had been born, I caught up the paraphernalia of the bed-making lesson and carried it with me.

The child led me over broken roadways … between tall, reeking houses whose laden fire-escapes, useless for their appointed purpose, bulged with household goods of every description. The rain added to the dismal appearance of the streets and to the discomfort of the crowds which thronged them, intensifying the odors which assailed me from every side. Through Hester and Division Streets we went to the end of Ludlow; past odorous fish-stands, for the streets were a market-place, unregulated, unsupervised, unclean; past evil-smelling, uncovered garbage cans….

All the maladjustments of our social and economic relations seemed epitomized in this brief journey and what was found at the end of it. The family to which the child led me was neither criminal nor vicious. Although the husband was a cripple, one of those who stand on street corners exhibiting deformities to enlist compassion, and masking the begging of alms by a pretense of selling; although the family of seven shared their two rooms with boarders—who were literally boarders, since a piece of timber was placed over the floor for them to sleep on—and although the sick woman lay on a wretched, unclean bed, soiled with a hemorrhage two days old, they were not degraded human beings, judged by any measure of moral values.

In fact, it was very plain that they were sensitive to their condition, and when, at the end of my ministrations, they kissed my hands (those who have undergone similar experiences will, I am sure, understand), it would have been some solace if by any conviction of the moral unworthiness of the family I could have defended myself as a part of a society which permitted such conditions to exist. Indeed, my subsequent acquaintance with them revealed the fact that miserable as their state was, they were not without ideals for the family life, and for society, of which they were so unloved and unlovely a part.

That morning's experience was a baptism of fire. Deserted were the laboratory and the academic work of the college. I never returned to them. On my way from the sick-room to my comfortable student quarters my mind was intent on my own responsibility. To my inexperience it seemed certain that conditions such as these were allowed because people did not know, and for me there was a challenge to know and to tell. When early morning found me still awake, my naive conviction remained that, if people knew things—and "things" meant everything implied in the condition of this family—such horrors would cease to exist, and I rejoiced that I had a training in the care of the sick that in itself would give me an organic relationship to the neighborhood in which this awakening had come.

Source: Wald, L. D. (1915). *The house on Henry Street*. New York, NY: Henry Holt.

What Wald found changed her life forever and secured a place for her in American nursing history. Wald (1915) said, "All the maladjustments of our social and economic relations seemed epitomized in this brief journey" (p. 6). Wald was profoundly affected by her observations; she and her colleague, Mary Brewster, quickly established the Henry Street Settlement in this same neighborhood in 1893. She quit medical school and devoted the remainder of her life to "visions of a better world" for the public's health. According to Wald, "Nursing is love in action, and there is no finer manifestation of it than the care of the poor and disabled in their own homes" (Wald, 1915, p. 14).

The Henry Street Settlement was an independent nursing service where Wald lived and worked. This later became the Visiting Nurse Association of New York City, which laid the foundation for the establishment of public health nursing in the United States. The health needs of the population were met through addressing social, economic, and environmental determinants of health, in a pattern after Nightingale. These nurses helped educate families about disease transmission and emphasized the importance of good hygiene. They provided preventive, acute, and long-term care. As such, Henry Street went far beyond the care of the sick and the prevention of illness: It aimed at rectifying those causes that led to the poverty and misery. Wald was a tireless social activist for legislative reforms that would provide a more just distribution of services for the marginal and disadvantaged in the United States (Donahue, 1985). Wald began with 10 nurses in 1893, which grew to 250 nurses serving 1,300 clients a day by 1916. During this same period, the budget grew from nothing to more than $600,000 a year, all from private donations.

Wald hired African American nurse **Elizabeth Tyler** in 1906 as evidence of her commitment to cultural diversity. Although unable to visit white clients, Tyler made her own way by "finding" African American families who needed her service. In 3 months, Tyler had so many African American families within her caseload that Wald hired a second African American nurse, Edith Carter. Carter remained at Henry Street for 28 years until her retirement (Carnegie, 1991). During her tenure at Henry Street, Wald demonstrated her commitment to racial and cultural diversity by employing 25 African American nurses over the years, and she paid them salaries equal to white nurses and provided identical benefits and recognition to minority nurses (Carnegie, 1991). This was exceptional during the early part of the 1900s, a time when African American nurses were often denied admission to white schools of nursing and membership in professional organizations and were denied opportunities for employment in most settings. Because hospitals of this era often set quotas for African American clients, those nurses who managed to graduate from nursing schools found themselves with few clients who needed or could afford their services. African American nurses struggled for the right to take the registration examination available for white nurses.

Wald submitted a proposal to the city of New York after learning of a child's dismissal from a New York City school for a skin condition. Her proposal was for one of the Henry Street Settlement nurses to serve free for 1 month in a New York school. The results of her experiment were so convincing that salaries were approved for 12 school nurses. From this, school nursing was born in the United States and became one of many community specialties credited to Wald (Dietz & Lehozky, 1963). In 1909, Wald proposed a program to the Metropolitan Life Insurance Company to provide nursing visits to their industrial policyholders. Statistics kept by the company documented the lowered mortality rates of policyholders attributed to the nurses' public health practice and clinical expertise. The program demonstrated savings for the company and was so successful that it lasted until 1953 (Hamilton, 1988).

Wald's other significant accomplishments include the establishment of the Children's Bureau, set up in 1912 as part of the U.S. Department of Labor. She also was an enthusiastic supporter of and participant in women's suffrage, lobbied for inspections of the workplace, and supported her employee, Margaret Sanger, in her efforts to give women the right to birth control. She was active in the American Red Cross and International Red Cross and helped form the Women's Trade Union League to protect women from sweatshop conditions.

Wald first coined the phrase "public health nursing" and transformed the field of community health nursing from the narrow role of home visiting to the population focus of today's community health nurse (Robinson, 1946). According to Dock and Stewart (1931), the title of public health nurse was purposeful: The role designation was designed to link the public's health to governmental responsibility, not private funding. As state departments of health and local governments began to employ more and more public health nurses, their role increasingly focused on prevention of illness in the entire community. Discrimination developed between the visiting nurse, who was employed by the voluntary agencies primarily to provide home care to the sick, and the public health nurse, who concentrated on preventive measures (Brainard, 1922).

Early public health nurses came closer than hospital-based nurses to the autonomy and professionalism that Nightingale advocated. Their work was conducted in the unconfined setting of the home and community, they were independent, and they enjoyed recognition as specialists in preventive health (Buhler-Wilkerson, 1985). Public health nurses from the beginning were much more holistic in their practice than their hospital counterparts. They were involved with the health of industrial workers, immigrants, and their families and were concerned about exploitation of women and children. These nurses also played a part in prison reform and care of the mentally ill (Heinrich, 1983).

Considered the first African American public health nurse, **Jessie Sleet Scales** was hired in 1902 by the Charity Organization Society, a philanthropic organization, to visit African American families infected by TB. Scales provided district nursing care to New York City's African American families and is credited with paving the way for African American nurses in the practice of community health (Mosley, 1996).

▪ Dorothea Linde Dix

Dorothea Linde Dix, a Boston schoolteacher, became aware of the horrendous conditions in prisons and mental institutions when asked to do a Sunday school class in the House of Correction at Cambridge, Massachusetts. She was appalled at what she saw and went about studying whether the conditions were isolated or widespread; she took 2 years off to visit every jail and almshouse from Cape Cod to Berkshire (Tiffany, 1890, p. 76). Her report was devastating. Boston was scandalized by the reality that the most progressive state in the Union was now associated with such appalling conditions. The shocked legislature voted to allocate funds to build hospitals. For the rest of her life, Dorothea Dix stood out as a tireless zealot for the humane treatment of the insane and imprisoned. She had exceptional savvy in dealing with legislators. She acquainted herself with the legislators and their records and displayed the "spirit of a crusader." For her contributions, Dix is recognized as one of the pioneers of the reform movement for mental health in the United States, and her efforts are felt worldwide to the present day (Dietz & Lehozky, 1963).

Dix was also known for her work in the Civil War, having been appointed superintendent of the female nurses of the Army by the secretary of war in 1861. Her tireless efforts led to the recruitment of more than 2,000 women to serve in the army during the Civil War. Officials had consulted with Nightingale concerning military hospitals and were determined not to make the same mistakes. Dix enjoyed far more sweeping powers than Nightingale in that she had the authority to organize hospitals, to appoint nurses, and to manage supplies for the wounded (Brockett & Vaughan, 1867). Among her most well-known nurses during the Civil War were the poet Walt Whitman and the author Louisa May Alcott (Donahue, 1985).

▪ Clara Barton

The idea for the International Red Cross was the brainchild of a Swiss banker, J. Henri Dunant, who proposed the formation of a neutral international relief society that could be activated in time of war. The International Red Cross was ratified by the Geneva Convention on August 22, 1864. Clara Barton, through her work in the Civil War, had come to believe that such an organization was desperately needed in the United States. However, it was not until 1882 that Barton was able to convince Congress to ratify the Treaty of Geneva, thus becoming the founder of the American Red Cross (Kalisch & Kalisch, 1986). Barton also played a leadership role in the Spanish-American War in Cuba, where she led a group of nurses to provide care for both U.S. and Cuban soldiers and Cuban civilians. At the age of 76, Barton went to President McKinley and offered the help of the Red Cross in Cuba. The president agreed to allow Barton to go with Red Cross nurses, but only to care for the Cuban citizens. Once in Cuba, the U.S. military saw what Barton and her nurses were able to accomplish with the Cuban military, and American soldiers pressured military officials to allow Barton's help. Along with battling yellow fever, Barton was able to provide care to both Cuban and U.S. military personnel and eventually expanded that care to Cuban citizens in Santiago. One of Barton's most famous clients was young Colonel Teddy Roosevelt, who led his Rough Riders and who later became the president of the United States. Barton became an instant heroine both in Cuba and in the United States for her bravery, tenaciousness, and for organizing services for the military and civilians torn apart by war. On August 13, 1898, the Spanish-American War came to an end. The grateful people of Santiago, Cuba, built a statue to honor Clara Barton in the town square, where it stands to this day. The work of Barton and her Red Cross nurses spread through the newspapers of the United States and in the schools of nursing. A congressional committee investigating the work of Barton's Red Cross staff applauded the work of these nurses and recommended that the U.S. Medical Department create a permanent reserve corps of trained nurses. These reserve nurses became the Army Nurse Corps in 1901. Clara Barton will always be remembered both as the founder of the American Red Cross and the driving force behind the creation of the Army Nurse Corps (Frantz, 1998).

■ Birth of the Midwife in the United States

Women have always assisted other women in the birth of babies. These "lay midwives" were considered by communities to possess special skills and some-what of a "calling." With the advent of professional nursing in England, registered nurses became associated with safer and more predictable child-birth practices. In England and in other countries where Nightingale nurses were prevalent, most registered nurses were also trained as midwives with a 6-month specialized training period. In the United States, the training of registered nurses in the practice of midwifery was prevented primarily by physicians. U.S. physicians saw midwives as a threat and intrusion into medical practice. Such resistance indirectly led to the proliferation of "granny wives" who were ignorant of modern practices, were untrained, and were associated with high maternal morbidity (Donahue, 1985).

The first organized midwifery service in the United States was the **Frontier Nursing Service** founded in 1925 by **Mary Breckenridge**. Breckenridge gradu-ated from the St. Luke's Hospital Training School in New York in 1910 and received her midwifery certificate from the British Hospital for Mothers and Babies in London in 1925. She had extensive experience in the delivery of babies and midwifery systems in New Zealand and Australia. In rural Appa-lachia, babies had been delivered for decades by granny midwives, who relied mainly on tradition, myths, and superstition as the bases of their practice. For example, they might use ashes for medication and place a sharp axe, blade up,

under the bed of a laboring woman to "cut" the pain. The people of Appala-
chia were isolated because of the terrain of the hollows and mountains, and
roads were limited to most families. They had one of the highest birth rates
in the United States. Breckenridge believed that if a midwifery service could
work under these conditions, it could work anywhere (Donahue, 1985).

Breckenridge had to use English midwives for many years and only began
training her own midwives in 1939 when she started the Frontier Graduate
School of Nurse Midwifery in Hyden, Kentucky, with the advent of World
War II. The nurse midwives accessed many of their families on horseback.
In 1935, a small 12-bed hospital was built at Hyden and provided delivery
services. The nurse midwives under the direction of Breckenridge were successful in lowering the highest maternal mortality rate in the United States (in
Leslie County, Kentucky) to substantially below the national average. These
nurses, as at Henry Street Settlement, provided health care for everyone in the
district for a small annual fee. A delivery had an additional small fee. Nurse
midwives provided primary care, prenatal care, and postnatal care, with an
emphasis on prevention (Wertz & Wertz, 1977).

Armed with the right to vote, in the Roaring Twenties American women
found the new freedom of the "flapper era"—shrinking dress hemlines, shortened hairstyles, and the increased use of cosmetics. Hospitals were used by
greater numbers of people, and the scientific basis of medicine became well
established because most surgical procedures were done in hospitals. Penicillin
was discovered in 1928, creating a revolution in the prevention of infectious
disease deaths (Donahue, 1985; Kalisch & Kalisch, 1986). The previously
mentioned Goldmark Report recommended the establishment of college- and
university-based nursing programs.

Mary D. Osborne, who functioned as supervisor of public health nursing
for the state of Mississippi from 1921 to 1946, had a vision for a collaboration with community nurses and granny midwives, who delivered 80% of the
African American babies in Mississippi. The infant and maternal mortality
rates were both exceptionally high among African American families, and
these granny midwives, who were also African American, were untrained
and had little education.

Osborne took a creative approach to improving maternal and infant
health among African American women. She developed a collaborative
network of public health nurses and granny midwives in which the nurses
implemented training programs for the midwives, and the midwives in turn
assisted the nurses in providing a higher standard of safe maternal and infant
health care. The public health nurses used Osborne's book, *Manual for
Midwives*, which contained guidelines for care and was used in the state until
the 1970s. They taught good hygiene, infection prevention, and compliance
with state regulations. Osborne's innovative program is credited with reducing
the maternal and infant mortality rates in Mississippi and in other states where
her program structure was adopted (Sabin, 1998).

■ The Nursing Profession Responds to the Great Depression and World War II

With the stock market crash of 1929 came the Great Depression, resulting in widespread unemployment of private-duty nurses and the closing of nursing schools with a simultaneous increase in need for charity health services for the population. Nursing students who had previously been the primary source to staff hospitals declined in number. Unemployed graduate nurses were hired to replace them for minimal wages, a trend that was to influence the profession for years to come (MacEachern, 1932).

Other nurses found themselves accompanying troops to Europe when the United States entered World War II. Military nurses were a critical presence at the invasion of Normandy in 1938, as well as in North Africa, Italy, France, and the Philippines, while Navy nurses provided care aboard hospital ships. More than 100,000 nurses volunteered and were certified for military service in the Army and Navy Nurse Corps. The resulting severe shortage of nurses on the home front resulted in the development of the **Cadet Nurse Corps**. **Frances Payne Bolton**, congressional representative from Ohio, is credited with the founding of the Cadet Nurse Corps through the Bolton Act of 1945. By the end of the war, more than 180,000 nursing students had been trained through this act, while advanced practice graduate nurses in psychiatry and public health nursing had received graduate education to increase the numbers of nurse educators (Donahue, 1985; Kalisch & Kalisch, 1986).

Ernie Pyle, a famous war correspondent in World War II, offered Americans a "front-seat view" through his detailed journalistic accounts of daily life on the war front. Pyle was the first journalist to put his own life in danger by reporting from the battlefront; he spent a great deal of time with soldiers during active combat and was killed during a sniper attack in Ie Shima, Japan. Chaplin Nathan Baxter Saucier was assigned to retrieve his body, conduct his service, and assist the soldiers with building his coffin. The funeral service lasted only about 10 minutes. Pyle was buried with his helmet on, at Chaplin Saucier's request. The Navy, Marine Corps, and Army were all represented at the service. Pyle, who died during the Battle of Okinawa in 1945, was a highly regarded and humanistic voice for those serving America during World War II. Here is an example of Pyle's accounts of life for nurses in a field hospital in Europe:

> The officers and nurses live two in a tent on two sides of a company street—nurses on one side, officers on the other.... The nurses wear khaki overalls because of the mud and dust. Pink female panties fly from a line among the brown warlike tents. On the flagpole is a Red Cross flag made from a bed sheet and a French soldier's red sash. The American nurses—and there were lots of them turned out just as you would expect: wonderfully. Army doctors and

patients too were unanimous in their praise of them. Doctors told me that in the first rush of casualties they were calmer than the men. For the first ten days they had to live like animals, even using open ditches for toilets but they never complained. One nurse was always on duty in each tentful of 20 men. She had medical orderlies to help her. The touch of femininity, the knowledge that a woman was around, gave the wounded man courage and confidence and a feeling of security. (Pyle, 1944)

Amid the Depression, many nurses found the expansion and advances in aviation as a new field for nurses. In efforts to increase the public's confidence in the safety of transcontinental air travel, nurses were hired in the promising new role of "nurse-stewardess" (Kalisch & Kalisch, 1986). Congress created an additional relief program, the Civil Works Administration, in 1933 that provided jobs to the unemployed, including placing nurses in schools, public hospitals and clinics, public health departments, and public health education community surveys and campaigns. The Social Security Act of 1935 was passed by Congress to provide old-age benefits, rehabilitation services, unemployment compensation administration, aid to dependent and/or disabled children and adults, and monies to state and local health services. The Social Security Act included Title VI, which authorized the use of federal funds for the training of public health personnel. This led to the placement of public health nurses in state health departments and the expansion of public health nursing as a viable career path.

While nursing was forging new paths for itself in various fields, during the 1930s Hollywood began featuring nurses in films. The only feature-length films to ever focus entirely on the nursing profession were released during this decade. *War Nurse* (1930), *Night Nurse* (1931), *Once to Every Woman* (1934), *The White Parade* (1934 Academy Award nominee for Best Picture), *Four Girls in White* (1939), *The White Angel* (1936), and *Doctor and Nurse* (1937) all used nurses as major characters. During the bleak years of the economic depression, young women found these nurse heroines who promoted idealism, self-sacrifice, and the profession of nursing over personal desires particularly appealing. No longer were nurses depicted as subservient handmaidens who worked as nurses only as a temporary pastime before marriage (Kalisch & Kalisch, 1986).

■ Science and Health Care, 1945–1960: Decades of Change

Dramatic technological and scientific changes characterized the decades following World War II, including the discovery of sulfa drugs, new cardiac drugs, surgeries, and treatment for ventricular fibrillation (Howell, 1996). The Hill-Burton Act, passed in 1946, provided funds to increase the construction of new hospitals. A significant change in the healthcare system was the expansion of private health insurance coverage and the dramatic increase in the birth rate, called the "baby boom" generation. Clinical research, both in medicine and in nursing, became an expectation of health providers, and more nurses sought advanced degrees. The *Journal of Nursing Research* was first published, heralding the arrival of nursing scholarship in the United States.

As a result of increased numbers of hospital beds, additional financial resources for health care, and the post–World War II economic resurgence, nursing faced an acute shortage and nurses confronted increasingly stressful working conditions. Nurses began showing signs of the strain through debates about strikes and collective bargaining demands.

The American Nurses Association (ANA) accepted African American nurses for membership, consequently ending racial discrimination in the dominant nursing organizations. The National Association of Colored Graduate Nurses was disbanded in 1951. Males entered nursing schools in record number, often as a result of previous military experience as medics. Prior to the 1950s and 1960s, male nurses also suffered minority status and were discouraged from nursing as a career. A fact seemingly forgotten by modern society, including Florence Nightingale and early U.S. nursing leaders, is that during medieval times more than one-half of the nurses were male. The Knights Hospitalers, Teutonic Knights, Franciscans, and many other male nursing orders had provided excellent nursing care for their societies. Saint Vincent de Paul had first conceived of the idea of social service. Pastor Theodor Fliedner, teacher and mentor of Florence Nightingale at Kaiserwerth in Germany; Ben Franklin; and Walt Whitman during the Civil War all either served as nurses or were strong advocates for male nurses (Kalisch & Kalisch, 1986).

> **Dramatic technological and scientific changes characterized the decades following World War II, including the discovery of sulfa drugs, new cardiac drugs, surgeries, and treatment for ventricular fibrillation.**

■ Years of Revolution, Protest, and the New Order, 1961–2000

During the social upheaval of the 1960s, nursing was influenced by many changes in society, such as the women's movement, the organized protest against the Vietnam conflict, civil rights movement, President Lyndon Johnson's "Great Society" social reforms, and increased consumer involvement in health care. Specialization in nursing, such as cardiac ICU, nurse anesthetist training, and the clinical specialist role for nursing became trends that affected both education and practice in the healthcare system. Medicare and Medicaid, enacted in 1965 under Title XVIII of the Social Security Act, provided access to health care for older adults, poor persons, and people with disabilities. The American Nurses Association took a courageous and controversial stand in that same year (1965) by approving its first position paper on nursing education, advocating for all nursing education for professional practice to take place in colleges and universities (American Nurses Association, 1965). Nurses returning from Vietnam faced emotional challenges in the form of post-traumatic stress disorder (PTSD) that affected their postwar lives.

With increased specialization in medicine, the demand for primary care healthcare providers exceeded the supply (Christman, 1971). As a response to this need for general practitioners, Dr. Henry Silver, MD, and Dr. Loretta Ford, RN, collaborated to develop the first nurse practitioner (NP) program in the United States at the University of Colorado (Ford & Silver, 1967). Nurse practitioners (NPs) were initially prepared in pediatrics with advanced role preparation in common childhood illness management and well-child care. Ford and Silver (1967) found that NPs could manage as much as 75% of the pediatric patients in community clinics, leading to the widespread use of and educational programs for nurse practitioners. The first state in 1971 to recognize diagnosis and treatment as part of the legal scope of practice for NPs was Idaho. Alaska and North Carolina were among the first states to expand the NP role to include prescriptive authority (Ford, 1979). By the new century, nurse practitioner programs were offered at the MSN level in family nursing; gerontology; adult, neonatal, mental health, and maternal-child areas and have expanded to include the acute care practitioner as well (Huch, 2001). Certification of nurse practitioners now occurs at the national level through the American Nurses Association and by many specialty organizations. NPs are licensed throughout the United States by state boards of nursing.

In the late 1980s, escalating healthcare costs resulting from the explosion of advanced technology and the increased life span of Americans led to the demand for healthcare reform. The nursing profession heralded healthcare reform with an unprecedented collaboration of more than 75 nursing associations, led by the American Nurses Association and the National League for Nursing, in the publication of *Nursing's Agenda for Health Care Reform*. In this document, the challenge of managed care was addressed in the context of cost containment and quality assurance of healthcare service for the nursing profession (American Nurses Association, 1991). Managed care is a market approach based on managed competition as a major strategy to contain healthcare costs, which is still the dominant approach used today (Lundy, Janes, & Hartman, 2001).

The New Century: An Era of Managed Care and Healthcare Reform

U.S. healthcare system reform continues to be the topic of political debate with the primary focus on federal coverage, access, and healthcare cost control. Healthcare organizations in a managed care environment, such as preferred provider organizations and health maintenance organizations, now see the economic and quality outcome benefits of caring for patients and managing their care over a continuum of settings and needs. Patients are followed more closely within the system, both during illness and wellness. Hospital stays are shorter, and more and more healthcare services are provided in outpatient facilities and through community-based settings, such as home health, occupational health, and school health (Lundy, Janes, & Hartman, 2009). And more of these healthcare services are provided by nurses.

The Nurse of the Future

With the roles of nurses in the healthcare system expected to expand in the future, focus is placed on raising educational levels and competencies of nurses and fostering interdisciplinary collaboration to increase access, safety, and quality of patient care. For example, the latest Institute of Medicine (IOM, 2011) report, titled *The Future of Nursing: Leading Change, Advancing Health*, specifically calls for interdisciplinary education, decreasing barriers to nursing scope of practice, and increasing educational levels of nurses. The Robert Wood Johnson Foundation sponsored the Quality and Safety Education for Nurses (QSEN) initiative with the overall goal of "preparing future nurses who will have the knowledge, skills and attitudes (KSAs) necessary to continuously improve the quality and safety of the healthcare systems within which they work" (QSEN, 2007). QSEN is directed to develop competencies of future nursing graduates in six key areas, including patient-centered care, evidence-based practice, quality improvement, teamwork and collaboration, safety, and informatics.

In 2006, the Massachusetts Department of Higher Education (MDHE) and Massachusetts Organization of Nurse Executives convened a working session of stakeholders titled Creativity and Connections: Building the Framework for the Future of Nursing Education and Practice. From this beginning, the *Nurse of the Future: Nursing Core Competencies* (MDHE, 2010, p. 2) was developed in response to the goals of creating a seamless progression through all levels of nursing education and development of consensus on competencies. This movement to facilitate creation of a core set of entry-level nursing competencies and seamless transition in nursing education is not singular and reflects the current focus in the profession to increase access, safety, and quality of health care.

www | CRITICAL THINKING QUESTION ✳

What do you think would be the response of historical nursing leaders such as Florence Nightingale, Lillian Wald, and Mary Breckenridge if they could see what the profession of nursing looks like today? ✳

Conclusion

Consensus regarding basic education and the entry level of registered nurses has not occurred. Changes in the advanced practice role challenge the nurse education and healthcare systems as the primary healthcare needs of the U.S. population compete with acute care for scarce resources. A global community demands that nurses remain committed to cultural sensitivity in care delivery.

The history of health care and nursing provides ample examples of the wisdom of our forebears in the advocacy of nursing in challenging settings and an unknown future. By considering the lessons of our past, the nursing profession is well prepared to provide a full range of quality, cost-effective services in the promotion of health throughout this century.

Classroom Activity 1

There are many theories about Nightingale's chronic illness, which caused her to be an invalid for most of her adult life. Many people have interpreted this as hypochondriacal, something of a melodrama of the Victorian times. Nightingale was rich and could take to her bed. Rumors have abounded among nursing students that she suffered from tertiary syphilis. She became ill during the Crimean War in May 1855 and was diagnosed with a severe case of Crimean fever. Today Crimean fever is recognized as Mediterranean fever and is categorized as brucellosis. She developed spondylitis, or inflammation of the spine. For the next 34 years, she managed to continue her writing and advocacy, often predicting her imminent death. Others have claimed that Nightingale suffered from bipolar disorder, causing her to experience long periods of depression alternating with remarkable bursts of productivity. Read about the various theories of her chronic disabling condition and reflect on your own conclusions about her mysterious illness. With supporting evidence, what are your conclusions about Nightingale's health condition? www

Sources: Dossey, B. (2000). *Florence Nightingale: Mystic, visionary, healer.* Philadelphia, PA: Lippincott Williams & Wilkins; Nightingale suffered bipolar disorder. (2004). *Australian Nursing Journal, 12,* 2.

Classroom Activity 2

What would Florence Nightingale's résumé or curriculum vitae look like? Check out Nightingale's curriculum vitae at www.countryjoe.com/nightingale/cv.htm. www

References

Abel, E. K. (1997). Take the cure to the poor: Patients' responses to New York City's tuberculosis program, 1894–1918. *American Journal of Public Health, 87,* 11.

American Nurses Association. (1965). *Educational preparation for nurse practitioners and assistants to nurses: A position paper.* New York, NY: Author.

American Nurses Association. (1991). *Nursing's agenda for health care reform: Executive summary.* Washington, DC: Author.

Andrews, G. (2003). Nightingale's geography. *Nursing Inquiry, 10*(4), 270–274.

Attewell, A. (1996). Florence Nightingale's health-at-home visitors. *Health Visitor, 6.9*(10), 406.

Barker, E. R. (1989). Care givers as casualties. *Western Journal of Nursing Research, 11*(5), 628–631.

Boorstin, D. J. (1985). *The discoverers: A history of man's search to know his world and himself.* New York, NY: Vintage.

Brainard, A. M. (1922). *The evolution of public health nursing.* Philadelphia, PA: Saunders.

Brockett, L. P., & Vaughan, M. C. (1867). *Women's work in the Civil War: A record of heroism: Patriotism and patience.* Philadelphia, PA: Seigler McCurdy.

Brooke, E. (1997). *Medicine women: A pictorial history of women healers.* Wheaton, IL: Quest Books.

Brown, E. L. (1936). *Nursing as a profession.* New York, NY: Russell Sage Foundation.

Brown, E. L. (1948). *Nursing for the future.* New York, NY: Russell Sage Foundation.

Brown, P. (1988). *Florence Nightingale.* Hats, UK: Exley Publications.

Buhler-Wilkerson, K. (1985). Public health nursing: In sickness or in health? *American Journal of Public Health, 75,* 1155–1156.

Bullough, V. L., & Bullough, B. (1978). *The care of the sick: The emergence of modern nursing.* New York, NY: Prodist.

Calabria, M. D. (1996). *Florence Nightingale in Egypt and Greece: Her diary and visions.* Albany, NY: State University of New York Press.

Carnegie, M. E. (1991). *The path we tread: Blades in nursing 1854–1990* (2nd ed.). New York, NY: National League for Nursing Press.

Cartwright, F. F. (1972). *Disease and history.* New York, NY: Dorset Press.

Christman, L. (1971). The nurse specialist as a professional activist. *Nursing Clinics of North America, 6*(2), 231–235.

Christy, T. E. (1975). The fateful decade: 1890–1900. *American Journal of Nursing, 75*(7), 1163–1165.

Cohen, M. N. (1989). *Health and the rise of civilization.* New Haven, CT: Yale University Press.

Cook, E. (1913). *The life of Florence Nightingale* (Vols. 1 and 2). London, England: Macmillan.

D'Antonio, P. (2002). Nurses in war. *Lancet, 360*(9350), 7–12.

Diamond, J. (1997). *Guns, germs, and steel: The fates of human societies.* New York, NY: W. W. Norton.

Dickens, C. (1844). *Martin Chuzzlewit.* New York, NY: Macmillan.

Dietz, D. D., & Lehozky, A. R. (1963). *History and modern nursing.* Philadelphia, PA: F. A. Davis.

Dock, L., & Stewart, I. (1931). *A short history of nursing from the earliest times to the present day* (3rd ed.). New York, NY: G. P. Putman's Sons.

Donahue, M. P. (1985). *Nursing: The finest art.* St. Louis, MO: Mosby.

Dossey, B. M. (2000). *Florence Nightingale: Mystic, visionary, healer.* Springhouse, PA: Springhouse.

Ford, L. C. (1979). A nurse for all seasons: The nurse practitioner. *Nursing Outlook, 27*(8), 516–521.

Ford, L. C., & Silver, H. K. (1967). The expanded role of the nurse in child care. *Nursing Outlook, 15*(8), 43–45.

Frantz, A. K. (1998). Nursing pride: Clara Barton in the Spanish American War. *American Journal of Nursing, 98*(10), 39–41.

Goldmark, J. C. (1923). Nursing and nursing education in the United States. New York, NY: Macmillan.

Hamilton, D. (1988). Clinical excellence, but too high a cost: The Metropolitan Life Insurance Company Visiting Nurse Service (1909–1953). *Public Health Nursing, 5,* 235–240.

Hanlon, J. J., & Pickett, G. E. (1984). *Public health administration and practice* (8th ed.). St. Louis, MO: Mosby.

Heinrich, J. (1983). Historical perspectives on public health nursing. *Nursing Outlook, 32*(6), 317–320.

Hine, D. C. (1989). *Black women in white: Racial conflict and cooperation in the nursing profession 1889–1950.* Bloomington, IN: Indiana University Press.

Howell, J. (1996). *Technology in the hospital.* Baltimore, MD: Johns Hopkins University Press.

Huch, M. (2001). Advanced practice nursing in the community. In K. S. Lundy & S. Janes (Eds.), *Community health nursing: Caring for the public's health* (pp. 968–980). Sudbury, MA: Jones and Bartlett.

Institute of Medicine. (2011). *The future of nursing: Leading change, advancing health.* Washington, DC: National Academy Press.

Kalisch, P. A., & Kalisch, B. J. (1986). *The advance of American nursing* (2nd ed.). Boston, MA: Little, Brown.

LeVasseur, J. (1998). Plato: Nightingale and contemporary nursing. *Image: Journal of Nursing Scholarship, 30*(3), 281–285.

Longfellow, H. W. (1857). Santa Filomena. *Atlantic Monthly, 1,* 22–23.

Lundy, K. S., Janes, S., & Hartman, S. (2001). Opening the door to health care in the community. In K. S. Lundy & S. Janes (Eds.), *Community health nursing: Caring for the public's health* (pp. 5–29). Sudbury, MA: Jones and Bartlett.

Lundy, K. S., Janes, S., & Hartman, S. (2009). Opening the door to health care in the community. In K. S. Lundy & S. Janes (Eds.), *Community health nursing: Caring for the public's health* (pp. 4–29). Sudbury, MA: Jones and Bartlett.

MacEachern, M. T. (1932). Which shall we choose: Graduate or student service? *Modern Hospital, 38,* 97–98, 102–104.

Massachusetts Department of Higher Education. (2010). *Nurse of the future: Nursing core competencies.* Retrieved from http://www.mass.edu/currentinit/documents/NursingCoreCompetencies.pdf

Montag, M. L. (1959). *Community college education for nursing: An experiment in technical education for nursing.* New York, NY: McGraw-Hill.

Monteiro, L. A. (1985). Florence Nightingale on public health nursing. *American Journal of Public Health, 75*(2), 181–185.

Mosley, M. O. P. (1996). Satisfied to carry the bag: Three black community health nurses' contribution to health care reform, 1900–1937. *Nursing History Review, 4,* 65–82.

Nightingale, F. (1860). *Notes on nursing: What it is and what it is not.* London, England: Harrison.

Nightingale, F. (1893). Sick-nursing and health-nursing. In B. Burdett-Coutts (Ed.), *Women's mission* (pp. 184–205). London, England: Sampson, Law, Marston and Co.

Nightingale, F. (1894). *Health teaching in towns and villages.* London, England: Spottiswoode & Co.

Nightingale, F. (1979). Cassandra. In M. Stark (Ed.), *Florence Nightingale's Cassandra.* Old Westbury, NY: Feminist Press.

Nutting, M. A., & Dock, L. L. (1907). *A history of nursing: The evolution of nursing systems from the earliest times to the foundation of the first English and American training schools for nurses.* New York, NY: G. P. Putnam's Sons.

The 100 people who made the millennium. (1997). *Life Magazine, 20*(10a).

Palmer, I. S. (1977). Florence Nightingale: Reformer, reactionary, researcher. *Nursing Research, 26*(2), 13–18.

Palmer, I. S. (1982). *Through a glass darkly: From Nightingale to now.* Washington, DC: American Association of Colleges of Nursing.

Pyle, E. (1944). *Here is your war: The story of G.I. Joe.* Cleveland, OH: World Publishing.

Quality and Safety Education for Nurses. (2007). Quality and safety competencies. Retrieved from http://www.qsen.org/competencies.php

Rathbone, W. (1890). *A history of nursing in the homes of the poor.* Introduction by Florence Nightingale. London, England: Macmillan.

Richardson, B. I. W. (1887). *The health of nations: A review of the works of Edwin Chadwick* (Vol. 2). London, England: Longmans, Green.

Roberts, M. (1954). *American nursing: History and interpretation.* New York, NY: Macmillan.

Robinson, V. (1946). *White caps: The story of nursing.* Philadelphia, PA: Lippincott.

Rosen, G. (1958). *A history of public health.* New York, NY: M.D. Publications.

Sabin, L. (1998). *Struggles and triumphs: The story of Mississippi nurses 1800–1950.* Jackson, MS: Mississippi Hospital Association Health, Research and Educational Foundation.

Sanger, M. (1928). *Motherhood in bondage.* New York, NY: Brentano's.

Seymer, L. (1954). *Selected writings of Florence Nightingale.* New York, NY: Macmillan.

Shryock, R. H. (1959). *The history of nursing: An interpretation of the social and medical factors involved.* Philadelphia, PA: Saunders.

Smith, E. (1934). *Mississippi special public health nursing project made possible by federal funds.* Paper presented at the 1934 annual Mississippi Nurses Association meeting, Jackson, MS.

Snow, J. (1855). *On the mode of communication of cholera* (2nd ed.). London, England: Churchill.

Stanmore, A. H. G. (1906). *Sidney Herbert of Lea: A memoir*. New York, NY: E. P. Dutton.

State board test pool examination. (1952). *American Journal of Nursing, 52*, 613.

Stewart, I. M. (1921). Developments in nursing education since 1918. *U.S. Bureau of Education Bulletin, 20*(6), 3–8.

Taylor, H. O. (1922). *Greek biology and medicine*. Boston, MA: Marshall Jones.

Tiffany, R. (1890). *The life of Dorothea Linda Dix*. Boston, MA: Houghton Mifflin.

Tooley, S. A. (1910). *The life of Florence Nightingale*. London, England: Cassell and Co.

Tyrell, H. (1856). *Pictorial history of the war with Russia 1854–1856*. London, England: W. and R. Chambers.

Vicinus, M., & Nergaard, B. (1990). *Ever yours: Florence Nightingale: Selected letters*. Cambridge, MA: Harvard University Press.

Wald, L. D. (1915). *The house on Henry Street*. New York, NY: Holt.

Wertz, R. W., & Wertz, D. C. (1977). *Lying-in: A history of childbirth in America*. New Haven, CT: Yale University Press.

Wheeler, W. (1999). Is Florence Nightingale holding us back? *Nursing 99, 29*(10), 22–23.

Williams, C. B. (1961). Stories from Scutari. *American Journal of Nursing, 61*, 88.

Winslow, C.-E. A. (1946). Florence Nightingale and public health nursing. *Public Health Nursing, 38*, 330–332.

Woodham-Smith, C. (1951). *Florence Nightingale*. New York, NY: McGraw-Hill.

Woodham-Smith, C. (1983). *Florence Nightingale*. New York, NY: Athenaeum.

Young, D. A. (1995). Florence Nightingale's fever. *British Medical Journal, 311*, 1697–1700.

Framework for Professional Nursing Practice

2

Kathleen Masters

Although the beginning of nursing theory development can be traced to Florence Nightingale, it was not until the second half of the 1900s that nursing theory caught the attention of nursing as a discipline. During the decades of the 1960s and 1970s, theory development was a major topic of discussion and publication. During the 1970s, much of the discussion was related to the development of one global theory for nursing. However, in the 1980s, attention turned from the development of a global theory for nursing as scholars began to recognize multiple approaches to theory development in nursing.

Because of the plurality in nursing theory, this information must be organized to be meaningful for practice, research, and further knowledge development. The goal of this chapter is to present an organized and practical overview of the major concepts, models, philosophies, and theories that are essential in professional nursing practice.

It can be helpful to define some terms that might be unfamiliar. A **concept** is a term or label that describes a phenomenon (Meleis, 2004). The phenomenon described by a concept can be either empirical or abstract. An empirical concept is one that can be either observed or experienced through the senses. An abstract concept is one that is not observable, such as hope or caring (Hickman, 2002).

Key Terms and Concepts

» **Concept**
» Conceptual model
» Propositions
» Assumptions
» Theory
» Metaparadigm
» Person
» Environment
» Health
» Nursing
» Philosophies

Learning Objectives

After completing this chapter, the student should be able to:

1. Identify the four metaparadigm concepts of nursing.
2. Identify and describe several theoretical works in nursing.
3. Begin the process of identifying theoretical frameworks of nursing that are consistent with a personal belief system.

A **conceptual model** is defined as a set of concepts and statements that integrate the concepts into a meaningful configuration (Lippitt, 1973; as cited in Fawcett, 1994). **Propositions** are statements that describe relationships among events, situations, or actions (Meleis, 2004). **Assumptions** also describe concepts or connect two concepts and represent values, beliefs, or goals. When assumptions are challenged, they become propositions (Meleis, 2004).

Conceptual models are composed of abstract and general concepts and propositions that provide a frame of reference for members of a discipline. This frame of reference determines how the world is viewed by members of a discipline and guides the members as they propose questions and make observations relevant to the discipline (Fawcett, 1994).

A **theory** "is an organized, coherent, and systematic articulation of a set of statements related to significant questions in a discipline that are communicated in a meaningful whole," according to Meleis (2007, p. 37). The primary distinction between a conceptual model and a theory is the level of abstraction and specificity. A conceptual model is a highly abstract system of global concepts and linking statements. A theory, in contrast, deals with one or more specific, concrete concepts and propositions (Fawcett, 1994).

A **metaparadigm** is the most global perspective of a discipline and "acts as an encapsulating unit, or framework, within which the more restricted ... structures develop" (Eckberg & Hill, 1979, p. 927). Each discipline singles out phenomena of interest that it will deal with in a unique manner. The concepts and propositions that identify and interrelate these phenomena are even more abstract than those in the conceptual models. These are the concepts that comprise the metaparadigm of the discipline (Fawcett, 1994).

The conceptual models and theories of nursing represent various paradigms derived from the metaparadigm of the discipline of nursing. Therefore, although each of the conceptual models might link and define the four metaparadigm concepts differently, the four metaparadigm concepts are present in each of the models.

> **The conceptual models and theories of nursing represent various paradigms derived from the metaparadigm of the discipline of nursing.**

The central concepts of the discipline of nursing are **person**, **environment**, **health**, and **nursing**. These four concepts of the metaparadigm of nursing are more specifically "The person receiving the nursing, the environment within which the person exits, the health–illness continuum within which the person falls at the time of the interaction with the nurse, and, finally, nursing actions themselves" (Flaskerud & Holloran, 1980, cited in Fawcett, 1994, p. 5).

Because concepts are so abstract at the metaparadigm level, many conceptual models have developed from the metaparadigm of nursing. Subsequently, multiple theories have been derived from each conceptual model in an effort to describe, explain, and predict the phenomena within the model.

Overview of Selected Nursing Theories

To apply nursing theory in practice, the nurse must have some knowledge of the theoretical works of the nursing profession. This chapter is not intended to provide an in-depth analysis of each of the theoretical works in nursing but rather provides an introductory overview of selected theoretical works to give you a launching point for further reflection and study as you begin your journey into professional nursing practice.

Theoretical works in nursing are generally categorized either as philosophies, conceptual models, theories, or middle-range theories depending on the level of abstraction. We begin with the most abstract of these theoretical works, the philosophies of nursing.

> **www CRITICAL THINKING QUESTION** ✳
>
> What are the specific competencies for nurses in relation to theoretical knowledge? ✳

■ Selected Philosophies of Nursing

Philosophies set forth the general meaning of nursing and nursing phenomena through reasoning and the logical presentation of ideas. Philosophies are broad and address general ideas about nursing. Because of their breadth, nursing philosophies contribute to the discipline by providing direction, clarifying values, and forming a foundation for theory development (Alligood, 2006).

Nightingale's Environmental Theory

Nightingale's philosophy includes the four metaparadigm concepts of nursing (Table 2-1), but the focus is primarily on the patient and the environment, with the nurse manipulating the environment to enhance patient recovery. Nursing interventions using Nightingale's philosophy are centered on her 13 canons, which follow (Nightingale, 1860/1969):

- Ventilation and warming: The interventions subsumed in this canon include keeping the patient and the patient's room warm and keeping the patient's

TABLE 2-1 Metaparadigm Concepts as Defined in Nightingale's Model

Person Recipient of nursing care **Environment** External (temperature, bedding, ventilation) and internal (food, water, and medications) **Health** Health is "not only to be well, but to be able to use well every power we have to use" (Nightingale, 1969, p. 24)	**Nursing** Alter or manage the environment to implement the natural laws of health

room well ventilated and free of odors. Specific instructions included "keep the air within as pure as the air without" (Nightingale, 1860/1969, p. 10).

- Health of houses: This canon includes the five essentials of pure air, pure water, efficient drainage, cleanliness, and light.
- Petty management: Continuity of care for the patient when the nurse is absent is the essence of this canon.
- Noise: Instructions include the avoidance of sudden noises that startle or awaken patients and keeping noise in general to a minimum.
- Variety: This canon refers to an attempt at variety in the patient's room to avoid boredom and depression.
- Taking food: Interventions include the documentation of the amount of food and liquids that the patient ingests.
- What food? Instructions include trying to include patient food preferences.
- Bed and bedding: The interventions in this canon include comfort measures related to keeping the bed dry and wrinkle free.
- Light: The instructions contained in this canon relate to adequate light in the patient's room.
- Cleanliness of rooms and walls: This canon focuses on keeping the environment clean.
- Personal cleanliness: This canon includes measures such as keeping the patient clean and dry.
- Chattering hopes and advices: Instructions in this canon include the avoidance of talking without reason or giving advice that is without fact.
- Observation of the sick: This canon includes instructions related to making observations and documenting observations.

The 13 canons are central to Nightingale's theory but are not all inclusive. Nightingale believed that nursing was a calling and that the recipients of nursing care were holistic individuals with a spiritual dimension; thus, the nurse was expected to care for the spiritual needs of the patients in spiritual distress. Nightingale also believed that nurses should be involved in health promotion and health teaching with the sick and with those who were well (Bolton, 2006).

Although Nightingale's theory was developed long ago in response to a need for environmental reform, the nursing principles are still relevant today. Even as some of Nightingale's rationales have been modified or disproved by advances in medicine and science, many of the concepts in her theory have not only endured, but have been used to provide general guidelines for nurses for more than 150 years (Pfettscher, 2006).

Virginia Henderson: Definition of Nursing and 14 Components of Basic Nursing Care

Henderson made such significant contributions to the discipline of nursing during her more-than-60-year career as a nurse, teacher, author, and researcher that some refer to her as the Florence Nightingale of the 20th century (Tomey, 2006). She is perhaps best known for her definition of nursing, which was first published in 1955 (Harmer & Henderson, 1955) and then published in 1966 with minor revisions. According to Henderson,

> The unique function of the nurse is to assist the individual, sick or well, in the performance of those activities contributing to health or its recovery (or to a peaceful death) that he would perform unaided if he had the necessary strength, will, or knowledge and to do this in such a way as to help him gain independence as rapidly as possible. (Henderson, 1966, p. 15)

In her work Henderson emphasized the art of nursing as well as empathetic understanding, stating that the nurse must "get inside the skin of each of her patients in order to know what he needs" (Henderson, 1964, p. 63). She believed that "the beauty of medicine and nursing is the combination of your heart, your head and your hands and where you separate them, you diminish them ..." (McBride, 1997, as cited by Gordon, 2001).

Henderson identified 14 basic needs on which nursing care is based. These needs include the following:

- Breathe normally.
- Eat and drink adequately.
- Eliminate bodily wastes.
- Move and maintain desirable postures.
- Sleep and rest.
- Select suitable clothes; dress and undress.
- Maintain body temperature within normal range by adjusting clothing and modifying the environment.
- Keep the body clean and well groomed and protect the integument.
- Avoid dangers in the environment, and avoid injuring others.
- Communicate with others in expressing emotions, needs, fears, or opinions.
- Worship according to one's faith.
- Work in such a way that there is a sense of accomplishment.
- Play or participate in various forms of recreation.
- Learn, discover, or satisfy the curiosity that leads to normal development and health and use the available health facilities (Henderson, 1966, 1991).

Although Henderson did not consider her work a theory of nursing, and did not explicitly state assumptions or define each of the domains of nursing, her work includes the metaparadigm concepts of nursing (Furukawa & Howe, 2002) (Table 2-2).

Jean Watson: Philosophy and Science of Caring

According to Watson's theory (1996), the goal of nursing is to help persons attain a higher level of harmony within the mind–body–spirit. Attainment of that goal can potentiate healing and health (Table 2-3). This goal is pursued through transpersonal caring guided by carative factors and corresponding caristas processes.

TABLE 2-2 Metaparadigm Concepts as Defined in Henderson's Philosophy and Art of Nursing	
Person Recipient of nursing care who is composed of biological, psychological, sociological, and spiritual components	**Health** Based upon the patient's ability to function independently (as outlined in 14 components of basic nursing care)
Environment External environment (temperature, dangers in environment); some discussion of impact of community on the individual and family	**Nursing** Assist the person, sick or well, in performance of activities (14 components of basic nursing care) and help the person gain independence as rapidly as possible (Henderson, 1966, p. 15)

TABLE 2-3 Metaparadigm Concepts as Defined in Watson's Philosophy and Science of Caring	
Person (human) A "unity of mind–body–spirit/nature" (Watson, 1996, p. 147); embodied spirit (Watson, 1989)	**Health (healing)** Harmony, wholeness, and comfort
Healing space and environment A nonphysical energetic environment; a vibrational field integral with the person where the nurse is not only in the environment but "the nurse IS the environment" (Watson, 2008, p. 26)	**Nursing** Reciprocal transpersonal relationship in caring moments guided by carative factors and caritas processes

Watson's theory for nursing practice is based on 10 carative factors (Watson, 1979). As Watson's work evolved, she renamed these carative factors into what she termed clinical caritas processes (Fawcett, 2005). *Caritas* means to cherish, to appreciate, and to give special attention. It conveys the concept of love (Watson, 2001). The 10 caritas processes are summarized here:

- Practice of loving kindness and equanimity for oneself and other
- Being authentically present and enabling and sustaining the deep belief system and subjective life world of self and the one being cared for
- Cultivating one's own spiritual practices; going beyond the ego self; deepening of self-awareness
- Developing and sustaining a helping–trusting, authentic caring relationship

- Being present to, and supportive of, the expression of positive and negative feelings as a connection with a deeper spirit of oneself and the one being cared for
- Creatively using oneself and all ways of knowing as part of the caring process and engagement in artistry of caring–healing practices
- Engaging in a genuine teaching–learning experience within the context of a caring relationship, while attending to the whole person and subjective meaning; attempting to stay within the other's frame of reference
- Creating a healing environment at all levels, subtle environment of energy and consciousness whereby wholeness, beauty, comfort, dignity, and peace are potentiated
- Assisting with basic needs, with an intentional caring consciousness; administering human care essentials, which potentiate alignment of the mind–body–spirit, wholeness, and unity of being in all aspects of care; attending to both embodied spirit and evolving emergence
- Opening and attending to spiritual, mysterious, and unknown existential dimensions of life, death, suffering; "allowing for a miracle" (Watson, 2008)

Watson (2001) refers to the clinical caritas processes as the "core" of nursing, which is grounded in the philosophy, science, and the art of caring. She contrasts the core of nursing with what she terms the "trim," a term she uses to refer to the practice setting, procedures, functional tasks, clinical disease focus, technology, and techniques of nursing. The trim, Watson explains, is not expendable, but it cannot be the center of professional nursing practice (Watson, 1997, p. 50).

Regarding the value system that is blended with these 10 carative factors, Watson (1985) states:

> Human care requires high regard and reverence for a person and human life…. There is high value on the subjective–internal world of the experiencing person and how the person (both patient and nurse) is perceiving and experiencing health–illness conditions. An emphasis is placed upon helping a person gain more self-knowledge, self control, and readiness for self-healing. (pp. 34, 35)

The carative factors described by Watson provide guidelines for nurse–patient interactions; however, the theory does not furnish instructions about what to do to achieve authentic caring–healing relationships. Watson's theory is more about being than doing, but it provides a useful framework for the delivery of patient-centered nursing care (Neil & Tomey, 2006).

Patricia Benner's Clinical Wisdom in Nursing Practice
Benner's work has focused on the understanding of perceptual acuity, clinical judgment, skilled know-how, ethical comportment, and ongoing experiential learning (Brykczynski, 2010, p. 141). Also important in Benner's philosophy is an understanding of ethical comportment. According to Day and Benner (2002),

good conduct is a product of an individual relationship with the patient that involves engagement in a situation combined with a sense of membership in a profession where professional conduct is socially embedded, lived, and embodied in the practices, ways of being, and responses to clinical situations and where clinical and ethical judgments are inseparable.

Benner's original domains and competencies of nursing practice were derived inductively from clinical situation interviews and observations of nurses in actual practice. From these interviews and observations, 31 competencies and 7 domains were identified and described. The 7 domains are the helping role, the teaching-coaching function, the diagnostic and patient monitoring function, effective management of rapidly changing situations, administering and monitoring therapeutic interventions and regimens, monitoring and ensuring the quality of healthcare practices, and organizational work role competencies (Benner, 1984/2001). Along with the identification of the competencies and domains of nursing, Benner identified five stages of skill acquisition based on the Dreyfus model of skill acquisition as applied to nursing along with characteristics of each stage. The stages identified included novice, advanced beginner, competent, proficient, and expert (Benner, 1984/2001).

Later, in an extension of her original work, Benner and her colleagues identified nine domains of critical care nursing. These domains are diagnosing and managing life-sustaining physiologic functions in unstable patients, using skilled know-how to manage a crisis, providing comfort measures for the critically ill, caring for patients' families, preventing hazards in a technological environment, facing death: end-of-life care and decision making, communicating and negotiating multiple perspectives, monitoring quality and managing breakdown, using the skilled know-how of clinical leadership and the coaching and mentoring of others (Benner, Hooper-Kyriakidis, & Stannard, 1999). In addition, the nine domains of critical care nursing practice are used as broad themes in data interpretation for the identification and description of six aspects of clinical judgment and skilled comportment. These six aspects are as follows:

- Reasoning-in-transition: Practical reasoning in an ongoing clinical situation
- Skilled know-how: Also known as embodied intelligent performance; knowing what to do, when to do it, and how to do it
- Response-based practice: Adapting interventions to meet the changing needs and expectations of patients
- Agency: One's sense of and ability to act on or influence a situation
- Perceptual acuity and the skill of involvement: The ability to tune into a situation and hone in on the salient issues by engaging with the problem and the person
- Links between clinical and ethical reasoning: The understanding that good clinical practice cannot be separated from ethical notions of good outcomes for patients and families (Benner et al., 1999).

TABLE 2-4 Metaparadigm Concepts as Defined in Benner's Philosophy

Person Embodied person living in the world who is a "self-interpreting being, that is, the person does not come into the world pre-defined but gets defined in the course of living a life" (Benner & Wrubel, 1989, p. 41)

Environment (situation) A social environment with social definition and meaningfulness

Health The human experiencee of health or wholeness

Nursing A caring relationship that includes the care and study of the lived experience of health, illness, and disease

Benner identifies and defines the four metaparadigm concepts of nursing in addition to the concepts previously discussed. The concepts of person, environment, health, and nursing as defined by Benner are summarized in Table 2-4.

■ Selected Conceptual Models and Grand Theories of Nursing

Conceptual models provide a comprehensive view and guide for nursing practice. They are organizing frameworks that guide the reasoning process in professional nursing practice (Alligood, 2006). At the level of the conceptual model, each metaparadigm concept is defined and described in a manner unique to the model, with the model providing an alternative way to view the concepts considered important to the discipline (Fawcett, 2005, pp. 17–18).

Martha Rogers's Science of Unitary Human Beings

According to Rogers (1994), nursing is a learned profession, both a science and an art. The art of nursing is the creative use of the science of nursing for human betterment.

Rogers's theory asserts that human beings are dynamic energy fields that are integrated with environmental energy fields so that the person and his or her environment form a single unit. Both human energy fields and environmental fields are open systems, pandimensional in nature and in a constant state of change. Pattern is the identifying characteristic of energy fields (Table 2-5).

Rogers identified the principles of helicy, resonancy, and integrality to describe the nature of change within human and environmental energy fields. Together, these principles are known as the principle of homeodynamics. The helicy principle describes the unpredictable but continuous, nonlinear evolution of energy fields, as evidenced by a spiral development that is a continuous, nonrepeating, and innovative patterning that reflects the nature

TABLE 2-5 Metaparadigm Concepts as Defined in Rogers's Theory

Person An irreducible, irreversible, pandimensional, negentropic energy field identified by pattern; a unitary human being develops through three principles: helicy, resonancy, and integrality (Rogers, 1992)

Environment An irreducible, pandimensional, negentropic energy field, identified by pattern and manifesting characteristics different from those of the parts and encompassing all that is other than any given human field (Rogers, 1992)

Health Health and illness as part of a continuum (Rogers, 1970)

Nursing Seeks to promote symphonic interaction between human and environmental fields, to strengthen the integrity of the human field, and to direct and redirect patterning of the human and environmental fields for realization of maximum health potential (Rogers, 1970)

of change. Resonancy is depicted as a wave frequency and an energy field pattern evolution from lower to higher frequency wave patterns and is reflective of the continuous variability of the human energy field as it changes. The principle of integrality emphasizes the continuous mutual process of person and environment (Rogers, 1970, 1992).

Rogers used two widely recognized toys to illustrate her theory and constant interaction of the human–environment process. The Slinky illustrates the openness, rhythm, motion, balance, and expanding nature of the human life process, which is continuously evolving (Rogers, 1970). The kaleidoscope illustrates the changing patterns that appear to be infinitely different (Johnson & Webber, 2010, p. 142).

Rogers (1970) identified five assumptions that support and connect the concepts in her conceptual model:

- Man is a unified whole possessing his own integrity and manifesting characteristics more than and different from the sum of his parts (p. 47).
- Man and environment are continuously exchanging matter and energy with one another (p. 54).
- The life process evolves irreversibly and unidirectionally along the space–time continuum (p. 59).
- Pattern and organization identify man and reflect his innovative wholeness (p. 65).
- Man is characterized by the capacity for abstraction and imagery, language and thought, sensation, and emotion (p. 73).

Rogers's model is an abstract system of ideas but is applicable to practice, with nursing care focused on pattern appraisal and patterning activities. Pattern appraisal involves a comprehensive assessment of environmental field patterns and human field patterns of communication, exchange, rhythms, dissonance, and harmony through the use of cognitive input, sensory input, intuition, and language. Patterning activities can include interventions such as meditation, imagery, journaling, or modifying surroundings. Evaluation is ongoing and requires a repetition of the appraisal process (Gunther, 2006).

Dorothea Orem's Self-Care Deficit Theory of Nursing

Orem describes her theory as a general theory that is made up of three related theories, the Theory of Self-Care, the Theory of Self-Care Deficit, and the Theory of Nursing Systems. The Theory of Self-Care describes why and how people care for themselves. The Theory of Self-Care Deficit describes and explains why people can be helped through nursing. The Theory of Nursing Systems describes and explains relationships that must exist and be maintained for nursing to occur. These three theories in relationship constitute Orem's general theory of nursing known as the Self-Care Deficit Theory of Nursing (Berbiglia, 2010; Orem, 1990; Taylor, 2006).

Theory of Self-Care

The Theory of Self-Care describes why and how people care for themselves and suggests that nursing is required in case of inability to perform self-care as a result of limitations. This theory includes the concepts of self-care agency, therapeutic self-care demand, and basic conditioning factors.

Self-care agency is an acquired ability of mature and maturing persons to know and meet their requirements for deliberate and purposive action to regulate their own human functioning and development (Orem, 2001, p. 492). The concept of self-care agency has three dimensions: development, operability, and adequacy. According to Orem (2001, p. 491), therapeutic self-care demand consists of the summation of care measures necessary to meet all of an individual's known self-care requisites. *Basic conditioning factors* refer to those factors that affect the value of the therapeutic self-care demand or self-care agency of an individual. Ten factors are identified: age, gender, developmental state, health state, pattern of living, healthcare system factors, family system factors, sociocultural factors, availability of resources, and external environmental factors (Orem, 2001).

Orem identifies three types of self-care requisites that are integrated into the theory of self-care and provide the basis for self-care. These include universal self-care requisites, developmental self-care requisites, and health deviation self-care requisites.

Universal self-care requisites are those found in all human beings and are associated with life processes. These requisites include the following needs:

- Maintenance of sufficient intake of air
- Maintenance of sufficient intake of water
- Maintenance of sufficient intake of food
- Provision of care associated with elimination processes and excrements

- Maintenance of a balance of activity and rest
- Maintenance of a balance between solitude and social interaction
- Prevention of hazards to human life, human functioning, and human well-being
- Promotion of human functioning and development within social groups in accordance with human potential, known limitations, and the human desire to be normal (Orem, 1985, pp. 90–91)

Developmental self-care requisites are related to different stages in the human life cycle and might include events such attending college, marriage, and retirement. Broadly speaking, the development self-care requisites include the following needs:

- Bringing about and maintenance of living conditions that support life processes and promote the processes of development—that is, human progress toward higher levels of organization of human structures and toward maturation
- Provision of care either to prevent the occurrence of deleterious effects of conditions that can affect human development or to mitigate or overcome these effects from various conditions (Orem, 1985, p. 96)

Health-deviation self-care requisites are related to deviations in structure or function of a human being. There are six categories of health-deviation requisites:

- Seeking and securing appropriate medical assistance
- Being aware of and attending to the effects and results of illness states
- Effectively carrying out medically prescribed treatments
- Being aware of and attending to side effects of treatment
- Modifying self-concept in accepting oneself in a particular state of health
- Learning to live with the effects of illness and medical treatment (Orem, 1985, pp. 99–100)

Theory of Self-Care Deficit

The Theory of Self-Care Deficit explains that maturing or mature adults deliberately learn and perform actions to direct their survival, quality of life, and well-being; put more simply, it explains why people can be helped through nursing. According to Orem, nurses use five methods to help meet the self-care needs of patients:

- Acting for or doing for another
- Guiding and directing
- Providing physical or psychological support
- Providing and maintaining an environment that supports personal development
- Teaching (Johnson & Webber, 2010; Orem, 1995, 2001)

Theory of Nursing Systems

The Theory of Nursing Systems describes and explains relationships that must exist and be maintained for the product (nursing) to occur (Berbiglia, 2010; Taylor, 2006). Three systems can be used to meet the self-requisites of the patient: the wholly compensatory system, the partially compensatory system, and the supportive-educative system.

- In the *wholly compensatory system,* the patient is unable to perform any self-care activities and relies on the nurse to perform care.
- In the *partially compensatory system,* both the patient and the nurse participate in the patient's self-care activities, with the responsibility for care shifting from the nurse to the patient as the self-care demand changes.
- In the *supportive-educative system,* the patient has the ability for self-care but requires assistance from the nurse in decision making, knowledge, or skill acquisition. The nurse's role is to promote the patient as a self-care agent.

The system selected depends on the nurse's assessment of the patient's ability to perform self-care activities and self-care demands (Johnson & Webber, 2010; Orem, 1995, 2001).

There are eight general propositions for the Self-Care Deficit Theory of Nursing (although each of the three individual theories also has its own set of propositions) (Meleis, 2004):

- Human beings have capabilities to provide their own self-care or care for dependants to meet universal, developmental, and health-deviation self-care requisites. These capabilities are learned and recalled.
- Self-care abilities are influenced by age, developmental state, experiences, and sociocultural background.
- Self-care deficits should balance between self-care demands and self-care capabilities.
- Self-care or dependent care is mediated by age, developmental stage, life experience, sociocultural orientation, health, and resources.
- Therapeutic self-care includes actions of nurses, patients, and others that regulate self-care capabilities and meet self-care needs.
- Nurses assess the abilities of patients to meet their self-care needs and their potential of not performing their self-care.
- Nurses engage in selecting valid and reliable processes, technologies, or actions for meeting self-care needs.
- Components of therapeutic self-care are wholly compensatory, partly compensatory, and supportive-educative.

In addition to these other concepts, the four metaparadigm concepts of nursing are identified in Orem's theory (Table 2-6). Orem's theory clearly differentiates the focus of nursing and is one of the nursing theories that is most commonly used in practice.

TABLE 2-6 Metaparadigm Concepts as Defined by Orem's Theory

Person (patient)   A person under the care of a nurse; a total being with universal, developmental needs, and capable of self-care

Environment   Physical, chemical, biologic, and social contexts within which human beings exist; environmental components include environmental factors, environmental elements, environmental conditions, and developmental environment (Orem, 1985)

Health   "A state characterized by soundness or wholeness of developed human structures and of bodily and mental functioning" (Orem, 1995, p. 101)

Nursing   Therapeutic self-care designed to supplement self-care requisites. Nursing actions fall into one of three categories: wholly compensatory, partly compensatory, or supportive–educative system (Orem, 1985)

Callista Roy's Adaptation Model

The Roy Adaptation Model presents the person as an adaptive system in constant interaction with the internal and the external environments. The main task of the human system is to maintain integrity in the face of environmental stimuli (Phillips, 2006). The goal of nursing is to foster successful adaptation (Table 2-7).

According to Roy and Andrews (1999), adaptation refers to "the process and outcome whereby thinking and feeling persons, as individuals or in groups, use conscious awareness and choice to create human and environmental integration" (p. 54). Adaptation leads to optimum health and well-being, to quality of life, and to death with dignity (Andrews & Roy, 1991). The adaptation level represents the condition of the life processes. Roy describes three levels: integrated, compensatory, and compromised life processes. An integrated life process can change to a compensatory process, which attempts to reestablish adaptation. If the compensatory processes are not adequate, compromised processes result (Roy, 2009, p. 33).

The processes for coping in the Roy Adaptation Model are categorized as "the regulator and cognator subsystems as they apply to individuals, and the stabilizer and innovator subsystems as applied to groups" (p. 33). A basic type of adaptive process, the regulator subsystem responds through neural, chemical, and endocrine coping channels. Stimuli from the internal and external environments act as inputs through the senses to the nervous system, thereby affecting the fluid, electrolyte, and acid–base balance, as well as the endocrine system. This information is all channeled automatically, with the body producing an automatic, unconscious response to it (p. 41).

The second adaptive process, the cognator subsystem, responds through four cognitive-emotional channels: perceptual and information processing, learning, judgment, and emotion. Perceptual and information processing includes activities of selective attention, coding, and memory. Learning involves imitation, reinforcement, and insight. Judgment includes problem solving and decision making. Defenses are used to seek relief from anxiety and make affective appraisal and attachments through the emotions (p. 41).

The cognator–regulator and stabilizer–innovator subsystems function to maintain integrated life processes. These life processes—whether integrated, compensatory, or compromised—are manifested in behaviors of the individual or group. Behavior is viewed as an output of the human system and takes the form of either adaptive responses or ineffective responses. These responses serve as feedback to the system, with the human system using this information to decide whether to increase or decrease its efforts to cope with the stimuli (Roy, 2009, p. 34).

Behaviors can be observed in four categories, or adaptive modes: physiologic-physical mode, self-concept–group identify mode, role function mode, and interdependence mode. Behavior in the *physiologic-physical mode* is the manifestation of the physiologic activities of all cells, tissues, organs, and systems making up the body. The *self-concept–group identity mode* includes the components of the physical self, including body sensation and body image, and the personal self, including self-consistency, self-ideal, and moral-ethical-spiritual self. The *role function mode* focuses on the roles of the person in society and the roles within a group, and the *interdependence mode* is a category of behavior related to interdependent relationships. This mode focuses on interactions related to the giving and receiving of love, respect, and value (Roy, 2009).

In the Roy Adaptation Model, three classes of stimuli form the environment: the focal stimulus (internal or external stimulus most immediately in the awareness of the individual or group), contextual stimuli (all other stimuli present in the situation that contribute to the effect of the focal stimulus), and residual stimuli (environmental factors within or outside human systems, the effects of which are unclear in the situation) (Roy, 2009, pp. 35–36).

The propositions of Roy's theory include the following:

- Nursing actions promote a person's adaptive responses.
- Nursing actions can decrease a person's ineffective adaptive responses.
- People interact with the changing environment in an attempt to achieve adaptation and health.
- Nursing actions enhance the interaction of persons with the environment.
- Enhanced interactions of persons with the environment promote adaptation (Meleis, 2004).

TABLE 2-7 Metaparadigm Concepts as Defined in Roy's Model

Person "An adaptive system with cognator and regulator subsystems acting to maintain adaptation in the four adaptive modes" (Roy, 2009, p. 12)

Environment "All conditions, circumstances, and influences surrounding and affecting the development and behavior of persons and groups, with particular consideration of mutuality of person and earth resources" (Roy, 2009, p. 12)

Health "A state and process of being and becoming an integrated and whole that reflects person and environment mutuality" (Roy, 2009, p. 12)

Nursing The goal of nursing is "to promote adaptation for individuals and groups in the four adaptive modes, thus contributing to health, quality of life, and dying with dignity by assessing behavior and factors that influence adaptive abilities and to enhance environmental factors" (Roy, 2009, p.12)

The Roy Adaptation Model is commonly used in nursing practice. To use the model in practice, the nurse follows Roy's six-step nursing process, which is as follows (Phillips, 2006):

- Assessing the behaviors manifested from the four adaptive modes (physiologic-physical mode, self-concept–group identity mode, role function mode, and interdependence mode)
- Assessing and categorizing the stimuli for those behaviors
- Making a nursing diagnosis based on the person's adaptive state
- Setting goals to promote adaptation
- Implementing interventions aimed at managing stimuli to promote adaptation
- Evaluating achievement of adaptive goals

Andrews and Roy (1986) point out that by manipulating the stimuli rather than the patient, the nurse enhances "the interaction of the person with their environment, thereby promoting health" (p. 51).

Betty Neuman's Systems Model

The Neuman Systems Model is a wellness model based on general systems theory in which the client system is exposed to stressors from within and without the system. The focus of the model is on the client system in relationship to stressors. The client system is a composite of interacting variables that include the physiologic variable, the psychological variable, the sociocultural variable, the developmental variable, and the spiritual variable (Neuman, 2002, pp. 16–17). Stressors are classified as intrapersonal, interpersonal, or extrapersonal depending on their relationship to the client system (p. 22).

The client system is represented structurally in the model as a series of concentric rings or circles surrounding a basic structure. These flexible concentric circles represent normal lines of defense and lines of resistance that function to preserve client system integrity by acting as protective mechanisms for the basic structure. The basic structure or central core consists of basic survival factors common to the species, innate or genetic features, and strengths and weaknesses of the system. The flexible line of defense forms the outer boundary of the defined client system; it protects the normal line of defense. The normal line of defense represents what the client has become or the usual wellness state. Adjustment of the five client system variables to environmental stressors determines its level of stability. The series of concentric broken circles surrounding the basic structure are known as lines of resistance. They become activated following invasion of the normal line of defense by environmental stressors (Neuman, 2002, pp. 16–18). The greater the quality of the client system's health, the greater protection is provided by the various lines of defense (Geib, 2006). An overview and diagram of the model are provided on the Neuman Systems Model website (neumansystemsmodel.org/NSMdocs/nsm_powerpoint_overview.htm). See also Table 2-8.

Basic assumptions of the Neuman Systems Model include the following (Meleis, 2004; Neuman, 1995):

- Nursing clients have both unique and universal characteristics and are constantly exchanging energy with the environment.
- The relationships among client variables influence a client's protective mechanisms and determine the client's response.
- Clients present a normal range of responses to the environment that represent wellness and stability.
- Stressors attack flexible lines of defense and then normal lines of defense.
- Nurses' actions are focused on primary, secondary, and tertiary prevention.

The Neuman Systems Model is health oriented, with an emphasis on prevention as intervention, and has been used in a wide variety of settings. Perhaps one of the greatest attractions to this model is the ease with which it

TABLE 2-8 Metaparadigm Concepts as Defined in Neuman's Model

Person (client system) A composite of physiological, psychological, sociocultural, developmental, and spiritual variables in interaction with the internal and external environment; represented by central structure, lines of defense, and lines of resistance (Neuman, 2002).

Environment All internal and external factors of influences surrounding the client system. Three relevant environments identified are the internal environment, the external environment, and the created environment (Neuman, 2002, p. 18).

Health A continuum of wellness to illness; equated with optimal system stability (Neuman, 2002, p. 23).

Nursing Prevention as intervention; concerned with all potential stressors.

> **Prevention as intervention is concerned with all potential stressors.**

can be used for families, groups, and communities as well as the individual client. The use of the model in practice requires only moderate adaptation of the nursing process with a focus on assessment of stressors and client system perceptions.

Imogene King's Interacting Systems Framework and Theory of Goal Attainment

King, in her Interacting Systems Framework, conceptualizes three levels of dynamic interacting systems that include personal systems (individuals), interpersonal systems (groups), and social systems (society). Individuals exist within personal systems, and concepts relevant to this system include body image, growth and development, perception, self, space, and time. Interpersonal systems are formed when two or more individuals interact. The concepts important to understanding this system include communication, interaction, role, stress, and transaction. Examples of social systems include religious systems, educational systems, and healthcare systems. Concepts important to understanding the social system include authority, decision making, organization, power, and status (King, 1981; Sieloff, 2006).

King's Theory of Goal Attainment was derived from her Interacting Systems Framework (Sieloff, 2006) and addresses nursing as a process of human interaction (Norris & Frey, 2006). The theory focuses on the interpersonal system interactions in the nurse–client relationship (Table 2-9). During the nursing process, the nurse and the client each perceives one another, makes judgments, and takes action that results in reaction. Interaction results, and if perceptual congruence exists, transactions occur (Sieloff, 2006). Outcomes are defined in terms of goals obtained. If the goals are related to patient behaviors, they become the criteria by which the effectiveness of nursing care can be measured (King, 1989, p. 156).

TABLE 2-9　Metaparadigm Concepts as Defined in King's Model

Person (human being)　A personal system that interacts with interpersonal and social systems.
Environment　Can be both external and internal. The external environment is the context "within which human beings grow, develop, and perform daily activities" (King, 1981, p. 18); the internal environment of human beings transforms energy to enable them to adjust to continuous external environmental changes (King, 1981, p. 5).

Health　"Dynamic life experiences of a human being, which implies continuous adjustment to stressors in the internal and external environment through optimum use of one's resources to achieve maximum potential for daily living" (King, 1981, p. 5).
Nursing　A process of human interaction; the goal of nursing is to help patients achieve their goals.

The propositions of King's Theory of Goal Attainment are as follows (King, 1981):

> **According to King, the goal of nursing is to help patients achieve their goals.**

- If perceptual accuracy is present in nurse–client interactions, transactions will occur.
- If the nurse and client make transactions, goals will be attained.
- If goals are attained, satisfactions will occur.
- If goals are attained, effective nursing care will occur.
- If transactions are made in the nurse–client interactions, growth and development will be enhanced.
- If role expectations and role performance as perceived by the nurse and client are congruent, transactions will occur.
- If role conflict is experienced by nurse or client or both, stress in nurse–client interactions will occur.
- If nurses with special knowledge and skills communicate appropriate information to clients, mutual goal setting and goal attainment will occur.

King's theory can be implemented in practice using the nursing process where assessment focuses on the perceptions of the nurse and client, communication of the nurse and client, and interaction of the nurse and client. Planning involves deciding on goals and agreeing on how to attain goals. Implementation focuses on transactions made, and evaluation focuses on goals attained using King's theory (King, 1992).

Johnson's Behavioral System Model

Johnson's model for nursing presents the client as a living open system that is a collection of behavioral subsystems that interrelate to form a behavioral system (Table 2-10). The seven subsystems of behavior proposed by Johnson include achievement, affiliative, aggressive, dependence, sexual, eliminative, and ingestive. Motivational drives direct the activities of the subsystems that are constantly changing because of maturation, experience, and learning (Johnson, 1980).

TABLE 2-10 Metaparadigm Concepts as Defined in Johnson's Theory

Person (human being) A biopsychosocial being who is a behavioral system with seven subsystems of behavior

Environment Includes internal and external environment

Health Efficient and effective functioning of system; behavioral system balance and stability

Nursing An external regulatory force that acts to preserve the organization and integrity of the patient's behavior at an optimal level under those conditions in which the behavior constitutes a threat to physical or social health or in which illness is found (Johnson, 1980, p. 214)

The achievement subsystem functions to control or master an aspect of self or environment to achieve a standard. This subsystem encompasses intellectual, physical, creative, mechanical, and social skills. The affiliative or attachment subsystem forms the basis for social organization. Its consequences are social inclusion, intimacy, and the formation and maintenance of strong social bonds. The aggressive or protective subsystem functions to protect and preserve the system. The dependency subsystem promotes helping or nurturing behaviors. The consequences include approval, recognition, and physical assistance. The sexual subsystem has the function of procreation and gratification and includes development of gender role identity and gender role behaviors. The eliminative subsystem addresses "when, how, and under what conditions we eliminate," whereas the ingestive subsystem "has to do with when, how, what, how much, and under what conditions we eat" (Johnson, 1980, p. 213).

The nursing process for the behavioral system model is known as Johnson's nursing diagnostic and treatment process. The components of the process include the determination of the existence of a problem, diagnosis and classification of problems, management of problems, and evaluation of behavioral system balance and stability. When using Johnson's model in practice, the focus of the assessment process is obtaining information to evaluate current behavior in terms of past patterns, determining the impact of the current illness on behavioral patterns, and establishing the maximum level of health. The assessment is specifically related to gathering information related to the structure and function of the seven behavioral subsystems as well as the environmental factors that affect the behavioral subsystems (Holaday, 2006). The ultimate goals of nursing using the model are to maintain or restore behavioral system balance (Johnson, 1980).

▪ Selected Theories and Middle-Range Theories of Nursing

Rosemary Parse's Humanbecoming Theory

Parse's theory was originally called man-living-health (Parse, 1981). In 1992, Parse changed the name to *human becoming,* and then in 2007 again changed the name to *humanbecoming* (Mitchell & Bournes, 2010) to coincide with Parse's evolution of thought. The Humanbecoming Theory consists of three major themes: meaning, rhythmicity, and transcendence (Parse, 1998). Meaning is the linguistic and imagined content of something and the interpretation that one gives to something. Rhythmicity is the cadent, paradoxical patterning of the human–universe mutual process. Transcendence is defined as reaching beyond with possibles or the "hopes and dreams envisioned in multidimensional experiences powering the originating of transforming" (Parse, 1998, p. 29). The three major principles of the Humanbecoming Theory flow from these themes.

The first principle of the Humanbecoming Theory states, "Structuring meaning multidimensionally is cocreating reality through the languaging of valuing and imaging" (Parse, 1998, p. 35). This principle proposes that persons structure or choose the meaning of their realities and that the choosing occurs at levels that are not always known explicitly (Mitchell, 2006). This means that one person cannot decide the significance of something for another person and does not even understand the meaning of the event unless that person shares the meaning through the expression of his or her views, concerns, and dreams.

The second principle states, "Cocreating rhythmical patterns of relating is living the paradoxical unity of revealing—concealing and enabling—limiting while connecting—separating" (Parse, 1998, p. 42). This principle means that persons create patterns in life, and these patterns tell about personal meanings and values. The patterns of relating that persons create involve complex engagements and disengagements with other persons, ideas, and preferences (Mitchell, 2006). According to Parse (1998), persons change their patterns when they integrate new priorities, ideas, hopes, and dreams.

The third principle of the Humanbecoming Theory states, "Cotranscending with the possibles is powering unique ways of originating in the process of transforming" (Parse, 1998, p. 46). This principle means that persons are always engaging with and choosing from infinite possibilities. The choices reflect the person's ways of moving and changing in the process of becoming (Mitchell, 2006).

Three processes for practice have been developed from the concepts and principles in the Humanbecoming Theory, including the following (Parse, 1998, pp. 69, 70):

- Illuminating meaning is explicating what was, is, and will be. Explicating is making clear what is appearing now through language.
- Synchronizing rhythms is dwelling with the pitch, yaw, and roll of the human–universe process. Dwelling with is immersing with the flow of connecting–separating.
- Mobilizing transcendence is moving beyond the meaning moment with what is not yet. Moving beyond is propelling with envisioned possibles of transforming.

In practice, nurses guided by the Humanbecoming Theory prepare to be truly present (Table 2-11) with others through focused attentiveness on the moment at hand through immersion (Parse, 1998).

TABLE 2-11 Metaparadigm Concepts as Defined in Parse's Theory

Person   An open being, more than and different than the sum of parts in mutual simultaneous interchange with the environment who chooses from options and bears responsibility for choices (Parse, 1987, p. 160)
Environment   Coexists in mutual process with the person

Health   Continuously changing process of becoming
Nursing   A learned discipline; the nurse uses true presence to facilitate the becoming of the participant

Madeleine Leininger's Cultural Diversity and Universality Theory

Leininger (1995) identified the main features of the Cultural Diversity and Universality Theory:

> Transcultural nursing is a substantive area of study and practice focused on comparative cultural care (caring) values, beliefs, and practices of individuals or groups of similar or different cultures with the goal of providing culture-specific and universal nursing care practices in promoting health or well-being or to help people face unfavorable human conditions, illness, or death in culturally meaningful ways. (p. 58)

Consistent with the focus of her theory, Leininger defined the metaparadigm concepts of nursing in a manner that causes the nurse to specifically consider culture in the delivery of competent nursing care (Table 2-12).

According to Leininger (2001), three modalities guide nursing judgments, decisions, and actions to provide culturally congruent care that is

TABLE 2-12 Metaparadigm Concepts as Defined in Leininger's Theory

Person   Human being, family, group, community, or institution
Environment   Totality of an event, situation, or experience that gives meaning to human expressions, interpretations, and social interactions in physical, ecological, sociopolitical, and/or cultural settings (Leininger, 1991)

Health   A state of well-being that is culturally defined, valued, and practiced (Leininger, 1991, p. 46)
Nursing   Activities directed toward assisting, supporting, or enabling with needs in ways that are congruent with the cultural values, beliefs, and lifeways of the recipient of care (Leininger, 1995)

beneficial, satisfying, and meaningful to the persons the nurse serves. These three modes include cultural care preservation or maintenance, cultural care accommodation or negotiation, and cultural care repatterning or restructuring. Culture care preservation or maintenance refers to those assistive, supportive, facilitative, or enabling professional actions and decisions that help people of a specific culture to maintain meaningful care values for their well-being, recover from illness, or deal with a handicap or dying. Culture care accommodation or negotiation refers to those assistive, supportive, facilitative, or enabling professional actions and decisions that help people of a specific culture or subculture adapt to or negotiate with others for meaningful, beneficial, and congruent health outcomes. Culture care repatterning or restructuring refers to the assistive, supportive, facilitative, or enabling professional actions and decisions that help patients reorder, change, or modify their lifeways for new, different, and beneficial health outcomes (Leininger & McFarland, 2006).

The nurse using Leininger's theory plans and makes decisions with clients with respect to these three modes of action. All three care modalities require coparticipation of the nurse and client working together to identify, plan, implement, and evaluate nursing care with respect to the cultural congruence of the care (Leininger, 2001).

Leininger developed the sunrise model, which she revised in 2004. She labeled this model as "an enabler," to clarify that although it depicts the essential components of the Cultural Diversity and Universality Theory, it is a visual guide for exploration of cultures.

Hildegard Peplau's Theory of Interpersonal Relations

In her theory, Peplau addresses all of nursing's metaparadigm concepts (Table 2-13), but she is primarily concerned with one aspect of nursing: how persons relate to one another. According to Peplau, the nurse–patient relationship is the center of nursing (Young, Taylor, & McLaughlin-Renpenning, 2001).

TABLE 2-13 Metaparadigm Concepts as Defined in Peplau's Theory

Person Encompasses the patient (one who has problems for which expert nursing services are needed or sought) and the nurse (a professional with particular expertise) (Peplau, 1992, p. 14)
Environment Forces outside the organism within the context of culture (Peplau, 1952, p. 163).

Health "Implies forward movement of personality and other ongoing human processes in the direction of creative, constructive, productive, personal, and community living" (Peplau, 1992, p. 12)
Nursing The therapeutic, interpersonal process between the nurse and the patient

Peplau (1952) originally described four phases in nurse–patient relationships that overlap and occur over the time of the relationship: orientation, identification, exploitation, and resolution. In 1997, Peplau combined the phase of identification and exploitation, resulting in three phases: orientation, working, and termination. Nevertheless, most other theorists still consider the phases of identification and exploitation to be subphases of the working phase. During the orientation phase, a health problem has emerged that results in a "felt need," and professional assistance is sought (p. 18). In the working phase, the patient identifies those who can help, and the nurse permits exploration of feelings by the patient. During this phase, the nurse can begin to focus the patient on the achievement of new goals. The resolution (termination) phase is the time when the patient gradually adopts new goals and frees himself or herself from identification with the nurse (Peplau, 1952, 1997).

Peplau (1952) also describes six nursing roles that emerge during the phases of the nurse–patient relationship: the role of the stranger, the role of the resource person, the teaching role, the leadership role, the surrogate role, and the counseling role. Over the course of Peplau's career, the nursing roles were refined to include teacher, resource, counselor, leader, technical expert, and surrogate. As a teacher, the nurse provides knowledge about a need or problem. In the role of resource, the nurse provides information to understand a problem. In the role of counselor, the nurse helps recognize, face, accept, and resolve problems. As a leader, the nurse initiates and maintains group goals through interaction. As a technical expert, the nurse provides physical care using clinical skills. And, as a surrogate, the nurse may take the place of another (Johnson & Webber, 2010, p. 125).

Peplau (1952) also described four psychobiological experiences: needs, frustration, conflict, and anxiety. According to Peplau, these experiences "all provide energy that is transformed into some form of action" (p. 71) and provide a basis for goal formation and nursing interventions (Howk, 2002).

Peplau, as one of the first theorists since Nightingale to present a theory for nursing, is considered a pioneer in the area of theory development in nursing. Prior to Peplau's work, nursing practice involved acting on, to, or for the patient such that the patient was considered an object of nursing actions. Peplau's work was the force behind the conceptualization of the patient as a partner in the nursing process (Howk, 2002, pp. 379–380). Although Peplau's book was first published in 1952, her model continues to be used extensively by clinicians and continues to provide direction to educators and researchers (Howk, 2002).

Nola Pender's Health Promotion Model

The Health Promotion Model is an attempt to portray the multidimensionality of persons interacting with their interpersonal and physical environments as they pursue health while integrating constructs from expectancy-value theory and social cognitive theory with a nursing perspective of holistic human functioning (Pender, 1996, p. 53). A summary of the metaparadigm concepts of nursing as defined by Pender are presented in Table 2-14.

There are three major categories to consider in Pender's health promotion model: (1) individual characteristics and experiences, (2) behavior-specific cognitions and affect, and (3) behavioral outcome. Personal factors include personal biological factors such as age, body mass index, pubertal status, menopausal status, aerobic capacity, strength, agility, or balance. Personal psychological factors include factors such as self-esteem, self-motivation, and perceived health status; personal sociocultural factors include factors such as race, ethnicity, acculturation, education, and socioeconomic status. Some personal factors are amenable to change, whereas others cannot be changed (Pender, Murdaugh, & Parsons, 2006, p. 52).

Behavior-specific cognitions and affect are behavior-specific variables within the Health Promotion Model. Such variables are considered to have motivational significance. In the Health Promotion Model, these variables are the target of nursing intervention because they are amenable to change. The behavior-specific cognitions and affect identified in the Health Promotion Model include (1) perceived benefits of action, (2) perceived barriers to action, (3) perceived self-efficacy, and (4) activity-related affect. Perceived benefits of action are the anticipated positive outcomes resulting from health behavior. Perceived barriers to action are the anticipated, imagined, or real blocks or personal costs of a behavior. Perceived self-efficacy refers to the judgment of personal capability to organize and execute a health-promoting behavior. It influences the perceived barriers to actions, such that higher efficacy results in lower perceptions of barriers. Activity-related affect refers to the subjective positive or negative feelings that occur before, during, and following behavior based on the stimulus properties of the behavior. Activity-related affect influences perceived self-efficacy, such that the more positive the subjective feeling, the greater the perceived efficacy (Pender et al., 2006; Sakraida, 2010, p. 438).

Commitment to a plan of action marks the beginning of a behavioral event. Interventions in the Health Promotion Model focus on raising consciousness related to health-promoting behaviors, promoting self-efficacy,

TABLE 2-14 Metaparadigm Concepts as Defined in Pender's Theory	
Person The individual, who is the primary focus of the model **Environment** The physical, interpersonal, and economic circumstances in which persons live **Health** A positive high-level state	**Nursing** The role of the nurse includes raising consciousness related to health-promoting behaviors, promoting self-efficacy, enhancing the benefits of change, controlling the environment to support behavior change, and managing barriers to change

enhancing the benefits of change, controlling the environment to support behavior change, and managing the barriers to change. Health-promoting behavior, which is ultimately directed toward attaining positive health outcomes, is the product of the Health Promotion Model (Pender et al., 2006, pp. 56–63).

Kristen Swanson's Theory of Caring

Swanson's Theory of Caring (1991, 1993, 1999a, 1999b) offers an explanation of what it means to practice nursing in a caring manner. In this theory, *caring* is defined as a "nurturing way of relating to a valued other toward whom one feels a personal sense of commitment and responsibility" (Swanson, 1991, p. 162). Swanson (1993) posits caring for a person's biopsychosocial and spiritual well-being is a fundamental and universal component of good nursing care.

Five additional concepts are integral to Swanson's Theory of Caring and represent the five basic processes of caring: maintaining belief, knowing, being with, doing for, and enabling.

- The concept of maintaining belief is sustaining faith in the other's capacity to get through an event or transition and face a future with meaning. This includes believing in the other's capacity and holding him or her in high esteem, maintaining a hope-filled attitude, offering realistic optimism, helping to find meaning, and standing by the one cared for, no matter what the situation (Swanson, 1991, p. 162).
- The concept of knowing refers to striving to understand the meaning of an event in the life of the other, avoiding assumptions, focusing on the person cared for, seeking cues, assessing meticulously, and engaging both the one caring and the one cared for in the process of knowing (Swanson, 1991, p. 162).
- The concept of being with refers to being emotionally present to the other. It includes being present in person, conveying availability, and sharing feelings without burdening the one cared for (Swanson, 1991, p. 162).

TABLE 2-15 Metaparadigm Concepts as Defined in Swanson's Theory of Caring

Person "Unique beings who are in the midst of becoming and whose wholeness is made manifest in thoughts, feelings, and behaviors" (Swanson, 1993, p. 352)

Environment "Any context that influences or is influenced by the designated client" (Swanson, 1993, p. 353)

Health Health and well-being is "to live the subjective, meaning-filled experience of wholeness. Wholeness involves a sense of integration and becoming wherein all facets of being are free to be expressed" (Swanson, 1993, p. 353)

Nursing Informed caring for the well-being of others (Swanson, 1991, 1993)

- The concept of doing for refers to doing for others what one would do for oneself, including anticipating needs, comforting, performing skillfully and competently, and protecting the one cared for while preserving his or her dignity (Swanson, 1991, p. 162).
- The concept of enabling refers to facilitating the other's passage through life transitions and unfamiliar events by focusing on the event, informing, explaining, supporting, validating feelings, generating alternatives, thinking things through, and giving feedback (Swanson, 1991, p. 162).

These caring processes are sequential and overlapping. In fact, they might not exist separate from one another because each is an integral component of the overarching structure of caring (Wojnar, 2010, p. 746). According to Swanson (1999b), knowing, being with, doing for, enabling, and maintaining belief are essential components of the nurse–client relationship, regardless of the context. A summary of the metaparadigm concepts of nursing as defined by Swanson are included in Table 2-15.

Katharine Kolcaba's Theory of Comfort

Comfort, as described by Kolcaba (2004, p. 255) in the Theory of Comfort, is the immediate experience of being strengthened by having needs for relief, ease, and transcendence addressed in four contexts—physical, psychospiritual, sociocultural, and environmental; it is much more than simply the absence of pain or other physical discomfort. Physical comfort pertains to bodily sensations and homeostatic mechanisms. Psychospiritual comfort pertains to the internal awareness of self, including esteem, sexuality, meaning in one's life, and one's relationship to a higher order or being. Sociocultural comfort pertains to interpersonal, family, societal relationships, and cultural traditions. Environmental comfort pertains to the external background of the human experience, which includes light, noise, color, temperature, ambience, and natural versus synthetic elements (Kolcaba, 2004, p. 258).

TABLE 2-16 Metaparadigm Concepts as Defined in Kolcaba's Theory of Comfort	
Person Recipients of care may be individuals, families, institutions, or communities in need of health care (Kolcaba, Tilton, & Drouin, 2006). **Environment** The environment includes any aspect of the patient, family, or institutional setting that can be manipulated by the nurse, a loved one, or the institution to enhance comfort (Dowd, 2010, p. 711).	**Health** Health is considered optimal functioning of the patient, the family, the healthcare provider, or the community (Dowd, 2010, p. 711). **Nuring** Nursing is the intentional assessment of comfort needs, design of comfort interventions to address those needs, and reassessment of comfort levels after implementation compared with baseline (Dowd, 2010, p. 711).

According to Kolcaba, comfort care encompasses three components: an appropriate and timely intervention to meet the comfort needs of patients, a mode of delivery that projects caring and empathy, and the intent to comfort. Comfort needs include patients' or families' desire for or deficit in relief, ease, or transcendence in the physical, psychospiritual, sociocultural, or environmental contexts of human experience. Comfort measures refer to interventions that are intentionally designed to enhance patients' or families' comfort (Kolcaba, 2004, p. 255).

The Theory of Comfort also addresses intervening variables—negative or positive factors over which nurses and institutions have little control but that affect the direction and success of comfort care plans. Examples of intervening variables are the presence or absence of social support, poverty, prognosis, concurrent medical or psychological conditions, and health habits (Kolcaba, 2004, p. 255).

An additional concept within the theory comprises the health-seeking behaviors of patients and families. Health-seeking behaviors are those behaviors that patients and families engage in either consciously or unconsciously while moving toward well-being. Health-seeking behaviors can be either internal or external and can include dying peacefully. It is posited that enhanced comfort results in engagement in health-seeking behaviors (Kolcaba, 2004, p. 255).

The metaparadigm concepts of nursing as defined by Kolcaba are summarized in Table 2-16.

Pamela Reed's Self-Transcendence Theory

Three major concepts are central to the Theory of Self-Transcendence: self-transcendence, well-being, and vulnerability. Self-transcendence is the capacity to expand self-boundaries intrapersonally, interpersonally, temporally, and transpersonally (Reed, 2008, p. 107). The capacity to expand self-boundaries intrapersonally refers to a greater awareness of one's philosophy, values, and dreams. The capacity to expand interpersonally relates to others and one's environment. The capacity to expand temporally refers to integration of one's past and future in a way that has meaning for the present. Finally, the capacity to expand transpersonally refers to the capacity to connect with dimensions beyond the typically discernible world (p. 107). Self-transcendence is a characteristic of developmental maturity that is congruent with enhanced awareness of the environment and a broadened perspective on life. Self-transcendence is expressed through behaviors such as sharing wisdom with others, integrating physical changes of aging, accepting death as a part of life, and finding spiritual meaning in life (Reed, 2008, pp. 107–108).

Well-being is the second major concept of Reed's theory. Well-being is a sense of feeling whole and healthy, according to one's own criteria for wholeness and health. The definition of well-being depends on the individual or population. Indeed, indicators of well-being are as diverse as human perceptions of health and wellness. Examples of indicators of well-being are life satisfaction, positive self-concept, hopefulness, happiness, and having meaning in life. Well-being is viewed as a correlate and an outcome of self-transcendence (Reed, 2008).

The third major concept, vulnerability, is the awareness of personal mortality and the likelihood of experiencing difficult life situations. Self-transcendence emerges naturally in health experiences when a person is confronted with mortality and immortality. Life events such as illness, disability, aging, childbirth, or parenting—all of which heighten a person's sense of mortality, inadequacy, or vulnerability—can trigger developmental progress toward a renewed sense of identity and expanded self-boundaries. According to Reed (2008, pp. 108–109), self-transcendence is evoked through life events and can enhance well-being by transforming losses and difficulties into healing experiences.

Additional concepts in Reed's theory include moderating-mediating factors and points of intervention. Moderating-mediating factors are personal and contextual variables such as age, gender, life experiences, and social environment that can influence the relationships between vulnerability and self-transcendence and between self-transcendence and well-being. Nursing activities that facilitate self-transcendence are referred to as points of intervention (Coward, 2010, p. 623). Two points of intervention are intertwined with the process of self-transcendence: Nursing actions can focus either directly on a person's inner resource for self-transcendence or indirectly on the personal and contextual factors that affect the relationship between vulnerability and self-transcendence and the relationship between self-transcendence and well-being (p. 621). The metaparadigm concepts of nursing as defined by Reed are summarized in Table 2-17.

TABLE 2-17   Metaparadigm Concepts as Defined in Reed's Self-Transcendence Theory

Person Persons are human beings who develop over the life span through interactions with other persons and within an environment (Coward, 2010, p. 622).	**Health** Well-being is a sense of feeling whole and healthy, according to one's own criteria for wholeness and health (Reed, 2008).
Environment The environment is composed of family, social networks, physical surroundings, and community resources (Coward, 2010, p. 622).	**Nursing** The role of nursing activity is to assist persons through interpersonal processes and therapeutic management of their environment to promote health and well-being (Coward, 2010, p. 622).

The American Association of Critical-Care Nurses' Synergy Model for Patient Care

The Synergy Model is a conceptual framework for designing practice competencies to care for critically ill patients with a goal of optimizing outcomes for patients and families. Optimal outcomes are realized when the competencies of the nurse match the patient and family needs.

The Synergy Model for Patient Care is the result of the American Association of Critical-Care Nurses (AACN) envisioning a new paradigm for clinical practice. In 1993, the AACN Certification Corporation convened a think tank that included nationally recognized experts to develop a conceptual framework for certified practice. The initial work resulted in the description of 13 patient characteristics based on universal needs of patients and 9 characteristics required of nurses to meet patient needs. The patient characteristics identified were compensation, resiliency, margin of error, predictability, complexity, vulnerability, physiologic stability, risk of death, independence, self-determination, involvement in care decisions, engagement, and resource availability. The characteristics of nurses were engagement, skilled clinical practice, agency, caring practices, system management, teamwork, diversity responsiveness, experiential learning, and being an innovator–evaluator. The think tank suggested that the synergy emerging from the interaction between the patient needs and the nurse characteristics should result in optimal outcomes for the patient and that these characteristics of the nurse would determine competencies for certified practice (Hardin, 2005, pp. 3–4).

In 1995, the AACN Certification Corporation decided to refine this model, to conduct a study of practice and job analysis of critical care nurses, and to test the validity of the concepts in critical care nurses. The group refined the patient characteristics into eight concepts, merged the nurse characteristics into eight concepts, and delineated a continuum for the characteristics. The eight patient characteristics identified in the current model are resiliency, vulnerability, stability, complexity, resource availability, participation in care,

---

TABLE 2-18 Metaparadigm Concepts as Defined in The Synergy Model for Patient Care

Person   Persons are viewed in the context of patients who are biological, social, and spiritual entities who are present at a particular developmental stage.

Environment   The concept of environment is not explicitly defined. However, included in the assumptions is the idea that environment is created by the nurses for the care of the patient.

Health   The concept of health is not explicitly defined. An optimal level of wellness as defined by the patient is mentioned as a goal of nursing care.

Nursing   The purpose of nursing is to meet the needs of patients and families and to provide safe passage through the healthcare system during a time of crisis (Hardin, 2005, p. 8).

participation in decision making, and predictability. The eight nurse characteristics are clinical judgment, advocacy, caring practices, collaboration, systems thinking, response to diversity, clinical inquiry, and facilitation of learning (Hardin, 2005, p. 4). Each patient characteristic is placed on a scale from one to five, with the level of each patient characteristic being critical in terms of the competency required of the nurse (Hardin, 2005, pp. 4–7). The eight nurse characteristics can be considered essential competencies for providing care for critically ill patients. All eight competencies reflect an integration of knowledge, skills, and experience of the nurse. Each nurse characteristic can be understood on a continuum from one to five (Hardin, 2005, pp. 5–6).

The Synergy Model delineates three levels of outcomes: outcomes derived from the patient, outcomes derived from the nurse, and outcomes derived from the healthcare system. Outcomes data derived from the patient include functional changes, behavioral changes, trust, satisfaction, comfort, and quality of life. Outcomes data derived from nursing competencies include physiologic changes, the presence or absence of complications, and the extent to which treatment objectives are attained (Curley, 1998). Outcomes data derived from the healthcare system include readmission rates, length of stay, and cost utilization (Hardin, 2005, pp. 8–9). The metaparadigm concepts of nursing as defined in the Synergy Model for Patient Care are summarized in Table 2-18.

Nurse of the Future: Nursing Core Competencies

Although not a theory of nursing, the *Nurse of the Future: Nursing Core Competencies* (Massachusetts Department of Higher Education, 2010) document addresses the knowledge base and relationships among concepts important to the practice of nursing. In the context of nursing knowledge, the concepts of patient, environment, health, and nursing are defined and are presented in Table 2-19.

TABLE 2-19 Metaparadigm Concepts as Defined in The Nurse of The Future: Nursing Core Competencies

Human being/patients   The recipient of nursing care or services. Patients may be individuals, families, groups, communities, or populations (AACN, 1998, p. 2 as cited in Massachusetts Department of Higher Education, 2010, p. 7).

Environment   "The atmosphere, milieu, or conditions in which an individual lives, works or plays" (ANA, 2004, p. 47 as cited in Massachusetts Department of Higher Education, 2010, p. 7).

Health   "An experience that is often expressed in terms of wellness and illness, and may occur in the presence or absence of disease or injury" (ANA, 2004, p. 5 as cited in Massachusetts Department of Higher Education, 2010, p. 8).

Nursing   ... "the protection, promotion, and optimization of health and abilities, prevention of illness and injury, alleviation of suffering through the diagnosis and treatment of human response, and advocacy in the care of individuals, families, groups, communities, and populations" (ANA, 2001, p. 5 as cited in Massachusetts Department of Higher Education, 2010, p. 8).

There are 10 Nurse of the Future core competencies:

- Patient-centered care: "The Nurse of the Future will provide holistic care that recognizes an individual's preferences, values, and needs and respects the patient or designee as a full partner in providing compassionate, coordinated, age and culturally appropriate, safe and effective care" (Massachusetts Department of Higher Education, 2010, p. 9).
- Professionalism: "The Nurse of the Future will demonstrate accountability for the delivery of standard-based nursing care that is consistent with moral, altruistic, legal, ethical, regulatory, and humanistic principles" (Massachusetts Department of Higher Education, 2010, p. 13).
- Leadership: "The Nurse of the Future will influence the behavior of individuals or groups of individuals within their environment in a way that will facilitate the establishment and acquisition/achievement of shared goals" (Massachusetts Department of Higher Education, 2010, p. 17).
- Systems-based practice: "The Nurse of the Future will demonstrate an awareness of and responsiveness to the larger context of the health care system, and will demonstrate the ability to effectively call on microsystem resources to provide care that is of optimal quality and value" (Massachusetts Department of Higher Education, 2010, p. 19).
- Informatics and technology: "The Nurse of the Future will use information and technology to communicate, manage, knowledge, mitigate error, and support decision making" (Quality and Safety Education for Nurses [QSEN], 2007, as cited in Massachusetts Department of Higher Education, 2010, p. 22).
- Communication: "The Nurse of the Future will interact effectively with patients, families, and colleagues, fostering mutual respect and shared decision making to enhance patient satisfaction and health outcomes" (Massachusetts Department of Higher Education, 2010, p. 27).
- Teamwork and collaboration: "The Nurse of the Future will function effectively within nursing and interdisciplinary teams, fostering open communication, mutual respect, shared decision making, team learning, and development" (adapted from QSEN, 2007, as cited in Massachusetts Department of Higher Education, 2010, p. 31).
- Safety: "The Nurse of the Future will minimize risk of harm to patients and providers through both system effectiveness and individual performance" (QSEN, 2007, as cited in Massachusetts Department of Higher Education, 2010, p. 34).
- Quality improvement: "The Nurse of the Future uses data to monitor the outcomes of care processes, and uses improvement methods to design and test changes to continuously improve the quality and safety of health care systems" (QSEN, 2007, as cited in Massachusetts Department of Higher Education, 2010, p. 36).

- Evidence-based practice: "The Nurse of the Future will identify, evaluate, and use the best current evidence coupled with clinical expertise and consideration of patients' preferences, experience and values to make practice decisions" (adapted from QSEN, 2007, as cited in Massachusetts Department of Higher Education, 2010, p. 37).

The committee that designed the *Nurse of the Future: Nursing Core Competencies* also identified several assumptions and principles to serve as a framework. The assumptions include: (1) education and practice partnerships are key in developing an effective model, (2) it is imperative that leaders in nursing education and practice develop collaborative models to facilitate a minimum of a baccalaureate degree in nursing for all nurses, (3) a more effective education system must be created that will allow preparation of the nursing workforce to respond to the current and future healthcare needs of populations, (4) the nurse of the future will be proficient in a core set of competencies, and (5) nurse educators in education and practice settings will need to use different teaching strategies to integrate Nurse of the Future core competencies into the curriculum (Massachusetts Department of Higher Education, 2010, pp. 3-4).

The art and science of nursing are based on a framework of caring and respect for human dignity. A compassionate approach to patient care mandates that nurses provide care in a competent manner. The *Nurse of the Future: Nursing Core Competencies* provides a framework for the provision of competent nursing care (Massachusetts Department of Higher Education, 2010, p. 7).

> **www | CRITICAL THINKING QUESTION ✳**
>
> Think about the definitions of the metaparadigm concepts and the assumptions or propositions of each of the theories presented. Which of the theories most closely matches your beliefs? ✳

Relationship of Theory to Professional Nursing Practice

How will theory affect your nursing practice? Using a theoretical framework to guide your nursing practice assists you as you organize patient data, understand and analyze patient data, make decisions related to nursing interventions, plan patient care, predict outcomes of care, and evaluate patient outcomes (Alligood & Tomey, 2002). Why? The use of a theoretical framework provides a systematic and knowledgeable approach to nursing practice. The framework also becomes a tool that assists you to think critically as you plan and provide nursing care.

How do you begin? Now that you know why nursing theory is important to your nursing practice, it is time to identify a theoretical framework that fits you and your practice.

> **The use of a theoretical framework provides a systematic and knowledgeable approach to your nursing practice.**

Alligood (2006) presented guidelines for selecting a framework for theory-based nursing practice. Following are the steps:

1. Consider the values and beliefs in nursing that you truly hold.
2. Write a philosophy of nursing that clarifies your beliefs related to person, environment, health, and nursing.
3. Survey definitions of person, environment, health, and nursing in nursing models.
4. Select two or three frameworks that best fit with your beliefs related to the concepts of person, environment, health, and nursing.
5. Review the assumptions of the frameworks that you have selected.
6. Apply those frameworks in a selected area of nursing practice.
7. Compare the frameworks on client focus, nursing action, and client outcome.
8. Review the nursing literature written by persons who have used the frameworks.
9. Select a framework and develop its use in your nursing practice.

---

www CASE STUDY 2-1

Mr. M. is 34-year-old Caucasian male who presents to the mental health clinic with depression and complaints of fatigue. An interview reveals that his wife and both of his children were killed in a traffic accident 6 months ago. The nurse knows that Mr. M. is vulnerable as a result of the loss of his family, but that self-transcendence is evoked through life events and that well-being can be enhanced by transforming losses and difficulties into healing experiences.

1. The nurse using Reed's Self-Transcendence Theory focuses nursing activity for Mr. M. on facilitating self-transcendence. Based on the assessment, what intrapersonal strategies might be appropriate?

2. Which interpersonal strategies might be appropriate during follow-up visits to facilitate connecting to others?

Conclusion

As demonstrated by the descriptions of the philosophies, conceptual models, and theories presented in this chapter, there is a wide variety of perspectives and frameworks from which to practice nursing. There is no one right or wrong answer. Various nursing theories represent different realities and address different aspects of nursing (Meleis, 2007). For this reason, the multiplicity of nursing theories presented in this chapter should not be viewed as competing theories, but rather as complementary theories that can provide insight into different ways to describe, explain, and predict nursing concepts and/or prescribe nursing care. Curley (2007, p. 3) describes this understanding in an interesting way by comparing the multiplicity of nursing theories to a collection of maps of the same region. Each map might display a different characteristic of the region, such as rainfall, topography, or air currents. Although all of the maps are accurate, the best map for use depends on the information needed or the question being asked. This is precisely the case with the nurse's choice of nursing theories for practice.

So, begin with whichever theoretical framework seems to "fit," and then practice using it as you provide nursing care. "The full realization of nursing theory–guided practice is perhaps the greatest challenge that nursing as a scholarly discipline has ever faced" (Cody, 2006). So, be patient; developing your nursing practice guided by nursing theory takes time and practice. All nursing theories require in-depth study over time to master them fully (this chapter provides only a brief introduction), but the incorporation of theory into your practice can transform your nursing practice. The end result of this process will be seen in the excellent nursing care that you can provide to patients over the course of your professional nursing career.

Classroom Activity 1

Divide into small groups and give each group a copy of the same case study. Assign a different nursing theory to each group, and ask the groups to develop a plan of care using the assigned nursing theory as the basis for practice. Each group should share its plan of care with the class. Discuss the differences and similarities in the foci of care based on each of the selected theories. www

Classroom Activity 2

Think about the metaparadigm concepts of nursing. Draw each of the concepts in relation to the other concepts to show your ideas of how each of the concepts interfaces with the others. Present your "conceptual model" to the class, and discuss your ideas about each of the concepts represented.

This activity works best if you use colored pencils, crayons, or markers and a large piece of paper or newsprint. Actual student examples are presented in Figure 2-1 and Figure 2-2. www

Figure 2-1   Student conceptual model

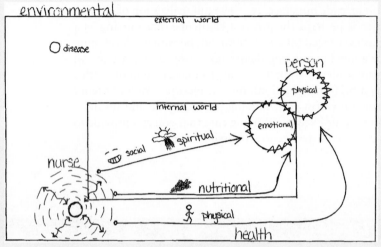

Source: Used with permission of Heather Grush.

Figure 2-2   Student conceptual model

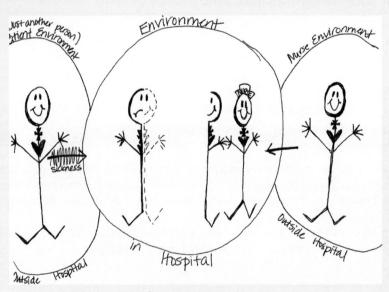

Source: Used with permission of Linzee McGinnis.

References

Alligood, M. R. (2006). Philosophies, models, and theories: Critical thinking structures. In M. R. Alligood & A. M. Tomey (Eds.), *Nursing theory: Utilization & application* (3rd ed., pp. 43–65). St. Louis, MO: Mosby.

Alligood, M. R., & Tomey, A. M. (2002). Significance of theory for nursing as a discipline and profession. In A. M. Tomey & M. R. Alligood (Eds.), *Nursing theorists and their work* (5th ed., pp. 14–31). St. Louis, MO: Mosby.

American Association of Colleges of Nursing. (1998). *The essentials of baccalaureate education for professional nursing practice.* Washington, DC: Author.

American Nurses Association. (2001). *Nursing scope and standards of practice.* Silver Springs, MD: Author.

American Nurses Association. (2004). *Nursing scope and standards of practice.* Silver Springs, MD: Author.

Andrews, H. A., & Roy, C., Sr. (1986). *Essentials of the Roy adaptation model.* Norwalk, CT: Appleton-Century-Crofts.

Andrews, H. A., & Roy, C., Sr. (1991). Essentials of the Roy adaptation model. In C. Roy Sr. & H. A. Andrews (Eds.), *The Roy adaptation model: The definitive statement* (pp. 2–25). Norwalk, CT: Appleton & Lange.

Benner, P. (1984/2001). *From novice to expert: Excellence and power in clinical nursing practice.* Upper Saddle River, NJ: Prentice Hall.

Benner, P., Hooper-Kyriakidis, P., & Stannard, D. (1999). *Clinical wisdom and interventions in critical care: A thinking-in-action approach.* Philadelphia, PA: Saunders.

Benner, P., & Wrubel, J. (1989). *The primacy of caring: Stress and coping in health and illness.* Menlo Park, CA: Addison-Wesley.

Berbiglia, V. A. (2010). Orem's self-care deficit theory in nursing practice. In M. R. Alligood (Ed.), *Nursing theory: Utilization and application* (4th ed., pp. 261–286). Maryland Heights, MO: Mosby.

Bolton, K. (2006). Nightingale's philosophy in nursing practice. In M. R. Alligood & A. M. Tomey (Eds.), *Nursing theory: Utilization & application* (3rd ed., pp. 89–102). St. Louis, MO: Mosby.

Brykczynski, K. A. (2010). Benner's philosophy in nursing practice. In M. R. Alligood (Ed.), *Nursing theory: Utilization and application* (4th ed., pp. 137–159). Maryland Heights, MO: Mosby.

Cody, W. K. (2006). Nursing theory–guided practice: What it is and what it is not. In W. K. Cody (Ed.), *Philosophical and theoretical perspectives for advanced nursing practice* (4th ed., pp. 119–121). Sudbury, MA: Jones and Bartlett.

Coward, D. D. (2010). Self-Transcendence Theory: Pamela G. Reed. In M. R. Alligood & A. M. Tomey (Eds.), *Nursing theorists and their work* (7th ed., pp. 618–637). Maryland Heights, MO: Mosby.

Curley, M. A. Q. (1998). Patient–nurse synergy: Optimizing patients' outcomes. *American Journal of Critical Care, 7*(1), 64–72.

Curley, M. A. Q. (2007). *Synergy: The unique relationship between nursing and patients.* Indianapolis, IN: Sigma Theta Tau International.

Day, L., & Benner, P. (2002). Ethics, ethical comportment, and etiquette. *American Journal of Critical Care, 11*(1), 76–79.

Dowd, T. (2010). Katharine Kolcaba: Theory of Comfort. In M. R. Alligood & A. M. Tomey (Eds.), *Nursing theorists and their work* (7th ed., pp. 706–721). Maryland Heights, MO: Mosby.

Eckberg, D. L., & Hill, L., Jr. (1979). The paradigm concept and sociology: A critical review. *American Sociological Review, 44,* 925–937.

Fawcett, J. (1994). *Analysis and evaluation of conceptual models of nursing.* Philadelphia, PA: F. A. Davis.

Fawcett, J. (2005). *Contemporary nursing knowledge: Analysis and evaluation of nursing models and theories* (2nd ed., pp. 553–585). Philadelphia, PA: F. A. Davis.

Flaskerud, J. H., & Holloran, E. J. (1980). Areas of agreement in nursing theory development. *Advances in Nursing Science, 3*(1), 1–7.

Furukawa, C. Y., & Howe, J. S. (2002). Definition and components of nursing: Virginia Henderson. In J. B. George (Ed.), *Nursing theories: The base for professional nursing practice* (5th ed., pp. 83–109). Upper Saddle River, NJ: Prentice Hall.

Geib, K. M. (2006). Neuman's systems model in nursing practice. In M. R. Alligood & A. M. Tomey (Eds.), *Nursing theory: Utilization & application* (3rd ed., pp. 229–254). St. Louis, MO: Mosby.

Gordon, S. C. (2001). Virginia Avenel Henderson: Definition of nursing. In M. Parker (Ed.), *Nursing theories and nursing practice.* Philadelphia, PA: F. A. Davis.

Gunther, M. (2006). Rogers' science of unitary human beings in nursing practice. In M. R. Alligood & A. M. Tomey (Eds.), *Nursing theory: Utilization & application* (3rd ed., pp. 283–306). St. Louis, MO: Mosby.

Hardin, S. R. (2005). Introduction to the AACN Synergy Model for Patient Care. In S. R. Hardin & R. Kaplow (Eds.), *Synergy for clinical excellence: The AACN Synergy Model for Patient Care* (pp. 3–10). Sudbury, MA: Jones and Bartlett.

Harmer, B., & Henderson, V. (1955). *Textbook of the principles and practice of nursing.* New York, NY: Macmillan.

Henderson, V. (1964). The nature of nursing. *American Journal of Nursing, 64,* 62–68.

Henderson, V. (1966). *The nature of nursing: A definition and its implications for practice, research, and education.* New York, NY: Macmillan.

Henderson, V. (1991). *The nature of nursing: Reflections after 25 years.* New York, NY: National League for Nursing Press.

Hickman, J. S. (2002). An introduction to nursing theory. In J. B. George (Ed.), *Nursing theories: A base for professional nursing practice* (5th ed., pp. 1–20). Upper Saddle River, NJ: Prentice Hall.

Holaday, B. (2006). Johnson's behavioral system model in nursing practice. In M. R. Alligood & A. M. Tomey (Eds.), *Nursing theory: Utilization & application* (3rd ed., pp. 157–180). St. Louis, MO: Mosby.

Howk, C. (2002). Hildegard E. Peplau: Psychodynamic nursing. In A. M. Tomey & M. R. Alligood (Eds.), *Nursing theorists and their work* (5th ed., pp. 379–398). St. Louis, MO: Mosby.

Johnson, B. M., & Webber, P. B. (2010). *An introduction to theory and reasoning in nursing* (3rd ed.). Philadelphia, PA: Lippincott Williams & Wilkins.

Johnson, D. (1980). The behavioral systems model for nursing. In J. Riehl & C. Roy (Eds.), *Conceptual models for nursing practice* (2nd ed., pp. 207–216). New York, NY: Appleton-Century-Crofts.

King, I. M. (1981). *A theory of nursing: Systems, concepts, process.* New York, NY: Wiley.

King, I. M. (1989). King's general systems framework and theory. In J. P. Riehl-Sisca (Ed.), *Conceptual models for nursing practice* (3rd ed., pp. 149–158). Norwalk, CT: Appleton & Lange.

King, I. M. (1992). King's theory of goal attainment. *Nursing Science Quarterly, 5*(1), 19–26.

Kolcaba, K. (2004). Comfort. In S. J. Peterson & T. S. Bredow (Eds.), *Middle range theories: Application to nursing research* (pp. 255–273). Philadelphia, PA: Lippincott Williams & Wilkins.

Kolcaba, K., Tilton, C., & Drouin, C. (2006). Comfort theory: A unifying framework to enhance the practice environment. *Journal of Nursing Administration, 36*(11), 538–544.

Leininger, M. (1991). *Culture care diversity and universality: A theory of nursing.* New York: National League for Nursing Press.

Leininger, M. (1995). Transcultural nursing perspectives: Basic concepts, principles, and culture care incidents. In M. M. Leininger (Ed.), *Transcultural nursing: Concepts, theories, research, and practices* (2nd ed., pp. 57–92). New York, NY: McGraw-Hill.

Leininger, M. (2001). *Culture care diversity and universality: A theory of nursing.* Sudbury, MA: Jones and Bartlett.

Leininger, M. M., & McFarland, M. R. (2006). *Culture care diversity and universality: A worldwide theory of nursing* (2nd ed.). Sudbury, MA: Jones and Bartlett.

Lippitt, G. L. (1973). *Visualizing change: Model building and the change process.* Fairfax, VA: NTL Learning Resources.

Massachusetts Department of Higher Education. (2010). *Nurse of the future: Nursing core competencies.* Retrieved from http://www.mass.edu/currentinit/documents/NursingCoreCompetencies.pdf

McBride, A. B. (Narrator). (1997). *Celebrating Virginia Henderson* (Video). (Available from Center for Nursing Press, 550 West North Street, Indianapolis, IN 46202).

Meleis, A. I. (2004). *Theoretical nursing: Development & progress* (3rd ed.). Philadelphia, PA: Lippincott.

Meleis, A. I. (2007). *Theoretical nursing: Development & progress* (4th ed.). Philadelphia, PA: Lippincott.

Mitchell, G. J. (2006). Rosemarie Rizzo Parse: Human becoming. In A. M. Tomey & M. R. Alligood (Eds.), *Nursing theorists and their work* (6th ed., pp. 522–559). St. Louis, MO: Mosby.

Mitchell, G. J., & Bournes, D. A. (2010). Rosemarie Rizzo Parse: Humanbecoming. In M. R. Alligood & A. M. Tomey (Eds.), *Nursing theorists and their work* (7th ed., pp. 503–535). Maryland Heights, MO: Mosby.

Neil, R. M., & Tomey, A. M. (2006). Jean Watson: Philosophy and science of caring. In A. M. Tomey & M. R. Alligood (Eds.), *Nursing theorists and their work* (6th ed., pp. 91–115). St. Louis, MO: Mosby.

Neuman, B. (1995). *The Neuman systems model* (3rd ed.). Norwalk, CT: Appleton & Lange.

Neuman, B. (2002). The Neuman systems model. In B. Neuman & J. Fawcett (Eds.), *The Neuman systems model* (4th ed., pp. 3–34). Upper Saddle River, NJ: Prentice Hall.

Nightingale, F. (1969). *Notes on nursing: What it is and what it is not.* New York, NY: Dover. (Original work published 1860).

Norris, D., & Frey, M. A. (2006). King's system framework and theory in nursing practice. In M. R. Alligood & A. M. Tomey (Eds.), *Nursing theory: Utilization & application* (3rd ed., pp. 181–205). St. Louis, MO: Mosby.

Orem, D. (1985). *Nursing: Concepts of practice* (3rd ed.). St. Louis, MO: Mosby.

Orem, D. (1990). A nursing practice theory in three parts, 1956–1989. In M. E. Parker (Ed.), *Nursing theories in practice* (pp. 47–60). New York, NY: National League for Nursing.

Orem, D. (1995). *Nursing: Concepts of practice* (5th ed.). St. Louis, MO: Mosby.

Orem, D. (2001). *Nursing concepts of practice* (6th ed.). St. Louis, MO: Mosby.

Parse, R. R. (1981). *Man–living–health: A theory of nursing.* New York, NY: Wiley.

Parse, R. R. (1987). *Nursing science: Major paradigms, theories, and critiques.* Philadelphia, PA: Saunders.

Parse, R. R. (1998). *The human becoming school of thought: A perspective for nurses and other health professionals.* Thousand Oaks, CA: Sage.

Pender, N. J. (1996). *Health promotion in nursing practice* (3rd ed.). Stamford, CT: Appleton & Lange.

Pender, N. J., Murdaugh, C. L., & Parsons, M. A. (2006). *Health promotion in nursing practice* (5th ed.). Upper Saddle River, NJ: Prentice Hall.

Peplau, H. (1952). *Interpersonal relations in nursing.* New York, NY: G. P. Putnam's Sons.

Peplau, H. E. (1992). Interpersonal relations: A theoretical framework for application in nursing practice. *Nursing Science Quarterly, 5,* 13–18.

Peplau, H. E. (1997). Peplau's theory of interpersonal relations. *Nursing Science Quarterly, 10*(4), 162–167.

Pfettscher, S. A. (2006). Florence Nightingale: Modern nursing. In A. M. Tomey & M. R. Alligood (Eds.), *Nursing theorists and their work* (6th ed., pp. 71–90). St. Louis, MO: Mosby.

Phillips, K. D. (2006). Sister Callista Roy: Adaptation model. In A. M. Tomey & M. R. Alligood (Eds.), *Nursing theorists and their work* (6th ed., pp. 355–385). St. Louis, MO: Mosby.

Quality and Safety Education for Nurses. (2007). Quality and safety competencies. Retrieved from http://www.qsen.org/competencies.php

Reed, P. G. (2008). Theory of self-transcendence. In M. J. Smith & P. R. Liehr (Eds.), *Middle range theory for nursing* (2nd ed., pp. 105–129). New York, NY: Springer.

Rogers, M. E. (1970). *An introduction to the theoretical basis of nursing.* Philadelphia, PA: F. A. Davis.

Rogers, M. E. (1992). Nursing science and the space age. *Nursing Science Quarterly, 5,* 27–34.

Rogers, M. E. (1994). The science of unitary human beings: Current perspectives. *Nursing Science Quarterly, 7,* 33–35.

Roy, C., Sr. (2009). *The Roy adaptation model* (3rd ed.). Upper Saddle River, NJ: Pearson.

Roy, C., Sr., & Andrews, H. A. (1999). *The Roy adaptation model* (2nd ed.). Stamford, CT: Appleton & Lange.

Sakraida, T. J. (2010). The health promotion model. In A. M. Tomey & M. R. Alligood (Eds.), *Nursing theorists and their work* (7th ed., pp. 434–453). St. Louis, MO: Mosby.

Sieloff, C. L. (2006). Imogene King: Interacting systems framework and middle range theory of goal attainment. In A. M. Tomey & M. R. Alligood (Eds.), *Nursing theorists and their work* (6th ed., pp. 297–317). St. Louis, MO: Mosby.

Swanson, K. M. (1991). Empirical development of a middle range theory of caring. *Nursing Research, 40*(3), 161–166.

Swanson, K. M. (1993). Nursing as informed caring for the well-being of others. *Image: The Journal of Nursing Scholarship, 25*(4), 352–357.

Swanson, K. M. (1999a). The effects of caring, measurement, and time on miscarriage impact and women's well-being in the first year subsequent to loss. *Nursing Research, 48*(6), 288–298.

Swanson, K. M. (1999b). What's known about caring in nursing: A literary meta-analysis. In A. S. Hinshaw, J. Shaver, & S. Freetham (Eds.), *Handbook of clinical nursing research* (pp. 31–60). Thousand Oaks, CA: Sage.

Taylor, S. G. (2006). Self-care deficit theory of nursing. In A. M. Tomey & M. R. Alligood (Eds.), *Nursing theorists and their work* (6th ed., pp. 267–296). St. Louis, MO: Mosby.

Tomey, A. M. (2006). Nursing theorists of historical significance. In A. M. Tomey & M. R. Alligood (Eds.), *Nursing theorists and their work* (6th ed., pp. 54–67). St. Louis, MO: Mosby.

Watson, J. (1979). *Nursing: The philosophy and science of caring.* Boston, MA: Little, Brown.

Watson, J. (1985). *Nursing: Human science and human care: A theory of nursing.* Sudbury, MA: Jones and Bartlett.

Watson, J. (1989). Watson's philosophy and theory of human caring in nursing. In J. P. Riehl-Sisca (Ed.), *Conceptual model for nursing practice* (3rd ed., pp. 219–236). Norwalk, CT: Appleton & Lange.

Watson, J. (1996). Watson's philosophy and theory of human caring in nursing. In J. P. Riehl-Sisca (Ed.), *Conceptual models for nursing practice* (pp. 219–235). Norwalk, CT: Appleton & Lange.

Watson, J. (1997). The theory of human caring: Retrospective and prospective. *Nursing Science Quarterly, 10*, 49–52.

Watson, J. (2001). Jean Watson: Theory of human caring. In M. E. Parker (Ed.), *Nursing theories and nursing practice* (pp. 343–354). Philadelphia, PA: F. A. Davis.

Watson, J. (2008). *Nursing: The philosophy and science of caring* (rev. ed.). Boulder, CO: University Press of Colorado.

Wojnar, D. M. (2010). Kristin M. Swanson: Theory of caring. In M. R. Alligood & A. M. Tomey (Eds.), *Nursing theorists and their work* (7th ed., pp. 741–752). Maryland Heights, MO: Mosby.

Young, A., Taylor, S. G., & McLaughlin-Renpenning, K. (2001). *Connections: Nursing research, theory, and practice.* St. Louis, MO: Mosby.

Philosophy of Nursing

Mary W. Stewart

3

What is truth? Where do our ideas about truth originate? Why does truth matter?

In a previous chapter, information was presented about the four principal domains of nursing: person, environment, health, and nursing. These concepts are the building blocks for all philosophies of nursing. As you are learning about these ideas, you are also learning that many nurses develop nursing theories or models. Think about it ... nurses creating theory! Yet, who better to describe our profession than professional nurses? All right, so maybe you are not that excited about this reality. Still, you have to admit that the ability to articulate nursing values and beliefs to guide us in our understanding of professional nursing is impressive. More than impressive, nursing theory is necessary.

In this chapter, we look more closely at nursing philosophy and its significance to professional nursing. We study the difference between beliefs and values and investigate the importance of values clarification. Finally, we examine guidelines for creating a personal philosophy of nursing.

Learning Objectives

After completing this chapter, the student should be able to:

1. Identify various philosophical views of truth.
2. Differentiate between values and beliefs.
3. Discuss the process of value clarification.
4. Explain the major components of nursing philosophy.
5. Articulate the purpose for having a personal philosophy of nursing.
6. Begin the development of a personal philosophy of nursing.

Philosophy

Though no single definition of *philosophy* is uncontroversial, philosophy is defined in the following ways by the *American Heritage Dictionary of the English Language* (2000):

- Love and pursuit of wisdom by intellectual means and moral self-discipline
- Investigation of the nature, causes, or principles of reality, knowledge, or values, based on logical reasoning rather than empirical methods
- A system of thought based on or involving such inquiry; for example, the philosophy of Hume
- The critical analysis of fundamental assumptions or beliefs
- The disciplines presented in university curriculums of science and the liberal arts, except medicine, law, and theology
- The discipline comprising logic, ethics, aesthetics, metaphysics, and epistemology
- A set of ideas or beliefs relating to a particular field or activity; an underlying theory; for example, an original philosophy of advertising
- A system of values by which one lives; for example, has an unusual philosophy of life

Examples of philosophies can be found in university catalogs, clinical agency manuals, and nursing school handbooks—and they are prolific on the Internet. Needless to say, people have strong values and beliefs about many topics. A written statement of philosophy is a good way to communicate to others what you see as truth.

Some people are anxious to prescribe their own system of values to others by implying what "should be." However, each person or group of persons is responsible for delineating their particular philosophy. At the same time, how the insider's philosophy fits with the outsider's view is also important, particularly in situations such as nursing. Because nursing is inextricably linked to society, those of us within the profession must consider how society defines the values and beliefs within nursing.

> **As society and individuals change, our philosophy of nursing changes to be congruent with new and renewed understanding.**

So, how do we please everyone all the time? The answer is simple: We don't. We do, however, consider our own values and beliefs, which are interdependent of society, as we convey our professional philosophy of nursing. Does the philosophy ever change? Absolutely. As society and individuals change, our philosophy of nursing changes to be congruent with new and renewed understanding. How did we ever get started on this journey? A brief look at the beginnings of philosophy can help answer that question.

Early Philosophy

As society and individuals change, our philosophy of nursing changes to be congruent with new and renewed understanding. In the beginning, the Greeks moved from seeking supernatural to natural explanations. One assumption by the early Greek philosophers was that "something" had always existed. They did not question how something could come from nothing. Rather, they wanted to know what the "something" was. The pre-Socratics took the first step toward science in that they abandoned mythological thought and sought reason to answer their questions.

Heraclitus, a pre-Socratic philosopher, is well known for his thesis, Everything Is in Flux. He moved from simply looking at "being" to "becoming." A popular analogy he used was that of a river, saying, "You cannot step into the same river twice, for different and again different waters flow." More emphasis was placed on the senses versus reasoning.

On the other hand, Parmenides, who followed Heraclitus, said these two things: (1) Nothing can change, and (2) our sensory perceptions are unreliable. He is called the first metaphysician, a "hard-core philosopher." Metaphysics is the study of reality as a whole, including beyond the natural senses. What is the nature of reality? The universe? He starts with what it means and then moves to how the world must ultimately be. He does not go with his sense or experience. Parmenides thought that everything in the world had always been and that there was no such thing as change. He did, of course, sense that things changed, but his reason told him otherwise. He believed that our senses give us incorrect information and that we can rely only on our reason for acquiring knowledge about the world. This is called rationalism.

Probably a name more familiar to us is Socrates (469–399 B.C.), famous for the "know thyself " philosophy that focused on man, not nature. Plato wrote about his teacher, "Socrates ... believed in the immortal soul—all natural phenomena are merely shadows of the eternal forms or ideas. The soul, which existed before the body, longs to return to the world of ideas." Plato was a rationalist—we know with our reason.

Aristotle (384–322 B.C.) followed Socrates and Plato. His father was a physician, apparently framing his own interest in the natural world. He is known for his contribution to logic. Aristotle believed that the highest degree of reality is what we perceive with our senses. Unlike Plato, Aristotle did not believe in forms as separate from the real objects! When an object has both form and matter, it is called a substance. Aristotle said happiness was man's goal and came through balance of the following: life of pleasure and enjoyment, life as a free and responsible citizen, and life as a thinker and philosopher.

During the Neoplatonism age in the third century, philosophy became known as the soul's vehicle to return to its intelligible roots. There was an extrarational approach to reach union with the One. Thinking was that truth, and certainty was not found in this world. This was a revival of the "other worldliness" thinking of Plato.

The birth of Christianity and Western philosophy came at the death of classicism. Augustine of Hippo (A.D. 354–430) became a Christian and was attracted to Neoplatonism, where existence is divine. In that period, evil was defined as an absence or incompleteness. Saint Thomas Aquinas (A.D. 1225–1274) is credited with bringing theology and philosophy together.

Throughout the centuries, from the Greeks to the present day, people have debated the same questions: What is man? What is God? How do God and man relate? How does man relate to man? One can become dizzy thinking about the possibilities. Humans have been asking questions for a very long time, and thankfully, that practice is not about to change. People have searched for truth and will continue to do so. Therefore, we should not strive to find absolute answers; rather, we should endeavor to be comfortable with the questioning. Table 3-1 provides an overview of the perspectives of truth through the ages. From the pre-Socratics to the

TABLE 3-1 Overview of the Perspectives of Truth Through the Ages

School of Thought	Meaning of Truth (Philosophers)
Classical philosophers	Truth corresponds with reality, and reality is achieved through our perceptions of the world in which we live. Truth could be found in the natural world—through our sensory experiences. (Heraclitus, Aristotle) Truth can be found in the natural world—through our rational intellect. (Parmenides, Plato) Truth is found when one knows self. (Socrates) Truth is not of this world. (Plotinus)
Theocratics	Truth comes through an understanding of God. Truth can be found through both the senses and the intellect. (St. Thomas Aquinas)
Empiricists	Truth is based on experience and relating to our experiences. (Bacon, Locke, Hume, Mill)
Rationalists	All things are knowable by man's deductive reasoning. (Descartes, Spinoza)
Idealists	Truth exists only in the mind. (Berkeley, Hegel, Kant)
Positivists	Truth is science and the facts that science discovers. (Comte, Mill, Spencer)
Early existentialists	Truth is found through man's faith in his existence as it relates to God. (Kierkegaard)

School of Thought	Meaning of Truth (Philosophers)
Pragmatists	Truth is relative and practical—if it works, then it is truth. (James, Peirce, Dewey)
Relativists	Truth is always dependent on the knower and the knower's context. (Kuhn, Laudan)
Phenomenologists	Truth is in human consciousness. (Husserl, Heidegger)
Existentialists	If truth can be found, it can be found only through man's search for self. (Sartre, Merleau-Ponty, Gadamer)
Poststructuralists/ Postmodernists	Truth (if there is truth) is not singular and is always historical. Truth can be found in the deconstruction of language. (Derrida) Truth is (evolves from) the outcome of events. (Foucault) Truth is created through dialogue with a purpose of emancipatory action. (Habermas, Freire) Truth is unique to gender. (Feminists)

poststructuralists and postmodern thinkers, ways of knowing and finding truth have changed.

Now, back to the real world: What is the purpose for this dialogue in a text on professional nursing? One of the critical theorists, Habermas, would say, "Communication is the way to truth." We have this discussion because it leads us to truth. In this case, the dialogue leads us to truth about nursing. What we hold as truth does not come through mere reading, studying, or debating. The truth comes through dialogue. Let's continue.

Paradigms

How do you see the world? Whether you know it or not, you have an established worldview or **paradigm**. A paradigm is the lens through which you see the world. Paradigms are also philosophical foundations that support our approaches to research (Weaver & Olson, 2006). The continuum of **realism** and **idealism** explains bipolar paradigms (Box 3-1). Most people today would agree that "somewhere in the middle" of these dichotomies lies truth.

Our philosophies are established from a lifelong process of learning and show us how we find truth. In other words, a philosophy is our method of knowing. The experiences we have with ourselves, others, and the environment provide structure to our thinking. Ultimately, our philosophies are demonstrated in the outcomes of our day-to-day living. Nurses' values and beliefs about the profession come from observation and experience (Buresh & Gordon, 2000).

> **BOX 3-1 THE CONTINUUM OF REALISM AND IDEALISM**
>
> Realism
> - The world is static.
> - Seeing is believing.
> - The social world is a given.
> - Reality is physical and independent.
> - Logical thinking is superior.
>
> Idealism
> - The world is evolving.
> - There is more than meets the eye.
> - The social world is created.
> - Reality is a conception perceived in the mind.
> - Thinking is dynamic and constructive.

Your worldview of nursing began long before you enrolled in nursing school. As far as you can remember, think back on your understanding of nursing. What did you think you would do as a nurse? Did you know a nurse? Did you have an experience with a nurse? What images of the nurse did you see on television or in the movies? Since that time, your worldview of nursing has changed. What experiences in school have changed your perspective of nursing? Undoubtedly, how you see nursing now will differ from your worldview in a few years—or even a few months.

www | CRITICAL THINKING QUESTION ✳

Where do you see yourself and your understanding of truth on the continuum of realism and idealism? ✳

Beliefs

A chief goal in this chapter is to provide a starting point for writing a personal philosophy of nursing. To do that, we must have a discussion of beliefs and values. *Beliefs* indicate what we value, and according to Steele (1979), beliefs have a faith component. Rokeach (1973) identifies three categories of beliefs: existential, evaluative, and prescriptive/proscriptive beliefs. Existential beliefs can be shown to be true or false. An example is the belief that the sun will come up each morning. Evaluative beliefs describe beliefs that make a judgment about whether something is good or bad. The belief that social drinking is immoral is an evaluative belief. Prescriptive and proscriptive beliefs refer to what people should (prescriptive) or should not (proscriptive) do. An example of a prescriptive or desirable belief is that everyone should vote. An example of an undesirable or proscriptive belief is that people should not be dishonest. Beliefs demonstrate a personal confidence in the validity of a person, object, or idea.

How would you define *person*? Look at the following attributes given to a person: (1) the ability to think and conceptualize, (2) the capacity to interact with others, (3) the need for boundaries, and (4) the use of language (Doheny, Cook, & Stopper, 1997). Would you agree? What about Maslow's description of humanness in terms of a hierarchy of needs with self-actualization at the top? Another possibility is that persons are the major focus of nursing. Do you see humans as good or evil?

www CRITICAL THINKING QUESTION ∗

What are your beliefs about the major concepts in nursing—person, environment, health, nursing? ∗

Consider a second concept in nursing: *environment*. How do you define the internal (within the person) and external (outside the person) environments? Is it important that nurses look beyond the individual toward the surroundings and structures that influence quality of human life? If yes, then how do you see the relationship between the internal and external environments? Is one dimension more important than the other? How do they interact with each other? Martha Rogers, a grand theorist in nursing, described the environment as continuous with the person, no boundaries, in constant exchange of energy. Would you agree?

Health is the third domain of nursing to ponder. Is health the same as the absence of illness? Is health perception? A person who is living and surviving may be described as "healthy." Would you support that as a comprehensive definition of health? Doheny et al. (1997) referred to health in the following way:

> Health is dynamic and ever changing, not a stagnant state. Health can be measured only in relative terms. No one is absolutely healthy or ill. In addition, health applies to the total person, including progression toward the realization and fulfillment of one's potential as well as maintaining physical, psychosocial health. (p. 19)

Maybe that definition is sufficient, but probably not. All definitions—including yours—have limitations. Definitions merely give us a way to express our beliefs.

Finally, consider common beliefs about *nursing*. Clarke (2006) posed that question in "So What Exactly Is a Nurse?" an article addressing the problematic nature of defining nursing. The American Nurses Association (ANA) provided a much used definition of nursing in 1980: "Nursing is the diagnosis and treatment of human responses to actual and potential health problems" (p. 9). Fifteen years later, the ANA (1995, p. 6) expanded its basic definition of nursing to include four fundamental aspects. Nursing is the following:

- Attention to the full range of human experiences and responses to health and illness without restriction to a problem-focused orientation
- Integration of objective data with an understanding of the subjective experience of the patient

- Application of scientific knowledge to the processes of diagnosis and treatment
- Provision of a caring relationship that facilitates health and healing

How would you define nursing? Understanding our beliefs and articulating them in definitions are beginning steps for developing a personal philosophy. Definitions tell us what things are. Our philosophy tells us how things are. One other piece must be addressed before we begin writing our personal philosophy: the topic of values.

Values

Values refer to what the normative standard should be, not necessarily to how things actually are. Values are the principles and ideals that give meaning and direction to our social, personal, and professional lives. Steele (1979) defines *value* as "an affective disposition towards a person, object, or idea" (p. 1). The values of nursing have been articulated by groups such as the ANA in the *Code of Ethics* (2001) and the American Association of Colleges of Nursing's (AACN) (2008) essentials for baccalaureate nursing education. The AACN essentials document calls for integration of professional nursing values in baccalaureate education; they are altruism, autonomy, human dignity, integrity, and social justice. Ways of teaching these values have been addressed in recent literature (Fahrenwald, 2003).

Nursing values have been identified as the fundamentals that guide our standards, influence practice decisions, and provide the framework used for evaluation (Kenny, 2002). Nevertheless, nursing has been criticized as not clearly articulating what our values are (Kenny, 2002). If nursing is to engage in the move to "interprofessional working," which is beyond uniprofessional and multiprofessional relationships, we have to define our values clearly. Interprofessional working validates what others provide in health care, and the relationships depend on mutual input and collaboration. Values in nursing need to be clearly articulated so that they can be discussed in the context of interprofessional partnership. We can then work together across traditional boundaries for the good of patients. Nursing offers something to health care that no one else does, but that *something* must first be clear to those of us in nursing. "It is not enough just to argue that caring is never value-free, and that values are a fundamental aspect of nursing. What is required is greater precision and clarity so that values can be identified by those within the profession and articulated beyond it" (Kenny, 2002, p. 66).

Statements such as those by the ANA and the AACN mentioned earlier are a step in the right direction. Others have identified nursing values using different language. Antrobus (1997) sees nursing values as humanistic and included (1) a nurturing response to someone in need, (2) a view of the whole individual, (3) an emphasis on the individual's perspective, (4) concentration on developing human potential, (5) an aim of well-being, and (6) maintenance of the nurse–patient relationship at the heart of the helping situation. Nursing values have also been listed as caregiving, accountability, integrity, trust, freedom, safety, and knowledge (Weis & Schank, 2000).

Rokeach (1973) makes the following assertions about values:

> **Nursing offers something to health care that no one else does, but that *something* must first be clear to those of us in nursing.**

- Each person has a few.
- All humans possess the same values.
- People organize values into systems.
- Values are developed in response to culture, society, and personality.
- Behaviors are manifestations or consequences of values.

The process of valuing involves three steps: (1) choosing values, (2) prizing values, and (3) acting on values (Chitty, 2001). To choose a value is an intellectual stage in which a person selects a value from identified alternatives. Second, prizing values involves the emotional or affective dimension of valuing. When we "feel" a certain way about our values, it is because we have reached this second step. Finally, we have to act on our intellectual choice and emotion. This third step includes behavior or action that demonstrates our value. Ideally, a genuine value is evidenced by consistent behavior.

Steele (1979) distinguished between intrinsic and extrinsic values. An intrinsic value is required for living (e.g., food and water), whereas an extrinsic value is not required for living and is originated external to the person. According to Simon and Clark (1975), the following criteria must be met in acquiring values:

- Must be freely chosen
- Must be selected from a list of alternatives
- Must have thoughtful consideration of each of the outcomes of the alternatives
- Must be prized and cherished
- Must involve a willingness to make values known to others
- Must precipitate action
- Must be integrated into lifestyle

Value acquisition refers to when a new value is assumed, and *value abandonment* is when a value is relinquished. *Value redistribution* occurs when society changes views about a particular value. Values are more dynamic than attitude because values include motivation as well as cognitive, affective, and behavioral components. Therefore, people have fewer values than attitudes (feelings or dispositions toward a person, object, or idea). In the end, values determine our choices.

According to Steele (1979), values can compete with each other on our "hierarchy of values." We typically have values that we hold about education, politics, gender, society, occupations, culture, religion, and so on. The values that are higher in the hierarchy receive more time, energy, resources, and attention. For change to occur there must be conflict among the value system. For example, if a patient values both freedom from pain and long life but is diagnosed with bone cancer, a conflict in values will occur. If professional responsibilities and religious beliefs conflict, the solution is not as simple as "right versus wrong." Rather, it is the choice between two goods. For example, suppose you have strong religious views about abortion. During your rotation, you are assigned to care for someone who elects to have an abortion. As a nurse, you must balance the value of the patient's choice with your personal value about elective abortions. These decisions are not easy.

Dowds and Marcel (1998) conducted a study involving 40 female nursing students who were taking a psychology class. The students completed the World Hypothesis Scale, which provided 12 items, each with four possible explanations of an event. Each of the four explanations represented a distinct way of thinking. A list of definitions and descriptions of the different ways of thinking includes the following:

- *Contextualism:* Understanding is embedded in context; meaning is subjective and open to change and dependent on the moment in time and the person's perspective.
- *Formism:* Understanding events in relationship to their similarity to an ideal or objective standard comes from categorization (e.g., the classification of plants and animals in biology).
- *Mechanism:* Understanding is in terms of cause-and-effect relationships, the common approach used by modern medicine.
- *Organicism:* Understanding comes from patterns and relationships; must understand the whole to understand the parts (e.g., cannot look at a child's language development without looking at his or her overall development history).

The students ranked the explanations in terms of their preferences for understanding the event. Nursing students chose mechanistic thinking significantly more than all other ways of thinking and chose contextualistic thinking significantly less than the other worldviews. No other comparisons were significant among or between the four worldviews. In other words, the nursing students did not choose options that allowed for more than one right answer. They resisted the options that allowed for ambiguity. What this tells us in relationship to values is that we can say that we value human response and the whole individual, but do we really? Human situations are dynamic, fluid, and open for multiple options. Nursing claims to respond to these contextual needs, but do we?

■ Values Clarification

Clarifying our values is an eye-opening experience. The process of **values clarification** can occur in a group or individually and helps us understand who we are and what is most important to us. The outcome of values clarification is positive because the outcome is growth. If the process occurs in a group, there must be trust within the group. No one should be embarrassed or intimidated. Everyone is respected.

www CRITICAL THINKING QUESTIONS ✳

Do you believe there is more than one right answer to situations? How do you value the whole individual? What barriers prevent us from responding to the contextual needs of our patients? ✳

Values clarification exercises help people discern their individual values. A simple approach to begin the process is considering your responses to statements such as "Patients have a right to know everything that is in the medical record." What is your immediate reaction? How do you feel about the options available in this situation? Have you acted on these beliefs in the past? Another statement to consider is this: "Everyone should have equal access to health care—regardless of income." Ask yourself the same questions. Other exercises involve real or hypothetical clinical situations. For example, a 19-year-old male with HIV disease is totally dependent. His parents remain at his bedside but do not say a word. Another example is a single mom who has recently been diagnosed with multiple sclerosis. What about a 70-year-old man who loses his wife of 42 years, only to remarry a woman who is soon diagnosed with dementia? Reflect. What questions do you have? Why are these people in these situations? Does that matter? What in the patient's life choices conflicts with your choices? Share this with your peers, your friends, and your teachers. In values clarification, one should consider the steps identified earlier as necessary for value acquisition: (1) choosing freely from among alternatives, (2) experiencing an emotional connection, and (3) demonstrating actions consistent with a stated value.

We act on values as the climax of the values clarification process. We are more aware, more empathetic to others, and have greater insight to ourselves and those around us for having gone through this process. Our words and actions are not so different, and we become more content with the individuals we are (i.e., self-actualization). Values clarification also allows us to be more open to accepting others' choice of values.

We must keep in mind that values vary from person to person. Returning to the concept of health, if we asked several people "What is health?" we would get different responses because it means different things to different people. Most likely we would find that others do not place health as high in their hierarchy of values as we do. This helps explain why some people go to the physician for every little ailment, whereas others wait until the situation is critical. Maintaining a nonjudgmental attitude about the values of others is crucial to the nurse–patient relationship.

In health care, we need to clarify values for both the consumer and provider in society. Referring once again to health, we recognize that although the majority of our society states that health is a right, not a privilege, everyone does not have health care. Is health positioned at the top of society's hierarchy of values? We also have to assess the individual's values for congruency with the societal values. As research gives us new options to consider, continual reassessment of values is essential. A questioning attitude is healthy and necessary.

As a profession, nursing is responsible for clarifying our values on a regular basis. Just as society places a value on health, society also determines the value of nursing in the provision of health. Additionally, nurses need to be involved in all levels where decisions based on values are made, particularly with ethical decisions. The values that nursing supports need to be communicated clearly to those making the policies that affect the health of our society.

Values clarification is done for the purpose of understanding self—to discover what is important and meaningful (Steele, 1979). Throughout life, the process continues as it gives direction to life. As you work through the course of values clarification, keep in mind that personal and professional values are not necessarily the same.

> **www | CRITICAL THINKING QUESTIONS** *
>
> Do I believe in health care for everyone? Does health care for everyone have value to me as a person? Does it have value to me as a nurse? What value does universal health care have to my patients? *

Developing a Personal Philosophy of Nursing

> **KEY COMPETENCY 3-1**
>
> Examples of Applicable *Nurse of the Future: Nursing Core Competencies*
>
> Professionalism:
>
> Knowledge (K7) Understands ethical principles, values, concepts, and decision making that apply to nursing and patient care
>
> Skills (S7c) Identifies and responds to ethical concerns, issues, and dilemmas that affect nursing practice
>
> Attitudes/Behaviors (A7c) Clarifies personal and professional values and recognizes their impact on decision making and professional behavior
>
> *Source:* Massachusetts Department of Higher Education (2010, p. 14).

Before we begin writing our individual nursing philosophies, consider the following comments about philosophy. According to Doheny et al. (1997), philosophy is defined as "beliefs of a person or group of persons" and "reveals underlying values and attitudes regarding an area" (p. 259). In this concise definition, these authors mentioned the building blocks of philosophy that we have discussed thus far: attitudes, beliefs, and values. Another definition that is not as concise reads, "Nursing philosophy is a statement of foundational and universal assumptions, beliefs, and principles about the nature of knowledge and truth (epistemology) and about the nature of the entities—nursing practice and human healing processes—represented in the metaparadigm (ontology)" (Reed, 1999, p. 483). Finally, philosophy "looks at the nature of things and aims to provide the meaning of nursing phenomena" (Blais, Hayes, Kozier, & Erb, 2002, p. 90).

In *Nursing's Agenda for the Future*, the ANA (2002) identified the need for nurses to "believe, articulate, and demonstrate the value of nursing" (p. 15). To do that, each professional nurse is responsible for clearly articulating a personal philosophy of nursing. Suggestions for developing personal professional philosophies have been presented in the literature (Brown & Gillis, 1999). The overall purpose of personal philosophy is to define how one finds truth. Because there are different ways of knowing, each person has a unique way of finding truth, in other words, identifying our individual philosophy. Therefore, your philosophy of nursing will be unique.

How do you start writing? A suggested guide for writing your personal philosophy of nursing is in Box 3-2.

When defining nursing, you may refer to definitions by professional individuals or groups. You may also choose to write an original definition, which is certainly acceptable. A final challenge would be this: Once you have used words to describe your personal philosophy, try drawing it. This exercise can enlighten you to gaps in your understanding and further clarify the picture for you.

Writing a philosophy does not have to be a difficult exercise. In fact, you have one already—you just need to practice putting it on paper. Keep in mind that your philosophy will change over time. In addition, composing a nursing philosophy will help you see yourself as an active participant in the profession.

Consider the scene if no one in nursing had a philosophy. What would happen? Unfortunately, we would find ourselves doing tasks without

---

BOX 3-2 GUIDE FOR WRITING A PERSONAL PHILOSOPHY OF NURSING

1. Introduction
   a. Who are you?
   b. Where do you practice nursing?

2. Define nursing.
   a. What is nursing?
   b. Why does nursing exist?
   c. Why do you practice nursing?

3. What are your assumptions or underlying beliefs about:
   a. Nurses?
   b. Patients?
   c. Other healthcare providers?
   d. Communities?

4. Define the major domains of nursing and provide examples:
   a. Person
   b. Health
   c. Environment

5. Summary
   a. How are the domains connected?
   b. What is your vision of nursing for the future?
   c. What are the challenges that you will face as a nurse?
   d. What are your goals for professional development?

considering the rationale and performing routines in the absence of purpose. Most likely, we would find ourselves devalued by our patients and fellow care providers.

Although our individual philosophies vary, there are similarities that link us in our universal philosophy as a profession. As a whole, we are kept on track by continually evaluating our attitudes, beliefs, and values. We can evaluate our efforts by reflecting on our philosophies. In the process of personal and professional reflection, we are challenged to reach global relevancy and to begin the development of a global nursing philosophy (Henry, 1998).

www CRITICAL THINKING QUESTIONS ✳

How does my personal philosophy fit with the context of nursing? Does it fit? What areas, if any, need assessing? ✳

KEY COMPETENCY 3-2

Examples of Applicable *Nurse of the Future: Nursing Core Competencies*

Professionalism:

Knowledge (K8A) Understands the responsibilities inherent in being a member of the nursing profession

Skills (S8a) Understands the history and philosophy of the nursing profession

Attitudes/Behaviors (A8b) Values and upholds altruistic and humanistic principles

Source: Massachusetts Department of Higher Education (2010, p. 15).

Conclusion

In this chapter, we have discussed one of the most ambiguous concepts in professional disciplines—nursing philosophy. The history of philosophy helps us to see that asking questions about humans, environment, health, and nursing is a continual process that leads to a better understanding of truth in our profession. Our own values and beliefs must be clarified so that we can authentically respond to the healthcare needs of our patients and to society as a whole. All along the way, our philosophies are changing. Therefore, we must constantly question the values of our profession, our society, and ourselves—aiming to better the health of all people worldwide.

Hegel, an early philosopher, said, "History is the spirit seeking freedom." On this path of searching for truth, we ask the same question, but in different contexts and with distinct experiences. The answers for one person do not provide the same satisfaction for another person. Through our individual and collective searching, we become *truth knowers*. Habermas, the supporter of dialogue, would suggest that the journey does not end with communication and questioning alone. When truth is revealed, oppressive forces are acknowledged, and the truth knowers are then responsible to move to action. Through that action comes a change in the social structure and the hope of rightness in the world.

Classroom Activity 1

Take about 15 minutes after the discussion related to developing a philosophy of nursing to begin answering the questions in Box 3-2. Jot down answers to the questions in Box 3-2. Ask questions as necessary while still in the classroom. This simple activity will make it easier when writing a personal philosophy of nursing. **www**

Classroom Activity 2

After thinking about your answers to the questions in Box 3-2 related to the metaparadigm concepts (person, health, environment, and nursing), draw each of these concepts as you define them on a separate piece of paper. Save your drawings, and think about them and refine them as you develop your philosophy of nursing.

This activity works best if you use colored pencils, crayons, or markers. An example is presented in Figure 3-1. [www]

Figure 3-1 Drawing of the concept of person

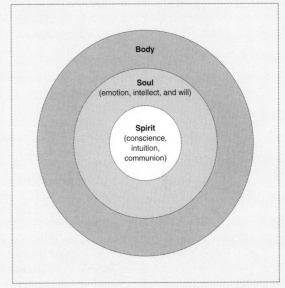

Source: Masters, 2006, as adapted from Nee, 1968

References

American Association of Colleges of Nursing. (2008). *The essentials of baccalaureate education for professional nursing practice.* Washington, DC: Author.

American Heritage Dictionary of the English Language (4th ed.). (2000). Boston, MA: Houghton Mifflin.

American Nurses Association. (1980). *Nursing: A social policy statement.* Washington, DC: Author.

American Nurses Association. (1995). *Nursing's social policy statement.* Washington, DC: Author.

American Nurses Association. (2001). *Code of ethics for nurses with interpretive statements.* Washington, DC: Author.

American Nurses Association. (2002, April). *Nursing's agenda for the future: A call to the nation.* Retrieved from http://ana.nursingworld.org/MainMenuCategories/HealthcareandPolicyIssues/HealthSystemReform/What-ANA-is-Doing/AgendafortheFuture.aspx

Antrobus, S. (1997). An analysis of nursing in context: The effects of current health policy. *Journal of Advanced Nursing, 45,* 447–453.

Blais, K. K., Hayes, J. S., Kozier, B., & Erb, G. (2002). *Professional nursing practice: Concepts and perspectives* (4th ed.). Upper Saddle River, NJ: Prentice Hall.

Brown, S. C., & Gillis, M. A. (1999). Using reflective thinking to develop personal professional philosophies. *Journal of Nursing Education, 38,* 171–176.

Buresh, B., & Gordon, S. (2000). *From silence to voice: What nurses know and must communicate to the public.* New York, NY: Cornell University Press.

Chitty, K. K. (2001). Philosophies of nursing. In K. K. Chitty (Ed.), *Professional nursing: Concepts and challenges* (pp. 199–217). Philadelphia, PA: Saunders.

Clarke, L. (2006). So what exactly is a nurse? *Journal of Psychiatric and Mental Health Nursing, 13,* 388–394.

Doheny, M. O., Cook, C. B., & Stopper, M. C. (1997). *The discipline of nursing: An introduction* (4th ed.). Stamford, CT: Appleton & Lange.

Dowds, B. N., & Marcel, B. B. (1998). Students' philosophical assumptions and psychology in the classroom. *Journal of Nursing Education, 37,* 219–222.

Fahrenwald, N. L. (2003). Teaching social justice. *Nurse Educator, 28,* 222–226.

Henry, B. (1998). Globalization, nursing philosophy, and nursing science. *Image: Journal of Nursing Scholarship, 30,* 302.

Kenny, G. (2002). The importance of nursing values in interprofessional collaboration. *British Journal of Nursing, 11*(1), 65–68.

Massachusetts Department of Higher Education. (2010). *Nurse of the future: Nursing core competencies.* Retrieved from http://www.mass.edu/currentinit/documents/NursingCoreCompetencies.pdf

Masters, K. (2006). *Drawing of concept of person.* Unpublished classroom exercise.

Nee, W. (1968). *The spiritual man.* New York, NY: Christian Fellowship Publishers.

Reed, P. G. (1999). A treatise on nursing knowledge development for the 21st century: Beyond postmodernism. In E. C. Polifroni & M. Welch (Eds.), *Perspectives on philosophy of science in nursing* (pp. 478–490). Philadelphia, PA: Lippincott.

Rokeach, M. (1973). *The nature of human values.* New York, NY: Free Press.

Simon, S. B., & Clark, J. (1975). *Beginning values clarification: A guidebook for the use of values clarification in the classroom.* San Diego, CA: Pennant Press.

Steele, S. (1979). *Values clarification in nursing.* New York, NY: Appleton-Century-Crofts.

Weaver, K., & Olson, J. K. (2006). Understanding paradigms used for nursing research. *Journal of Advanced Nursing, 53,* 459–469.

Weis, D., & Schank, M. J. (2000). An instrument to measure professional nursing values. *Journal of Nursing Scholarship, 32,* 201–204.

Foundations of Ethical Nursing Practice

4

Karen Rich and Janie B. Butts

Scientific and technological advances, economic realities, pluralistic worldviews, and global communication make it impossible for nurses to ignore important ethical issues in the world community, their individual lives, and their work. As controversial and sensitive ethical issues continue to challenge nurses and other healthcare professionals, many professionals have begun to develop an appreciation for personal philosophies of ethics and the diverse viewpoints of others.

Often ethical directives are not clearly evident, which leads some people to argue that ethics can be based merely on personal opinions. However, if nurses are to enter into the global dialogue about ethics, they must do more than practice ethics based simply on their personal opinions, their intuition, or the unexamined beliefs that are proposed by other people. It is important for nurses to have a basic understanding of the various concepts, theories, approaches, and principles used in ethics throughout history and to identify and analyze ethical issues and dilemmas that are relevant to nurses in this century. Mature ethical sensitivities are critical to professional nursing practice.

Learning Objectives

After completing this chapter, the student should be able to:

1. Discuss the meaning of key terms associated with ethical nursing practice.
2. Compare and contrast ethical theories and approaches that might be used in nursing practice.
3. Discuss each of the popular bioethical principles as they relate to nursing practice: autonomy, beneficence, nonmaleficence, and justice.
4. Justify the importance of the *Code of Ethics for Nurses* for professional nursing practice.
5. Explain how nurses can identify and analyze dilemmas that occur in nursing practice.

Ethics in Everyday Life

Ethics, a branch of philosophy, means different things to different people. When the term is narrowly defined according to its original use, ethics is the study of ideal human behavior and ideal ways of being. The approaches to ethics and the meanings of ethically related concepts have varied over time among philosophers and ethicists. As a philosophical discipline of study,

> **Mature ethical sensitivities are critical to professional nursing practice.**

ethics is a systematic approach to understanding, analyzing, and distinguishing matters of right and wrong, good and bad, and admirable and deplorable as they exist along a continuum and as they relate to the well-being of and the relationships among sentient beings. Ethical determinations are applied through the use of formal theories, approaches, and codes of conduct.

As contrasted with the term *ethics*, **morals** are specific beliefs, behaviors, and ways of being based on personal judgments derived from one's ethics. One's morals are judged to be good or bad through systematic ethical analysis. Because the word *ethics* is used when one might literally be referring to a situation of morals, the process-related conception of ethics is sometimes overlooked today. People often use the word *ethics* when referring to a collection of actual beliefs and behaviors, thereby using the terms *ethics* and *morals* in essentially synonymous ways.

Bioethics

The terms *bioethics* and *healthcare ethics* are sometimes used interchangeably in the literature. **Bioethics** is a specific domain of ethics that is focused on moral issues in the field of health care. Callahan (1995) calls it "the intersection of ethics and the life sciences—but also an academic discipline" (p. 248). Bioethics has evolved into a discipline all its own as a result of life-and-death moral dilemmas encountered by physicians, nurses, other healthcare professionals, patients, and families.

In his book *The Birth of Bioethics*, Albert Jonsen (1998) designates a span of 40 years, from 1947 to 1987, as the era when bioethics was evolving as a discipline. This era began with the Nuremberg Tribunal in 1947, when Nazi physicians were charged and convicted for the murderous and tortuous war crimes that these physicians labeled as scientific experiments during the early 1940s. The 10 judgments in the final court ruling of the Nazi trial provided the basis for the worldwide Nuremberg Code of 1947. This code became a document to protect human subjects during research and experimentation.

The 1950s and 1960s were preliminary years before the actual birth of bioethics. A transformation was occurring during these years as technology advanced. In this era, a new ethic was emerging about life and extension of life through technology. The development of the polio vaccine, organ transplantation, life support, and many other advances occurred. Scientists and physicians were forced to ask questions: "Who should live?" "Who should die?" "Who should decide?" (Jonsen, 1998, p. 11). Many conferences and workshops during the 1960s and 1970s addressed issues surrounding life and death.

By 1970, the public, physicians, and researchers were referring to these phenomena as bioethics (Johnstone, 1999). Today, bioethics is a vast interdisciplinary venture that has engrossed the public's interest from the time of its conception. The aim of bioethicists today is to continue to search for answers to deep philosophical questions about life, death, and the significance of human beings and to help guide and control public policy (Kuhse & Singer, 1998).

Nursing Ethics

"It is the real-life, flesh-and-blood cases that raise fundamental ethical questions" (Fry & Veatch, 2000, p. 1) in nursing. **Nursing ethics** sometimes is viewed as a subcategory of the broader domain of bioethics, just as medical ethics is a subcategory of bioethics. However, controversy continues about whether nursing has unique moral problems in professional practice. Nursing ethics, similar to all healthcare ethics, usually begins with cases or problems that are practice based.

Many nursing ethicists distinguish issues of nursing ethics from broader bioethical issues that nurses encounter. These nursing ethicists view nursing ethics as a separate field because of the unique variety of ethical problems that surface in relationships between nurses and patients, families, physicians, and other professionals who are a part of the healthcare team. The key criteria for distinguishing issues of nursing ethics from bioethics are that nurses are the primary agents in the scenario, and ethical issues are viewed from a nursing rather than a medical perspective.

> The key criteria for distinguishing issues of nursing ethics from bioethics are that nurses are the primary agents in the scenario, and ethical issues are viewed from a nursing rather than a medical perspective.

Moral Reasoning

In general, reasoning involves using abstract thought processes to solve problems and to formulate plans (Angeles, 1992). More specifically, **moral reasoning** pertains to making decisions about how humans ought to be and act. Deliberations about moral reasoning go back to the days of the ancient Greeks when Aristotle, in *Nicomachean Ethics*, discussed the intellectual virtue of wisdom as being necessary for deliberation about what is good and advantageous in terms of moving toward worthy ends (Broadie, 2002).

Moral reasoning can be described by what Aristotle (Broadie, 2002) called the intellectual virtue of wisdom (phronesis), also known as prudence. Virtue is an excellence of intellect or character. The virtue of wisdom is focused on the good achieved from being wise, that is, knowing how to act in a particular situation, practicing good deliberation, and having a disposition consistent with excellence of character (Broadie, 2002). Therefore, prudence involves more than having good intentions or meaning well. It includes knowing "what is what" but also transforming that knowledge into well-reasoned decisions. Deliberation, judgment, and decision are the steps in transforming knowledge into action. Prudence becomes truth in action (Pieper, 1966).

In more recent times, Lawrence Kohlberg, in 1981, reported his landmark research about moral reasoning based on 84 boys he had followed for more than 20 years. Kohlberg defined six stages ranging from immature to mature moral development. Interestingly, Kohlberg did not include any women in his research but expected that his six-stage scale could be used to measure moral development in both males and females. When the scale was applied to women, they seemed to score only at the third stage of the sequence, a stage in which Kohlberg described morality in terms of interpersonal relationships and helping others. Kohlberg viewed this third stage of development as deficient in regard to mature moral reasoning.

In light of Kohlberg's exclusion of females in his research and the negative implications of women being placed within the third stage of moral reasoning, Carol Gilligan raised the concern of gender bias. Gilligan, in turn, published an influential book in 1982, *In a Different Voice*, in which she argued that women's moral reasoning is different but is not deficient (Gilligan, 1993; Grimshaw, 1993; Thomas, 1993). The distinction that is usually made between the ethics of Kohlberg and Gilligan is that Kohlberg's is a male-oriented ethic of justice and Gilligan's is a more feminine ethic of care. The Kohlberg–Gilligan justice–care debate is still at the heart of feminist ethics.

Often the work of nurses does not involve independent moral reasoning and decision making in regard to the well-publicized issues in bioethics, such as withdrawing life support. Independent moral reasoning and decision making for nurses usually occurs more in the day-to-day care and relationships between nurses and their patients and between nurses and their coworkers. Nurses' moral reasoning is similar to the findings of Gilligan and is often based on caring and the needs of good interpersonal relationships. However, this does not negate what nurses can learn from studying Aristotle and his virtue of phronesis. Nurses' moral reasoning needs to be deliberate and practically wise to facilitate patients' well-being.

Values in Nursing

Values are emphasized in the American Nurses Association (ANA, 2001) *Code of Ethics for Nurses with Interpretive Statements*. *Values* refer to a group's or individual's evaluative judgments about what is good or what makes something desirable. Professional values are integral to moral reasoning. Values in nursing encompass appreciating what is important for both the profession and nurses personally, as well as what is important for patients.

In the *Code of Ethics for Nurses with Interpretive Statements* (discussed in more detail later in this chapter), the ANA (2001) includes statements about **wholeness of character**, which pertains to knowing the values of the nursing profession and one's own authentic moral values, integrating these two belief systems, and expressing them appropriately. **Integrity** is an important feature of wholeness of character. According to the code, maintaining integrity involves acting consistently with personal values and the values of the profession. In a healthcare system often burdened with constraints and self-serving groups and organizations, threats to integrity can be a serious pitfall for nurses. When nurses are asked and pressured to do things that conflict with their values, such as to falsify records, deceive patients, or accept verbal abuse from others, emotional and moral suffering can occur. A nurse's values must guide moral reasoning and actions, even when other people challenge the nurse's beliefs. When compromise is necessary, the compromise must not be such that it compromises personal or professional values.

> **Values in nursing encompass appreciating what is important for both the profession and nurses personally, as well as what is important for patients.**

Recognizing the essential dignity of oneself and each patient is another value that is basic to nursing and is given priority in moral reasoning. Pullman (1999) describes two conceptions of dignity. One type, called **basic dignity**, is intrinsic, or inherent, and dwells within all humans, with all humans being ascribed this moral worth. The other type, called **personal dignity**, often mistakenly equated with autonomy, is an evaluative type. Judging others and describing behaviors as dignified or undignified are of an evaluative nature. Personal dignity is a socially constructed concept that fluctuates in value from community to community, as well as globally. Most often, however, personal dignity is highly valued.

Ethical Theories and Approaches

Within each ethical theory or approach, a normative framework exists that includes foundational statements. Individuals who apply a particular theory or approach know what beliefs and values are right and wrong and what is and is not acceptable according to the particular ethical system. Normative ethical theories function as moral guides in answering the question: "What ought I do or not do?" Theory helps to provide guidance in moral thinking and reasoning and justification for moral actions. Optimally, ethical theories and approaches should

> **Theory helps to provide guidance in moral thinking and reasoning and justification for moral actions.**

help people to discern commonplace morality and strengthen moral judgments "in the face of moral dilemmas" (Mappes & DeGrazia, 2001, p. 5).

■ Virtue Ethics

Since the time of Aristotle (384–322 B.C.), **virtues**, *arête* in Greek, refer to excellences of intellect or character. Aristotle, the Greek philosopher, was one of the most influential thinkers in regard to virtue ethics. Virtue ethics pertains to questions of "What sort of person must I be to achieve my life's purpose?" and "What makes one a good or excellent person?" rather than "what is right or good to do based on my duty or to achieve good consequences?" Virtues are intellectual and character traits or habits that are developed throughout one's life. The idea behind virtue ethics is that when people are faced with complex moral dilemmas or situations, they will choose the right course of action because doing the right thing comes from a virtuous person's basic character. Aristotle believed that for a person to develop moral character, personal effort, training, and practice must occur. Examples of virtues include benevolence, compassion, courage, justice, generosity, truthfulness, wisdom, and patience.

■ Natural Law Theory

Saint Thomas Aquinas (1225–1274), who had a great influence on natural law theory as disseminated by Roman Catholic writers of that century, was himself influenced by Aristotle's work. Most versions of natural law theory today have their basis in Aquinas's basic philosophy. According to natural law theory, the rightness of actions is self-evident from the laws of nature, which in most cases is orchestrated by a law-giver God. Morality is determined not by customs and human preferences but is commanded by the law of reason, which is implanted in nature and human intellect. Natural law ethicists believe that behavior that is contrary to their views of the laws of nature is immoral. Examples include artificial means of birth control and homosexual relationships.

■ Deontology

Deontology refers to actions that are duty based, not based on their rewards, happiness, or consequences. One of the most influential philosophers for the deontologic way of thinking was Immanuel Kant, an 18th-century German philosopher. In his classic work, *Groundwork of the Metaphysics of Morals*, Kant (1785/2003) attempted to define a person as a rational human being with freedom, moral worth, and ideally having a good will, meaning that a person should act from a sense of duty. Because of their rationality, Kant believed, humans have the freedom to make moral judgments. Therefore, Kant argued that people ought to follow a universal framework of moral maxims, or rules, to guide right actions because it is only through performing dutiful actions that people have moral worth. Even when individuals do not want to act from duty, Kant stated that they are required to do so if they want to be ethical. Maxims apply to everyone universally and become the laws for guiding conduct. According to Kant, moral actions should be ends in themselves, not the means to ends. In fact, when people use others as a means to an end, such as deliberately using another person to reach one's personal goals, they are not treating other people with the dignity that they deserve.

Kant distinguished between two types of duties: hypothetical imperatives and categorical imperatives. Hypothetical imperatives are duties or rules that people ought to observe if certain ends are to be achieved. Hypothetical imperatives are sometimes called "if–then" imperatives, which are conditional: for instance, "If I want to pass my nursing course, then I should be diligent in my studies."

However, Kant stated that moral actions must be based on unconditional reasoning. Where moral actions are concerned, duties and laws are absolute and universal. Kant called these moral maxims, or duties, categorical imperatives. When acting according to a categorical imperative, one should ask this question: "If I perform this action, would I will that it becomes a universal law?" No action can ever be judged as right, according to Kant, if the action cannot have the potential to become a binding law for all people. For example, Kant's ethics would impose the categorical imperative that one can never tell a lie for any reason because if a person lies in any instance, the person cannot rationally wish that permission to lie should universally become a law for everyone.

■ Utilitarianism

Contrasted with deontology, the ethical approach of **utilitarianism** is to promote the greatest good that is possible in situations (i.e., the greatest good for the greatest number). British utilitarianism was promoted by Jeremy Bentham (1789/1988) in his book *An Introduction to the Principles of Morals and Legislation*. Bentham's thoughts on utilitarianism were that each form of happiness is equal and that each situation or action should be evaluated according to its production of happiness, good, or pleasure. John Stuart Mill (1863/2002) challenged Bentham's view when in his book, *Utilitarianism*, he clearly points out that experiences of pleasure and happiness do have different qualities and are not equal. For example, Mill stated that intellectual pleasures of humans have more value than physical pleasures of nonhuman animals.

Utilitarians place great emphasis on what is best for groups, not individual people. In doing so, the focus is on moral acts that produce the most good in terms of the most happiness. By aiming for the most happiness, this theory focuses on good consequences, utility (usefulness), or good ends. Although happiness is the goal, it should be kept in mind that utilitarianism is not based merely on subjective preferences or judgments of happiness. Commonsense ethical directives agreed upon by groups of people are usually applied.

■ Ethic of Care

The **ethic of care** has a history in feminist ethics, which has a focus in the moral experiences of women. In the ethic of care approach, personal relationships and relationship responsibilities are emphasized. Important concepts in this approach are compassion, empathy, sympathy, concern for others, and caring for others. Carol Gilligan with her study on gender differences in moral development (see the Moral Reasoning section earlier in this chapter) has had an influence on the ethic of care approach.

www CRITICAL THINKING QUESTIONS ✳

Think about the ethical theories and approaches discussed in this section and think about moral conflicts you have experienced in the past. Have you used one of these approaches to resolve a conflict? Which approach or approaches have you used? ✳

People who uphold the ethic of care think in terms of particular situations and individual contexts, not in terms of impersonal universal rules and principles. In resolving moral conflicts and understanding a complex situation, a person must use critical thinking to inquire about relationships, circumstances, and the problem at hand. The situation must be brought to light with "caring, consideration, understanding, generosity, sympathy, helpfulness, and a willingness to assume responsibility" (Munson, 2004, p. 788).

■ Ethical Principlism

Ethical principlism, a popular approach to ethics in health care, involves using a set of ethical principles that is drawn from the common or widely shared conception of morality. The four principles that are most commonly used in bioethics are autonomy, beneficence, nonmaleficence, and justice. In 1979, Tom Beauchamp and James Childress published the first edition of *Principles of Biomedical Ethics*, which featured these four principles. Currently, the book is in its sixth edition, and the four principles have become an essential foundation for analyzing and resolving bioethical problems.

These principles, which are closely associated with rule-based ethics, provide a framework to support moral behavior and decision making. However, the principles neither form a theory nor provide a well-defined decision-making model. The framework of principlism provides a prima facie model. As a prima facie model, principles are applied based on rules and justifications for moral behavior. Often, more than one principle is relevant in ethical situations, and no conflict occurs. However, if relevant principles conflict in any situation, judgment must be used in weighing which principle should take precedence in guiding actions.

> **The four principles that are most commonly used in bioethics are autonomy, beneficence, nonmaleficence, and justice.**

Autonomy

The word *autonomy* is a derivative of "the Greek *autos* ('self') and *nomos* ('rule, governance, or law')" (Beauchamp & Childress, 2009, p. 99). **Autonomy** then involves one's ability to self-rule and to generate personal decisions independently. Some people argue that autonomy has a top priority among the four principles. However, there is no general consensus about this issue, and many people argue that other principles, such as beneficence, should take priority. Ideally, when using a framework of principlism, no one principle should automatically be assumed to rule supreme.

The principle of autonomy sometimes is described as respect for autonomy (Beauchamp & Childress, 2009). In the domain of health care, respect for a patient's autonomy includes situations such as obtaining informed consent for treatment; facilitating patient choice regarding treatment options; accepting patients' refusal of treatment; disclosing medical information, diagnoses, and treatment options to patients; and maintaining confidentiality. It is important to note that a patient's right to respect for autonomy is not unqualified. In cases of endangering or harming others, for example, through communicable diseases or acts of violence, people lose their basic rights to self-determination.

Beneficence

The principle of **beneficence** consists of deeds of "mercy, kindness, and charity" (Beauchamp & Childress, 2001, p. 166). Beneficence in nursing implies that nurses take actions to benefit patients and to facilitate their well-being. Beneficent nursing actions include obvious interventions such as lifting side rails on the patient's bed to prevent falls. More subtle actions also might be considered to be beneficent and kind actions, such as taking time to make phone calls for a frail, older patient who is unable to do so herself.

Occasionally, nurses can experience ethical conflicts when confronted with having to make a choice between respecting a patient's right to self-determination (autonomy) and the principle of beneficence. Nurses might decide to act in ways that they believe are for a patient's "own good" rather than allowing patients to exercise their autonomy. The deliberate overriding of a patient's autonomy in this way is called **paternalism**. An example of a paternalistic action is for a nurse to decide that a patient must try to ambulate in the hall, even though the patient moans and complains of being too tired from his morning whirlpool treatment. In that case, the nurse is aware that the patient wants to wait until a later time but insists otherwise. Nurses must weigh carefully the value of paternalistic actions and determine whether they are truly in the patient's best interest. Justified paternalism often involves matters of patient safety.

> **Nurses might decide to act in ways that they believe are for a patient's "own good" rather than allowing patients to exercise their autonomy. The deliberate overriding of a patient's autonomy in this way is called paternalism.**

Nonmaleficence

Nonmaleficence, the injunction to "do no harm," is often paired with beneficence, but a difference exists between the two principles. Beneficence requires taking action to benefit others, whereas nonmaleficence involves refraining from action that might harm others. Nonmaleficence has a wide scope of implications in health care that includes most notably avoiding negligent care, as well as making decisions regarding withholding or withdrawing treatment and regarding the provision of extraordinary or heroic treatment.

Justice

The fourth major principle, **justice,** is a principle in healthcare ethics, a virtue, and the foundation of a duty-based ethical framework of moral reasoning. In other words, the concept of justice is quite broad in the field of ethics. Justice refers to the fair distribution of benefits and burdens. In regard to principlism, justice most often refers to the distribution of scarce healthcare resources. Most of the time, difficult resource allocation decisions are based on attempts to answer questions regarding who has a right to health care and who will pay for healthcare costs.

Professional Ethics and Codes

Professional nursing began in England in the 1800s at the school Florence Nightingale founded, where profession-shaping ethical precepts were communicated (Kuhse & Singer, 1998). Nightingale's achievement was a landmark in nursing even though graduates in the early days of the school were below average (Dossey, 2000). For the first 30 to 40 years in Nightingale's school, male physicians trained the probationers because not enough educated women were available to teach nursing. Because of this strong medical influence, early nursing education was focused on technical training rather than on the art and science of nursing as Nightingale would have preferred.

By the end of the 1800s, modern nursing was established, and by the early 1890s, ethics in nursing was being discussed seriously (Dossey, 2000; Kuhse & Singer, 1998). The Nightingale Pledge, first administered in 1893, was written under the chairmanship of Lystra Gretter, the principal of a Detroit nursing school, and the origination of the pledge helped to establish nursing as an art and a science (Dossey, 2000). The International Council of Nurses (ICN), which has been a pioneer in developing a code of nursing ethics, was established in 1899. By 1900, the first book on nursing ethics, *Nursing Ethics: For Hospital and Private Use,* was written by the American nursing leader Isabel Hampton Robb (Kuhse & Singer, 1998).

Historically, a primary consideration in nursing ethics has been the determination of who is the focus of nurses' work. Until the 1960s, this focus was on the physician, which is not surprising based on the fact that over the years most nurses have been women and most doctors have been men (Kuhse & Singer, 1998). The focus on nurses' obedience to physicians remained at the forefront of nursing responsibilities into the 1960s with this assumption still being reflected in the *ICN Code of Nursing Ethics* in 1965. By 1973, however, the focus of nurses' primary responsibility within the ICN's code changed from the physician to the patient, where it remains to this day.

No code can provide absolute or complete rules that are free of conflict and ambiguity. Because codes are unable to provide exact directives for ethical decision making and action in all situations, some ethicists believe that virtue ethics provides a better approach to ethics because the emphasis is on an agent's character rather than on rules, principles, and laws (Beauchamp & Childress, 2009). Proponents of virtue ethics consider that if a nurse's character is not virtuous, the nurse cannot be depended on to act in good or moral ways even with a professional code as a guide. Professional codes do serve a useful purpose in providing direction to healthcare professionals. Ultimately, one must remember that codes do not eliminate moral dilemmas and are of no use without professionals' motivation to act morally.

> **Ultimately, one must remember that codes do not eliminate moral dilemmas and are of no use without professionals' motivation to act morally.**

■ The *Code of Ethics for Nurses*

The ANA first adopted its code in 1950 (Daly, 2002). Although it has always been implied that the code reflected ethical provisions, the word *ethics* was not added to the title until the 1985 code was replaced with its sixth and latest revision in 2001 (Fowler & Benner, 2001). The ANA's (2001) *Code of Ethics for Nurses with Interpretative Statements* contains general moral provisions and standards for nurses to follow, but specific guidelines for clinical practice, education, research, and administration are contained within the accompanying interpretive statements. See Appendix B for ANA's *Code of Ethics for Nurses*.

The code is considered to be nonnegotiable in regard to nursing practice. Some of the significant positions and changes in the 2001 code include a return to the use of the word *patient*, rather than *client*; an application of the code to nurses in all roles, not just clinical roles; conceding that research is not the only method that contributes to professional development; reaffirming a stance against nurses' participation in euthanasia; emphasizing that nurses owe the same duties to self as to others; and recommending that members who represent nursing associations are responsible for expressing nursing values, maintaining professional integrity, and participating in public policy development (ANA, 2001; Fowler & Benner, 2001).

> **The ANA *Code of Ethics for Nurses* is considered to be nonnegotiable in regard to nursing practice.**

Fowler (Fowler & Benner, 2001) and Daly (2002), nursing leaders involved in revising the code completed in 2001, have proposed that the new code is clearly patient focused whether the patient is considered to be "an individual, family, group, or community" (Daly, 2002, p. 98). The nurse's loyalty must be foremost to the patient even though institutional politics is a frequent influence in today's nursing environment.

With the expanding role of nurse administrators and advanced practice nurses, each nurse must be cognizant of conflicts of interest that could potentially have a negative effect on relationships with patients and patient care. Often nurses have overlooked the responsibility to the patient by nurses who are not in clinical roles. Nurse researchers, administrators, and educators are indirectly but still involved in affecting patient care. According to Fowler and Benner (2001), "It is not the possession of nursing credentials, degrees, and position that makes a nurse a nurse; rather it is this very commitment to the patient" (p. 435). Therefore, the code applies to all nurses regardless of their role.

One issue that created a vigorous debate with the 2001 revision of the code involved the ethical implications of collective bargaining in nursing (Daly, 2002). Ultimately, the nurses who formulated the revisions decided that it was important for the code to contain provisions supporting nurses who work to ensure that the environment in which they work is conducive to quality patient care and that nurses are able to fulfill their moral requirements. Collective bargaining was determined to be an appropriate avenue for more than just negotiating for better salaries and benefits. It also can be used to improve the moral level of the environment in which nurses work.

■ The *ICN Code of Ethics for Nurses*

In 1953, the International Council of Nurses (ICN) adopted its first *Code of Ethics for Nurses*. The most recent revision and review of the code occurred in 2006. The code has been revised and reaffirmed many times. The four principal elements contained within the ICN code involve standards related to nurses and people, practice, the profession, and coworkers. These elements form a framework to guide nursing conduct and are elaborated within the code with practice applications for practitioners and managers, educators and researchers, and national nurses' associations. The *ICN Code of Ethics for Nurses* is available online at www.icn.ch/icncode.pdf.

■ A Common Theme of ANA and ICN Codes

A theme common to the codes of the ANA (2001) and ICN (2006) is a focus on the importance of nurses delivering compassionate patient care aimed at alleviating suffering. This emphasis is threaded throughout the codes but begins with the patient being the central focus of a nurse's work. Nurses are to support patients in self-determination and are to protect the moral environment in which patients receive care. The interests of various nursing associations and healthcare institutions must not be placed above those of patients. Although opportunities in the healthcare environment to exhibit compassion are not unique to nurses, nurses must always uphold the moral agreement that they make with communities when they join the nursing profession. Nursing care includes the important responsibilities of promoting health and preventing illness, but the heart of nursing care has always involved caring for patients who are experiencing varying degrees of physical, psychologic, and spiritual suffering.

> **A theme common to the codes of the ANA (2001) and ICN (2006) is a focus on the importance of nurses delivering compassionate patient care aimed at alleviating suffering.**

In the *Code of Ethics for Nurses with Interpretative Statements*, the ANA (2001) emphasizes the importance of moral respect for all human beings, including nurses' respect for themselves. Self-respect also can be thought of as personal regard. Personal regard involves nurses extending attention and care to their own requisite needs. Nurses who do not regard themselves as worthy of care usually cannot fully care for others.

Ethical Analysis and Decision Making in Nursing

Ethical issues and dilemmas are ever present in healthcare settings. Many times, ethical issues are so prevalent in practice that nurses do not even realize that they are making minute-by-minute ethical decisions (Chambliss, 1996; Kelly, 2000). Whether or not they are cognizant of the ethical matters at the time that the decisions are made, nurses use their critical thinking skills to respond to many of these everyday decisions. Personal values, professional values and competencies, ethical principles, and ethical theories and approaches are variables that must be considered when an ethical decision is made. Answers to the questions "What is the right thing to do for my patient?" and "What sort of nurse do I want to be?" are important to professional nursing practice.

> **KEY COMPETENCY 4-2**
>
> Examples of Applicable *Nurse of the Future: Nursing Core Competencies*
>
> Professionalism:
>
> Skills (S7a) Incorporates American Nurses Association's *Code of Ethics* into daily practice; (S7f) Applies a professional nursing code of ethics and professional guidelines to clinical practice
>
> Attitudes/Behaviors (A7b) Values acting in accordance with codes of ethics and accepted standards of practice
>
> *Source:* Massachusetts Department of Higher Education (2010, p. 14).

■ Ethical Dilemmas and Conflicts

An **ethical dilemma** is a situation in which an individual is compelled to make a choice between two actions that will affect the well-being of a sentient being and both actions can be reasonably justified as being good, neither action is readily justifiable as good, or the goodness of the actions is uncertain. One action must be chosen, thereby generating a quandary for the person or group who must make the choice.

> **Many times, ethical issues are so prevalent in practice that nurses do not even realize that they are making minute-by-minute ethical decisions.**

In addition to general, situational ethical dilemmas, dilemmas can arise from conflicts between nurses, other healthcare professionals, the healthcare organization, and the patient and family. A dilemma might involve nurses making a choice between staying to work an extra shift during a situation of inadequate staffing and going home to rest after a very tiring 8 hours of work. Nurses in this situation might believe that patients will not receive safe or good care if they do not stay to work the extra shift, but these nurses also might not provide safe care if they stay at the hospital because of already being tired from a particularly hard day of work.

■ Moral Suffering

Many times nurses experience disquieting feelings of anguish or uneasiness consistent with what might be called moral suffering. **Moral suffering** can be experienced when nurses attempt to sort out their emotions when they find themselves in situations that are morally unsatisfactory or when forces beyond their control prevent them from influencing or changing these perceived unsatisfactory moral situations. Suffering can occur because nurses believe that situations must be changed to bring well-being to themselves and others or to alleviate the suffering of themselves and others.

Moral suffering can arise, for example, from disagreements with institutional policy, such as a mandatory overtime or on-call policy that nurses believe does not allow adequate time for their psychological well-being. Nurses also might disagree with physicians' orders that the nurses believe are not in patients' best interest, or they might disagree with the way a family treats a patient or makes patient care decisions. These are but a few examples of the many types of encounters that nurses can have with moral suffering.

Another important, but often unacknowledged, source of moral suffering involves nurses freely choosing to act in ways that they, themselves, know is not morally commendable. A difficult situation that may cause moral suffering for a nurse would be covering up a patient care error made by a valued nurse best friend. On the other hand, nurses might experience moral suffering when they act courageously by doing what they believe is morally right despite anticipated disturbing consequences. Sometimes, doing the right thing or acting as a virtuous person would act is difficult.

Some people view suffering as something to accept and to transform, if possible. Others react to situations with fear, bitterness, and anxiety. It is important to remember that wisdom and inner strength are often most increased during times of greatest difficulty.

www CRITICAL THINKING QUESTIONS ✳

Has there ever been a time when you have experienced the dilemma of having to make a choice that you know will affect the well-being of another individual? Have you ever experienced moral suffering? ✳

■ Using a Team Approach

When trying to navigate ethically laden situations, patients and families can experience extreme anguish and suffering. Physicians, nurses, and other healthcare providers might explain to a patient or family that to continue the patient's treatment would be nonbeneficial and futile while patients or family members insist on continued treatment. When patients are weakened by disease and illness and families are reacting to the pain and suffering of their loved one, decisions regarding treatment can become sensitive and challenging for everyone concerned. Members of the healthcare team might question the decision-making capacity of the patient or family. The patient's or family's decision might conflict with the physician's or healthcare team's opinions regarding treatment. Nurses who care for patients and interact with families sometimes find themselves caught in the middle of these conflicts.

It is important to note that most problematic ethical decisions in health care are not made unilaterally—not by physicians, nurses, or any other single person. Still, nurses are an integral part of the larger team of decision makers. Although nurses often make ethical decisions independently, many ethical dilemmas require nurses to participate interdependently with others in decision making. In analyzing healthcare ethics and decision making, nurses participate in extensive dialogue with others through committees, clinical team conferences, and other channels. Nurses are part of the larger team approach to ethical analysis. Commonly, the team is called an ethics consultation team or ethics committee.

Members of the team usually are physicians, nurses who represent their patients, an on-staff chaplain, nurses who regularly participate on the consultative team, a social worker, administrative personnel, possibly a legal representative, a representative for the patient in question or surrogate decision maker, and others drafted by the team. The number and membership of the ethics team vary among organizations and specific cases. When ethical disputes arise among any members of a patient's healthcare team, including disputes with patients and families, nurses often are the ones who seek an ethics consultation. It is within the right and duty of nurses to seek help and advice from the team if they encounter moral dilemmas or experience moral suffering.

In healthcare settings, moral reasoning to resolve an ethical dilemma is often a case-based, or bottom-up, inductive, casuistry approach. This approach begins with relevant facts about a particular case and moves toward a resolution through a structured analysis. A practical case-based ethical analysis approach that is used commonly by nurses and other healthcare professionals is the Four Topics Method or, often called in jargon, the 4-Box Approach (Table 4-1) (Jonsen, Siegler, & Winslade, 2006, p. 11). The Four Topics Method, developed by Albert Jonsen, Mark Siegler, and William Winslade, was published first in 1982 in their book *Clinical Ethics: A Practical Approach to Ethical Decisions in Clinical Medicine*, which is in its sixth edition.

This case-based approach facilitates critical thinking about the issues and problems of a particular situation and facilitates construction of the case through information gathering in a structured format. Each problematic ethical case is analyzed according to four topics: medical

KEY COMPETENCY 4-3

Examples of Applicable *Nurse of the Future: Nursing Core Competencies*

Professionalism:

Skills (S7e) Recognizes moral distress and seeks resources for resolution

Source: Massachusetts Department of Higher Education (2010, p. 14).

> **In healthcare settings, moral reasoning to resolve an ethical dilemma is often a case-based, or bottom-up, inductive, casuistry approach.**

TABLE 4-1 Four Topics Method for Analysis in Clinical Ethics Cases

Medical Indications

The Principles of Beneficence and Nonmaleficence

1. What is the patient's medical problem? history? diagnosis? prognosis?
2. Is the problem acute? chronic? critical? emergent? reversible?
3. What are the goals of treatment?
4. What are the probabilities of success?
5. What are the plans in case of therapeutic failure?
6. In sum, how can this patient be benefited by medical and nursing care, and how can harm be avoided?

Quality of Life

The Principles of Beneficence and Nonmaleficence and Respect for Autonomy

1. What are the prospects, with or without treatment, for a return to normal life?
2. What physical, mental, and social deficits is the patient likely to experience if treatment succeeds?
3. Are there biases that might prejudice the provider's evaluation of the patient's quality of life?
4. Is the patient's present or future condition such that his or her continued life might be judged undesirable?
5. Is there any plan and rationale to forgo treatment?
6. Are there plans for comfort and palliative care?

Patient Preferences

The Principle of Respect for Autonomy

1. Is the patient mentally capable and legally competent? Is there evidence of incapacity?
2. If competent, what is the patient stating about preferences for treatment?
3. Has the patient been informed of benefits and risks, understood this information, and given consent?
4. If incapacitated, who is the appropriate surrogate? Is the surrogate using appropriate standards for decision making?
5. Has the patient expressed prior preferences, e.g., advance directives?
6. Is the patient unwilling or unable to cooperate with medical treatment? If so, why?
7. In sum, is the patient's right to choose being respected to the extent possible in ethics and law?

Contextual Features

The Principles of Loyalty and Fairness

1. Are there family issues that might influence treatment decisions?
2. Are there provider (physicians and nurses) issues that might influence treatment decisions?
3. Are there financial and economic factors?
4. Are there religious and cultural factors?
5. Are there limits on confidentiality?
6. Are there problems of allocations of resources?
7. How does the law affect treatment decisions?
8. Is clinical research or teaching involved?
9. Is there any conflict of interest on the part of the providers or the institution?

Source: Jonsen, A. R., Siegler, M., & Winslade, W. J. (2006). *Clinical ethics: A practical approach to ethical decisions in clinical medicine* (6th ed.). New York: McGraw-Hill. Reprinted with permission of The McGraw-Hill Companies.

indications, patient preferences, quality of life, and contextual features (Jonsen et al., 2006). Nurses and other healthcare professionals on the team gather information in an attempt to answer the questions in each of the four boxes.

The Four Topics Method promotes a dialogue among the patient, family, and members of the healthcare ethics team. Each patient's case is unique and should be considered as such, but the subject matter concerning the dilemma involves common threads among cases, such as withdrawing or withholding treatment and right to life. Applicability of the four fundamental bioethical principles—autonomy, beneficence, nonmaleficence, and justice—is considered along with data generated by using the Four Topics Method in analyzing a patient's case. In Table 4-1, each box includes principles appropriate for each of the four topics. The additional principles of fairness and loyalty are included in the contextual features section.

---

www **CASE STUDY** ■ **MS. CRANFORD**

You are a student nurse who is caring for Ms. Cranford. She is an 87-year-old mentally competent woman who has lived alone since her husband died 10 years ago. She was admitted to the hospital with chest pain, feeling faint, a pulse of 48, and a blood pressure of 98/56. The physician and nurses stabilized Ms. Cranford with medications and intravenous fluids but later informed Ms. Cranford and her only son that she would need a heart pacemaker to regulate her heartbeat. After the physician explained the procedure and risks involved, Ms. Cranford pondered the situation for a long while before discussing it with her son and the physician. Her medical history includes long-term adult-onset diabetes, chronic renal failure, and arterial insufficiency. She feels very tired. She decides that she does not want a pacemaker. Once Ms. Cranford tells her son her wishes, he is quite upset, and thus, he meets with the physician to discuss the options. The physician and Ms. Cranford's son revisited this issue with her in an attempt to persuade her to change her mind, but she continues to refuse the recommended treatment. She and her son argue. The physician tries to explain to Ms. Cranford that the pacemaker is for her benefit, in her "best interest," and involves very minimal risks to her.

She feels as if they are "ganging up" on her. Once the registered nurse becomes aware of the problem, you and the nurse visit with Ms. Cranford and her son to assess and evaluate the ethical issues involved with her case.

Case Study Questions

Imagine that you are a nurse on the ethics committee consulted about Ms. Cranford's case. Answer the following questions:

1. What are the central ethical issues and questions in this case?

2. Which principles are in conflict in this case?

3. What did the physician mean by "best interest" for Ms. Cranford?

4. Use the Four Topics Method to discuss issues, to identify additional information that might be needed, and to analyze this case. What are your recommendations on behalf of the ethics committee?

5. What is the role of the nurses caring for Ms. Cranford in resolving this situation with the ethics team, her other healthcare providers, Ms. Cranford, and her son? ■

Intense emotional conflicts between healthcare professionals and the patient and family can occur and hurt feelings can result. Nurses need to be sensitive and open to the needs of patients and families, particularly during these times. As information is passed back and forth among healthcare professionals and patients and families, an attitude of respect is indispensable in keeping the lines of communication open. Nurses play an essential role in the decision-making process in bioethical cases because of their traditional roles as patient advocate, caregiver, and educator. Nurses must attempt to maximize the values and needs of patients and families. A key component in preserving patient autonomy, respect, and dignity is for the nurse to have all of the essential information necessary for wise and skillful decisions.

Conclusion

With any type of ethical matters in health care, a nurse must ask "What is good in terms of how one wants to be?" and "What is good in terms of what one ought to do?" Becoming ethically savvy does not just happen in nursing. Nurses must consciously cultivate ethical habits and use theoretical knowledge about how to navigate ethical dilemmas. Moral suffering cannot be eliminated from nursing practice; however, the cultivation of wisdom and skill in decision making can help to alleviate some of its effects.

References

American Nurses Association. (2001). *Code of ethics for nurses with interpretive statements.* Washington, DC: Author.

Angeles, P. A. (1992). *The Harper Collins dictionary of philosophy* (2nd ed.). New York, NY: Harper Perennial.

Beauchamp, T. L., & Childress, J. F. (1979). *Principles of biomedical ethics.* New York, NY: Oxford University Press.

Beauchamp, T. L., & Childress, J. F. (2001). *Principles of biomedical ethics* (5th ed.). New York, NY: Oxford University Press.

Beauchamp, T. L., & Childress, J. F. (2009). *Principles of biomedical ethics* (6th ed.). New York, NY: Oxford University Press.

Bentham, J. (1988). *The principles of morals and legislation.* Loughton, Essex, England: Prometheus. (Original work published 1789).

Broadie, S. (2002). Commentary. In C. Rowe (Trans.), *Aristotle: Nicomachean ethics: Translation, introduction, and commentary.* New York, NY: Oxford University Press.

Callahan, D. (1995). Bioethics. In W. T. Reich (Ed.), *Encyclopedia of bioethics: Revised edition* (Vol. 1, pp. 247–256). New York, NY: Simon & Schuster Macmillan.

Chambliss, D. F. (1996). *Beyond caring: Hospitals, nurses, and the social organization of ethics.* Chicago, IL: University of Chicago Press.

Daly, B. J. (2002). Moving forward: A new code of ethics. *Nursing Outlook, 50,* 70–99.

Dossey, B. M. (2000). *Florence Nightingale: Mystic, visionary, healer.* Springhouse, PA: Springhouse.

Fowler, M. D., & Benner, P. (2001). Implementing a new code of ethics for nurses: An interview with Marsha Fowler. *American Journal of Critical Care, 10*(6), 434–437.

Fry, S., & Veatch, R. M. (2000). *Case studies in nursing ethics* (2nd ed.). Sudbury, MA: Jones and Bartlett.

Gilligan, C. (1993). *In a different voice: Psychological theory and women's development.* Cambridge, MA: Harvard University Press.

Grimshaw, J. (1993). The idea of a female ethic. In P. Singer (Ed.), *A companion to ethics* (pp. 491–499). Oxford, England: Blackwell.

International Council of Nurses. (2006). *The ICN code of ethics for nurses.* Geneva, Switzerland: Author. Retrieved from http://www.icn.ch/icncode.pdf

Johnstone, M. J. (1999). *Bioethics: A nursing perspective* (3rd ed.). Sydney, Australia: Harcourt Saunders.

Jonsen, A. (1998). *The birth of bioethics.* New York, NY: Oxford University Press.

Jonsen, A. R., Siegler, M., & Winslade, W. J. (2006). *Clinical ethics: A practical approach to ethical decisions in clinical medicine* (6th ed.). New York, NY: McGraw-Hill.

Kant, I. (2003). *Groundwork of the metaphysics of morals.* New York, NY: Oxford University Press. (Original work published 1785).

Kelly, C. (2000). *Nurses' moral practice: Investing and discounting self.* Indianapolis, IN: Sigma Theta Tau International.

Kuhse, H., & Singer, P. (1998). What is bioethics? A historical introduction. In H. Kuhse & P. Singer (Eds.), *A companion to bioethics* (pp. 3–11). Oxford, England: Blackwell.

Mappes, T. A., & DeGrazia, D. (2001). *Biomedical ethics* (5th ed.). Boston, MA: McGraw-Hill.

Massachusetts Department of Higher Education. (2010). *Nurse of the future: Nursing core competencies.* Retrieved from http://www.mass.edu/currentinit/documents/NursingCoreCompetencies.pdf

Mill, J. S. (2002). *Utilitarianism* (G. Sher, Trans.). Indianapolis, IN: Hackett Publishing. (Original work published 1863).

Munson, R. (2004). *Intervention and reflection: Basic issues in medical ethics* (7th ed.). Victoria, Australia: Thomson Wadsworth.

Pieper, J. (1966). *The four cardinal virtues.* Notre Dame, IN: University of Notre Dame Press.

Pullman, D. (1999). The ethics of autonomy and dignity in long-term care. *Canadian Journal on Aging, 18*(1), 26–46.

Thomas, L. (1993). Morality and psychological development. In P. Singer (Ed.), *A companion to ethics* (pp. 464–475). Oxford, England: Blackwell.

Social Context of Professional Nursing

5

Rowena W. Elliott and Mary W. Stewart

When you hear the word *nurse*, what images, thoughts, perceptions, and assumptions come to mind? Ask yourself, "Why did I have those perceptions and assumptions about nurses?" The answer to your question reveals much about the social context of nursing or how society views nurses and the nursing profession. For many, the image that first comes into view is one of a white female who is dressed in a meticulously ironed white uniform with white hose, white shoes, and wearing a stiff white cap. For those of us in nursing, we recognize that this traditional American view of nursing is rarely seen in the real world of professional nursing. So, how do we communicate the true image of nursing in the 21st century?

In this chapter, we explore the social context of professional nursing and identify major influences that affect nursing in today's society. This quest for a deeper understanding of nursing challenges us to identify our individual responsibilities in educating our patients and the public about professional nursing. The end result is not necessarily an immediate change in the picture that comes to mind when one says "nursing." However, we might begin to see nursing and those of us committed to nursing in new, more accurate ways.

Key Terms and Concepts

- » **Stereotypes**
- » Multiculturalism
- » Access to care
- » Capitalistic society
- » Nurse-managed centers
- » Incivility
- » Violence
- » Mental health
- » Global aging
- » Nursing shortage
- » Consumerism
- » Complementary and alternative medicine
- » Disaster preparedness

Learning Objectives

After completing this chapter, the student should be able to:

1. Describe the social context of professional nursing.

2. Identify factors that influence the public's image of professional nursing.

3. List ways that nurses can promote an accurate image of professional nursing in the media.

4. Discuss the gender gap in nursing.

5. Recognize strategies to broaden the cultural and ethnic diversity in nursing.

6. Evaluate current barriers to health care in our society.

7. Analyze present trends in society that influence professional nursing.

8. Suggest research needs related to the future of nursing in our society.

Public Image of Nursing

The public values nursing. According to a Gallup poll in 2011, nurses received the top ranking for being the most trusted profession in 11 of the past 12 years (Jones, 2012). The only year when nurses did not rank number one was in 2001 when firefighters took the top spot after the September 11th terrorist attacks. When asked to defend this nationwide trust of nurses, people often respond with anecdotal stories of personal experiences with nurses. Popular stories include those of relatives or friends who are nurses and positive experiences with nurses in a clinical setting. The fact that nurses serve society seems to have an automatically positive impact on society's value of nursing. Although the trust is evident, there remains a gap between the public's perception of the nursing profession and the reality of nursing. For example, the general public might think that it requires only 2 years of schooling to become a registered nurse (RN), with the "training" consisting primarily of learning to administer medications, providing personal care, and sitting at the bedside. However, reality provides a stark revelation that nurses are educated at the baccalaureate, master's, and doctoral levels and work in areas of education, research, and independent clinical practice.

Nurses are aware of the gaps in society's knowledge of nursing. Hence, nurses should take the lead in making sure the public has an accurate picture of the vast knowledge and expertise that are present in the 3 million RNs in the United States (U.S. Department of Health and Human Services [USDHHS], 2010). So, where do we start? We must first begin with the realization that all nurses are not the same. As previously stated, many well-educated persons do not understand the various educational programs available to become a registered nurse. Likewise, knowledge about the differences in preparation and responsibility of licensed practical nurses (LPNs), registered nurses (RNs), and advanced practice nurses (e.g., nurse practitioners) is lacking.

> **Nurses should take the lead in making sure the public has an accurate picture of the vast knowledge and expertise that are present in the 3 million RNs in the United States.**

As you are preparing to be a professional nurse, ask yourself, "How do I clarify and communicate the significance of professional nursing?" First, become familiar with the scope of practice of professional nurses and understand the multifaceted roles for which you are being educated. Second, be able to identify the unique place that professional nurses have in the healthcare system. This comes by acquiring knowledge of the nursing profession and being aware of the roles, responsibilities, and contributions of other healthcare professionals. Most important, it is imperative you share your story of nursing. Although the public holds nurses in high regard, they know very little about what nurses actually do (Buresh & Gordon, 2000). Without articulating more clearly and loudly on our profession's behalf, we might be at a loss when trying to defend our place in the current healthcare system.

Suzanne Gordon, an award-winning journalist, has dedicated much of her career to telling the stories of nursing. Not a nurse herself, Gordon writes to empower nurses to find their voice and be heard. Gordon is committed to obtaining a first-hand account from nurses as they face the real challenges of being a nurse that include (1) inconvenient problems of improving patient safety (Gordon, Buchanan, & Bretherton, 2008), (2) challenges of standing up for themselves, their patients, and the nursing profession (Gordon, 2010), and (3) the effect of cutting healthcare costs on patient care (Gordon, 2005), to name a few. If a journalist can commit to sharing "our" stories, that should provide a spark of motivation in us to share our experiences, triumphs, and defeats.

When nurses are asked about the nurse's reluctance to promote nursing effectively, the responses are riddled with excuses such as a lack of time, resources, and support from colleagues. Professional nurses work in very demanding, stressful, and taxing jobs. Frequently, we are so consumed with the responsibilities of our work that we fail to notice what we are actually getting accomplished. Additionally, we rarely take time to become fully aware of and celebrate what our nursing colleagues are doing within the profession. Professional nursing organizations exist to communicate and support these achievements. However, only a small percentage of registered nurses are actually members of their professional nursing associations.

Better insight into professional nursing must start with nurses at all levels of practice and education. Once we have obtained the necessary insight, we can provide a clear picture of the nursing profession to society. When these two actions are taken, the public image of nursing will be directly reflective of the reality of nursing. We want to maintain the positive impression the public now holds of nursing and sustain the earned trust, but nursing and the public deserve a great deal more than that. All of us should be convinced of the expertise that professional nursing offers: mastery of complicated technologic skills; appreciation for the whole person; commitment to public health for all people; a keen knowledge of anatomy, physiology, pathophysiology, biochemistry, pharmacology, and other disciplines; the ability to think critically and connect the dots in today's ever-changing healthcare system; and proficiency in communication. The list continues.

Social change will take place one nurse at a time and one person at a time. By reflecting on the changes in racial relationships, for example, we know that transformation has not come solely because of the civil rights movement in the 1960s. Granted, that was a period of radical change to which we are all indebted. Nonetheless, real change in race relationships in our society has come from exposure and experience. Someone once said, "Ignorance is only removed by experience." Is it any different for our image as nurses?

KEY COMPETENCY 5-1

Examples of Applicable *Nurse of the Future: Nursing Core Competencies*

Professionalism:

Knowledge (K5b) Understands the culture of nursing and the healthcare system

Skills (S5b) Promotes and maintains a positive image of nursing

Source: Massachusetts Department of Higher Education (2010, p. 14).

Media's Influence

It is obvious that the media (television, radio, Internet) play a major role in how society views professional nursing. Historically, the nurse has been portrayed in the media in a variety of ways. First, the nurse appears as a young, seductive female whose principal qualification is the length of her slender legs and the amount of cleavage showing through her uniform. Needless to say, this nurse is usually depicted as one who is not educated and lacks common sense and intelligence. Another popular view of the nurse as portrayed by the media is an unattractive, overweight, and mean female. Her intelligence is not questioned, but her compassion for others is highly debatable. This nurse is shown as threatening and uncaring. Neither of these views is accurate, and probably no one would argue with this. At the same time, we continue to be perplexed when asked to define or describe the professional nurse.

In their book *From Silence to Voice: What Nurses Know and Must Communicate to the Public*, Buresh and Gordon (2006) state that "a profession's public status and credibility are enhanced by having its expertise acknowledged in the journalistic media" (p. 1). Buresh and Gordon also cite the study "Who Counts in News Coverage of Health Care," where the data show that many professional groups had a greater voice on health issues compared to nurses. Physicians were quoted the most in media, followed by government, business, education, public relations, and so forth. This is significant and shocking because nurses are the largest group of healthcare professionals, yet, we are the most silent group. As nurses, we have been complacent about refuting the negative stereotypes portrayed in the media. Furthermore, we have been lax in articulating our expertise to the media.

> **www CRITICAL THINKING QUESTION** ✳
>
> How can you, as a student nurse, tell society what professional nurses do? ✳

Buresh and Gordon (2006) describe three communication challenges faced by the nursing profession that need to be addressed:

1. Not enough nurses are willing to talk about their work.
2. When nurses and nursing organizations do talk about their work, too often they intentionally project an inaccurate picture of nursing by using a "virtue" instead of a "knowledge" script.
3. When nursing groups give voice to nursing, they sometimes bypass, downplay, or even devalue the basic nursing work that occurs in direct care of the sick while elevating an image of "elite" nurses in advanced practice, administration, and academia. (p. 4)

Nurses should face the **stereotypes** present in our society and erase the lines that define us. To do this, we must first recognize our value to society and ourselves. When introducing ourselves in the professional role, we should do so with confidence and clarity. For example, we can say, "Good morning, Mr. Smith. I'm Susan Jones, your registered nurse." This introduction should be accompanied by a kind and self-assured handshake. Such day-to-day engagement is important. We must tell the world what we do.

In *From Silence to Voice*, the authors identify the following actions to promote the real image of nursing:

- Educate the public in daily life.
- Describe the nurse's work.
- Make known the agency—independent thinker—of the RN.
- Deal with the fear of angering the physician.
- Accept thanks from others.
- Be ready to take advantage of openings to promote nursing.
- Respond to queries with real-life stories from nursing.
- Tell the details.
- Avoid using nursing jargon.
- Be prepared ahead of time to tell your story.
- Do not suppress your enthusiasm.
- Reflect the nurse's clinical judgment and competency.
- Connect your work to pressing contemporary issues.
- Respect patient confidentiality.
- Deal with and confront the fear of failure.

In an effort to address the challenges faced by nursing, Buresh and Gordon (2006) provide a history and understanding of modern media and provide examples of how to interconnect with them. Knowing how news media work, how to write a letter to the editor, present oneself on television or radio, and converse with community groups are among the guidelines provided. Being proactive is essential and it comes at a time when healthcare costs and cuts demand that only the fundamental players are left standing. Society needs to know that nurses are definitely fundamental players.

Sigma Theta Tau International commissioned the 1997 Woodhull Study on Nursing and the Media, which reported the lack of representation that nurses have in the media (Sigma Theta Tau International, 1998). In approximately 20,000 articles from 16 major news publications, nurses were cited only 3% of the time. Among the healthcare industry publications, only 1% of the references were nurses. Although nurses are highly relevant participants in patients' stories, they were neglected in almost every case. Key study recommendations from the Woodhull Study include the following:

- Nurses and media should be proactive in establishing ongoing dialogue.
- If the aim is to provide comprehensive coverage of health care, the media should include information by and about nurses.
- Training should be provided to nurses on how to speak about business, management, and policy issues.
- *Health care* needs to be clearly identified as the umbrella term for specific disciplines, such as medicine and nursing.

- Nurses with doctoral degrees should be identified correctly as doctors, and those with medical doctorate (MD) degrees should be identified as physicians.
- Language needs to reflect the diverse options for health care by avoiding phrases such as, "Consult your doctor." Rather, media need to state, "Consult your primary healthcare provider."

In recent years, we have seen more accurate portrayals of nurses supported in the media. Instead of portraying sexual prowess or disrespect and anger, nurses have been presented as intelligent, competent, and essential to patient care. Johnson & Johnson continues the Campaign of Nursing's Future to raise public awareness of professional nursing. This positive promotion has supported student and faculty recruitment into the profession. Johnson & Johnson has taken additional steps to recognize the courageous efforts of many nurses, including those who were intensely engaged in responding during national crises such as Hurricane Katrina. Nurses must continually evaluate the portrayal of nurses in the media. After all, if the image is inaccurate, we have a responsibility to correct it.

The Gender Gap

■ Women in Nursing and the Socialization of That Tradition

In Western culture, women have traditionally been socialized as the more passive of the sexes—to avoid conflict and yield to authority. The implications of this conventional thought are still evident in nursing practice today. Many nurses lack confidence in dealing with conflict and communicating with those in authority. For some, it is a matter of short supply of energy and too many other commitments. Others perceive assertiveness as clashing with people's expectations. We should ask ourselves, "Isn't the reward of knowing we do a good job enough?"

For female nurses who assume multiple personal and professional roles, career is often not at the top of our priorities. This can be attributed to the fact that the role of women in past society was primarily geared toward family responsibility, not career. Many women who chose nursing did so without the expectation of a long-term commitment to the profession. Rather, nursing was a "good job" when and if a woman needed to work. This centeredness on service continues in nursing today, albeit with less intensity than in the past.

The women's movement in the 1960s empowered intelligent career-seeking women to professions other than the traditional ones of teaching and nursing. After some years of competing for students, nursing saw a return of interest in the 1980s and 1990s. At this point, more women chose nursing as a career because nursing provided a natural complement to their gifts and not because it was one of only a few options available to them (Chitty & Campbell, 2001). As the message of varied opportunities for women and men in nursing is shared, the social status of all nurses can be elevated.

Another facet of women in nursing is the changing demographic of women entering the nursing profession. In the United States, a larger number of women from underrepresented groups are becoming nurses. According to U.S. Department of Health and Human Services (2010), approximately 170,235 registered nurses living in the United States obtained their initial nursing education in another country or U.S. territory. There was an increase from 3.7% in 2004 to 5.6% in 2008. About 50% of the internationally educated RNs living in the United States in 2008 were from the Philippines, 11.5% were from Canada, and 9.3% were from India.

Whether the swell is the result of an influx of minority nurses from other countries or increased recruiting efforts aimed at underrepresented groups, this shift has a direct impact on culture, values, and beliefs when educating and working with individuals from different cultures. It is up to us as nurses to be culturally aware and sensitive to differences while fostering a productive and professional working environment.

■ Men in Nursing

At the start of the new millennium, men represented approximately 5.4% of the registered nurse population in the United States (Trossman, 2003). By 2004, men comprised 5.8% of the RN population, and then 6.6% in 2008 (USDHHS, 2010). This steady increase can be attributed to recruitment campaigns focused on attracting men into nursing. For example, the Oregon Center for Nursing (2003) created a poster of men in nursing with the slogan "Are you man enough to be a nurse?" The Mississippi Hospital Association published an all-male calendar with monthly features of men in nursing, ranging from men who were nursing students to practicing professionals in a variety of roles. The calendar was used as a recruiting tool to help encourage men, young and old, to consider the extensive opportunities in nursing. It was distributed to nursing programs as part of a health careers recruitment information kit (Health Careers Center, 2012). These strategies help diminish the stigma associated with men in nursing.

The American Nurses Association (ANA) inducted the first man into its Hall of Fame in 2004 (American Nurses Association [ANA], 2007). Dr. Luther Christman was recognized for his 65-year career and contributions to the profession, including the founding of the American Assembly for Men in Nursing. In 2007, the ANA established the Luther Christman Award to recognize the contributions of men in nursing. Current literature also helps to keep the discussion of men in nursing at the forefront. In 2006, *Men in Nursing* journal was launched as the first professional journal dedicated to addressing the issues and topics facing the growing number of men who work in the nursing field.

Although a seemingly recent topic, men have served in nursing roles throughout history. In the 13th century, men played a vital role in providing nursing care to vulnerable individuals. John Ciudad (1495–1550) opened a hospital in Grenada, Spain, so that he (along with friends) could provide care to the mentally ill, homeless, and abandoned children (Blais, Hayes, Kozier, & Erb, 2001). Saint Camillus de Lellis (1550–1614) was the founder of the Nursing Order of Ministers of the sick. Men in this order were charged with providing care to alcoholics and those affected by the plague (Blais et al., 2001). In the United States, in the 1700s James Derham was an African American man who worked as a nurse in New Orleans and was subsequently able to buy his freedom and become the first African American physician in the United States.

However, despite her many contributions to the nursing profession, Florence Nightingale did not encourage the participation of men in nursing. She believed that traits such as nurturance, gentleness, empathy, and compassion were needed to provide care and that these traits existed primarily in women. Nightingale opposed men being nurses and stated that their "hard and horny" hands were not fit to "touch, bathe, and dress wounded limbs, however gentle their hearts may be" (Chung, 2001). There still remain some unsubstantiated stereotypes of men who pursue a career in nursing.

Even with negative societal perceptions and stereotypes, men are now more open to pursuing nursing as a career choice (Berlin, Stennett, & Bednash, 2004). In the fall of 2003, the percentage of men enrolled in undergraduate schools of nursing was 8.4%. In 2011, the percentage increased to 15% largely as a result of diminishing misconceptions and increased recruiting efforts (National League for Nursing, 2012). Men prefer distinct practice areas, including high-technology, fast-paced, and intense environments. Emergency departments, intensive care units, operating rooms, and nurse anesthesiology are examples of areas to which men are often attracted (American Society of Registered Nurses, 2008; Gibbs & Waugaman, 2004). Some speculate that men make these choices to avoid potential role strain if they were to choose other areas, such as obstetrics and pediatrics (Chitty & Campbell, 2001), and because they prefer areas that require more technical expertise (American Society of Registered Nurses, 2008).

There is some debate that men in nursing have an advantage over their female peers. It is not unusual for patients to assume that a male nurse is a physician or a medical student. On the other hand, men in nursing have been mistaken for orderlies. However, the percentage of men in leadership roles in nursing is much higher than the percentage of men in nursing overall. This is partly because male nurses are more oriented and motivated to upgrade their professional status (American Society of Registered Nurses, 2008). As a result, women in nursing are challenged to learn how to promote themselves within the profession.

What issues and challenges do men face in nursing? According to research conducted by Armstrong (2002) and Keogh and O'Lynn (2007), male nurses are unfairly stereotyped in the profession as homosexuals, low achievers, and feminine. These false assumptions and perceptions deter other men from entering the profession, create gender-based barriers in nursing schools, and decrease retention rates of male nurses once they are licensed.

Also, because most nursing faculty are female, most nursing textbooks are written by females, most leaders in nursing are female, men might have to learn new ways of thinking and understanding to find a comfortable place of belonging in the nursing profession. For example, a male nursing student was having difficulty answering questions on a nursing examination. When the student shared a sample question with his wife (who was not a nurse), she answered the question correctly (Brady & Sherrod, 2003).

As a consequence of gender bias, some patients might refuse or feel reluctant to allow men in the nursing role to care for them (American Society of Registered Nurses, 2008; Cardillo, 2001). During labor and delivery, patients and their partners might request a female nurse to be at the bedside. Overall, the presence of a male nurse alone in the room with a patient is out of the ordinary. On the other hand, male nurses are assumed to be physically stronger and willing to do the heavier tasks of nursing care, such as lifting and moving patients (Cardillo, 2001). Still, many men and women are learning to appreciate and enjoy the emerging culture in the profession (Meyers, 2003). The old biases continue to disappear as patients and providers become more educated about the need for gender diversity in nursing.

> **www | CRITICAL THINKING QUESTIONS** ✳
>
> What advantages do women have in nursing? What advantages do men have in the profession? What are the risks of being gender exclusive? ✳

Cultural and Ethnic Diversity

In addition to gender diversity, we are also privileged as a profession to experience a diversity of race, age, and socioeconomic backgrounds. However, this multiculturalism can lead to people feeling threatened, especially if the culture within the profession does not encourage mutual respect and acceptance (Waters, 2004).

Even though most registered nurses are Caucasian women, more minorities are being represented in schools of nursing. The American Association of Colleges of Nursing reported that in the fall of 2003 12.2% of students enrolled in baccalaureate programs were African American, which represented a 0.9% increase from earlier and the largest minority population in nursing. American Indians or Alaska Natives at 0.6% represent the lowest minority population, and their numbers revealed no change in the same time frame. The Hispanic nursing population grew slightly from 5.1% to 5.4% (Berlin, Stennett, & Bednesh, 2003, 2004).

In 2011, 12% of students enrolled in a baccalaureate program were African American, followed by 8% Asians or Pacific Islanders, 1% American Indians or Alaska Natives, 6%, Hispanics, and 6% identified as Other. In associate degree nursing programs, 9% were African American, 4% Asian or Pacific Islander, 1% American Indian or Alaska Native, 6% Hispanic, and 7% identified as Other. Of the remaining diploma programs in the United States, 30% of students were African American, 5% Asian or Pacific Islander, 1% American Indian or Alaska Native, 10% Hispanic, and 27% identified as Other (National League for Nursing, 2012).

As the general population of healthcare consumers becomes increasingly diverse, there is a greater need for culturally competent care (Jacob & Carnegie, 2002). To provide such nursing care, we must strive for a nursing population that more accurately represents the communities we serve. Partnerships among healthcare agencies and other community agencies are vital to increased understanding of various cultures.

The National Advisory Council on Nurse Education and Practice (NACNEP) was established to advise the secretary of the U.S. Department of Health and Human Services and Congress on policy issues related to Title VIII programs administered by the Health Resources and Services Administration. NACNEP identified the need to increase racial and ethnic diversity of the RN workforce as an issue. In its third report, NACNEP recommended that the country "expand the resources available to develop models that will effectively recruit and graduate sufficient numbers of racial/ethnic students to reflect the nation's diverse population" (National Advisory Council on Nurse Education and Practice [NACNEP], 2003). More details about the council's advocacy of a national action agenda to address nursing workforce diversity are available at www.diversitynursing.com.

The Joint Commission and the National Committee for Quality Assurance identify the need for healthcare professionals to recognize and respect cultural differences, including dialects, regional differences, and slang (Levine, 2012). In an effort to respond to this national message, many hospitals and healthcare agencies have initiated the use of interactive patient-engagement technology as part of their education programs. These services are provided in several languages, including Russian, Spanish, and Mandarin. Nurses know that illness and associated stress, pain, and fear can hinder patients' comprehension when learning about their condition and treatment plan. Language barriers compound the problem, resulting in major obstacles to learning and subsequent issues with adhering to the treatment plan. As nursing focuses more on cultural behaviors, norms, and practices, healthcare outcomes can move in a positive direction (Levine, 2012).

Dr. Madeleine Leininger, nurse theorist and anthropologist, began the field of transcultural nursing. In her work, Dr. Leininger has advanced nursing's thinking to include individuals from all cultures and to understand the significance of cultural context (Leininger, 1991). Being culturally competent, that is, having the ability to interact appropriately with others through cultural understanding, is an expectation for people entering the nursing profession (Grant & Letzring, 2003). Nurses should always keep in mind that there is a difference between *learning of* another culture and *learning from* another culture.

■ Efforts to Recruit and Retain Minorities in Nursing

In a recent literature review of ethnic diversity in the nurse workforce, Otto and Gurney (2006) explore two aspects: academic and career factors that influence diversity; and recruitment, retention, and other strategies to diversify the workforce. Only a small amount of scholarly research investigates ethnic diversity in nursing. However, some progress is being made. In a 2000 national survey, New York State reported a minority RN population similar to the overall minority population in the state. Authors also report that in one study, 56% of hospital units had a nursing team that represented at least three different ethnic groups (Otto & Gurney, 2006).

Kavanagh (2001) indicates that failure to recognize the issue of ethnic diversity ignores health issues and potential resources. Historically, ethnic minorities have experienced disparities and lack of equal opportunities for education, provision of health care, and access to health care. Jacob and Carnegie (2002) suggest the following strategies to promote minorities in the nursing workforce:

- Raise the awareness level of diversity issues through educational offerings in the workplace and through organizational meetings.
- Seek experts on cross-cultural nursing issues from reputable sources, such as the Transcultural Nursing Society and professional nursing organizations that represent various minority populations.
- Use mentoring programs where people are matched based on their cultural backgrounds.
- Use technology and media to connect with people of different cultures.

In 2012, *Minority Nurse Magazine* recognized efforts to recruit and retain minorities by developing the TAKE PRIDE Campaign. The purpose of this campaign is to recognize and reward healthcare facilities and nursing schools for their commitment to diversity. The campaign recognizes those entities and individuals who take the following steps toward diversity:

- Faculty and staff recruitment and retention efforts aimed at underrepresented groups
- Collaborative hiring practices

KEY COMPETENCY 5-2

Examples of Applicable *Nurse of the Future: Nursing Core Competencies*

Patient-Centered Care:

Knowledge (K4) Describes how diverse cultural, ethnic, spiritual and socioeconomic backgrounds function as sources of patient, family, and community values

Skills (S4b) Implements nursing care to meet holistic needs of patient on socioeconomic, cultural, ethnic, and spiritual values and beliefs influencing health care and nursing practice

Attitudes/Behaviors (A4b) Recognizes impact of personal attitudes, values, and beliefs regarding delivery of care to diverse clients

Source: Massachusetts Department of Higher Education (2010, p. 10).

- Diversity initiative and accessible organizations on site
- Cultural competency training and resources (diverse foods, translators)
- Partnerships with other diversity organizations

An additional strategy aimed at recruitment and retention is an increase in scholarly nursing research to demonstrate the value of a diverse workforce (Otto & Gurney, 2006). Analysis of recruitment and retention interventions is also necessary. Finally, professional nurses must be aware of the legislative process and actively engage in the political arena to influence policy and legislation, ensuring diversity in nursing (Otto & Gurney, 2006). In 2011, the U.S. Department of Health and Human Services provided $3.6 million for 11 awards to fund the Nursing Workforce Diversity Award. These awards fund nursing education for individuals from disadvantaged backgrounds, including racial and ethnic minority populations (USDHHS, 2010). For this type of funding to continue, nurses need to have an active voice in the legislative process and communicate the need for such programs.

Access to Health Care

Many Americans have health insurance coverage and access to some of the best healthcare professionals in the nation. However, a large number of individuals experience disparities in our healthcare system. These disparities, or unfair differences in access, can result in poor quality and quantity of health care. According to the Agency for Healthcare Research and Quality (AHRQ, 2010), individuals who are at greatest risk for experiencing healthcare disparities are racial and ethnic minorities and those with a low socioeconomic status. Lack of health insurance was the most significant contributing factor to a decrease in disease prevention (cancer screenings, dental care, vaccinations, etc.). Although lack of health insurance has a major effect on access to health care, other factors, such as continuity of care, economic barriers, geographic barriers, and sociocultural barriers, have a detrimental effect on the health and quality of life of individuals and are discussed in the following subsections.

■ Continuity of Care

Individuals who have a provider or facility where they receive routine care are more likely to receive preventive health care (AHRQ, 2010). These individuals usually have better health outcomes and experience reduced disparities. In 2008, the percentage of people with a specific source of ongoing care was significantly lower for poor people than for high-income people (77.5% compared with 92.1%). The AHRQ also notes that having a routine provider of care correlates with a greater trust in the provider and increased likelihood that the person coordinates care with the provider. In this regard, one role and responsibility of the nurse is to educate the community and patients on the importance of continuity of care with a routine healthcare provider and/or facility.

■ Economic Barriers

Undoubtedly, poverty poses the greatest risk to health care. The United States has a long-standing reputation for providing the highest quality health care to persons in the highest socioeconomic strata. Likewise, the lowest quality health care is provided to those at the other end of the

www **CRITICAL THINKING QUESTION** ✳

Who is entitled to health care? ✳

socioeconomic continuum (Jacob & Carnegie, 2002). As the largest segment of the healthcare industry, registered nurses can have a positive impact on the change required in this established system. Recognizing the stronghold that poverty currently has on the health care of citizens is a beginning to the much needed work in the fight for equality.

Although stereotypes communicate that poverty is limited to certain groups, we understand that poverty affects people of all cultures and ethnicities. We must recognize the impact that poverty has on healthcare practices. "Universally, the greatest threat to positive health status is poverty" (Kavanagh, 2001, p. 315). Our most vulnerable could be saved if poverty was eradicated. There would be no more homeless people, no more uninsured, and no more choices between food and medicine. Until that time, nursing continues to face the challenge of meeting the needs of all people. This is especially difficult as private insurance companies, Medicare, and Medicaid cut spending. Fewer and fewer healthcare providers accept government funds as payment. Individuals are being turned away if they do not have private insurance or cash. This results in a domino effect on emergency departments and hospitals that spend millions of dollars to cover the expenses of indigent patients.

■ Geographic Barriers

Those living in rural areas have unique concerns regarding **access to care**. As many rural hospitals close as a result of lack of financing, more communities find themselves struggling to find primary care providers who will work in those areas. State and national efforts attempt to provide more service to these areas, but the demand outweighs the supply.

Urban dwellers are not immune to geographic barriers. Large cities have economically depressed sections with fewer healthcare providers than the more affluent areas. Dependency on public transportation is another factor to be managed. Finally, most rural and many urban communities do not support a full range of healthcare services in one location. These variables affect patients' access to care and their continuation in prescribed treatment plans. It is imperative for the nurse to collaborate with other members of the healthcare team to become aware of various services available to enhance the health and quality of life of patients.

■ Sociocultural Barriers

The need for cultural and ethnic diversity in the nursing workforce has been discussed. Moreover, healthcare settings are challenged to provide an environment where people of various sociocultural backgrounds are respected. For example, having translators on site or within easy contact is critical for ensuring safe care to non-English-speaking clients. Written materials should also be provided in appropriate languages and at an appropriate reading level. It is not feasible or cost effective to provide educational materials and products to patients who will not use them because they are in a foreign language or too advanced. Specifically, consent forms for surgery and other procedures must be available in the client's language. To ignore the need for language-appropriate literature leads to patient harm, as well as disrespect for the uniqueness of others.

One subculture that has garnered much attention in recent years is the military patient population. The Department of Defense operates and finances health care through TRICARE, a comprehensive healthcare coverage program for members of the uniformed services, their families, and survivors. With national resources decreasing and demands for health care of our military population on the rise, nurses play a pivotal role in influencing the direction of care for this special group.

In an effort to address the needs of the military population and their families specifically, First Lady Michelle Obama led the "Joining Forces" national initiative to mobilize all sectors of the community to give service members, veterans, and their families the support they deserve, especially in regard to employment, education, and wellness. According to Joining Forces (White House, 2012), military service members, veterans, and their families have made significant contributions to the nation's safety and security. This contribution comes at great cost to each veteran and family. The profession of nursing has a long and established history of meeting and supporting the physical and mental health needs of our nation's military service members, veterans, and their families. The profession of nursing has pledged to inspire and prepare each nurse to recognize the unique health and wellness concerns of the population. One hundred fifty nursing organizations and 500 nursing schools pledged their support to help educate nurses on post-traumatic stress disorder (PTSD) and traumatic brain injury (TBI) in the coming years. Although each organization and nursing school has its unique mission and vision, various strategies to be employed include (1) increasing nurse awareness of PTSD and TBI, (2) recognizing the signs and symptoms in patients, and (3) integrating PTSD and TBI content in nursing school curricula, to name a few. The American Nurses Association, American Academy of Nurse

Practitioners, American Association of Colleges of Nursing, and the National League for Nursing took the lead in seeking nationwide support from nursing organizations and schools of nursing.

■ Healthcare Delivery in the United States

Economic variables pervade how our nation values health care. Individuals who are unable to secure a health insurance plan are at great risk for inadequate care. Further, insurance companies now dictate to care providers what is permissible by determining covered benefits. The confusing patterns of payment for health care are prohibitive and further increase the stress of individuals in poor health conditions. In addition to the complexity of healthcare payment options, the availability of charitable care in this country is shrinking.

Even though we live in a **capitalistic society**, nursing in the United States has been seemingly protected against the details of healthcare finance. We have focused our attention on patients and aspects of their care. The changing economy, uncertainty of the Affordable Care Act of 2010, new pharmaceutical regulations, and evolving roles of the registered nurse have forced us to reconsider and restructure the very nature of our delivery systems. In addition to participating in new, creative, and innovative healthcare delivery styles, nurses represent the intermediary between patients and the healthcare system. Part of the responsibility that comes with that role is being knowledgeable about healthcare finance and educating others about the current vocabulary in charges, reimbursement, and coverage. Moreover, nurses should be involved in the policy-making processes that regulate the healthcare system. We are in an unprecedented time of change in our nation's health care. Professional nurses should be at the forefront, leading the charge to ensure adequate health care for all people.

■ Nurse-Managed Centers

Nurse-managed centers increase access to health care in a cost-effective way (Turkeltaub, 2004). Also called nursing-managed clinics and nurse practice arrangements, these healthcare delivery options meet needs in communities across the country. Based on the philosophy of primary care and education, nurses offer vital services at a lower cost. Nurse-managed health clinics are led by advanced practice nurses, most of whom are nurse practitioners acting as primary care providers for patients. They provide primary care, health promotion services, and disease prevention services to patients least likely to receive ongoing healthcare services. This population includes patients of all ages who are uninsured, underinsured, living in poverty, or members of racial and ethnic minority groups.

Provisions in the Affordable Care Act allow the advanced practice nurse to deliver more primary care services. Additionally, the Institute of Medicine Report *The Future of Nursing: Leading Change, Advancing Health* (Institute of Medicine Report [IOM], 2010) strongly recommends that each nurse work to the fullest extent of his or her education. Implementation of these provisions and recommendations will definitely expand the roles and responsibilities of the nurse so that patients receive the full benefit of quality health care.

In addition to providing care and cure, nurse-managed centers enhance relationships with the community. Faculty performing advanced practice and community nursing provide role models for the community while making clinical experiences available for students. In 2002, 18 grants to support nurse-managed centers were funded through the Health Resources and Services Administration's Bureau of Health Professions, Division of Nursing. As a result, 36 access points to care were provided for underserved populations. Service delivery options include school-based clinics, homeless shelters, correctional facilities, mobile health units, shelters, and public housing units (Turkeltaub, 2004).

In 2010, the U.S. Department of Health and Human Services provided $14.8 million to support grants to 10 nurse-managed clinics as part of the Affordable Care Act's Nurse-Managed Health Clinic Grant Program. The purpose of the grants was to augment efforts to increase primary care access. The clinics were expected to provide primary care to more than 94,000 patients and train more than 900 advanced practice nurses by the end of the grant period. Unfortunately, Congress and the Obama administration elected not to renew these grants in 2011 in an effort to cut federal spending.

Nurse-managed clinics provide services that are primarily preventative. The Institute of Medicine's report on the future of nursing states, "Nurse-managed health clinics offer opportunities to expand access; provide quality, evidence-based care; and improve outcomes for individuals who may not otherwise receive needed care. These clinics also provide the necessary support to engage individuals in wellness and prevention activities." Because the funding was cut, it is imperative that nurses at all levels strongly voice to local, state, and federal legislators the positive impact nurse-managed clinics have on decreasing disparities and improving the lives of individuals.

> **www CRITICAL THINKING QUESTIONS ✳**
>
> What barriers to health care do you see in your community? How are the underprivileged served in our current healthcare system? What actions should be taken to ensure universal access to health care? ✳

Trends

At any time in history, societal trends affect the nursing profession. Major current movements include incivility, violence in the workplace, mental health needs, global aging, imbalance of supply and demand of nursing professionals, consumerism, complementary and alternative care, technologic changes, disaster preparedness, and nursing research. Discussion of these issues allows us to see more clearly the professional landscape and some of our challenges.

■ Incivility

Incivility, or "bullying," has been exposed in the media to a great extent in the past few years. This heightened attention is partly the result of media coverage of suicide attempts and homicides that were instigated by harassment at the physical, verbal, and electronic levels. Incivility is seen in every area of society, including high school, college, and even on the job. Nursing is not immune to this behavior. Greater light has been shed on the incidence and prevalence of bullying in nurse-to-nurse, faculty-to-student, and even student-to-faculty interactions. Rocker (2008) reports that some of the behaviors include criticism, humiliation in front of others, undervaluing of effort, and teasing. It is also reported that bullying contributes to burnout, school dropout, isolation, and even attempted suicides. Bullying is costly to organizations because it contributes to increased leave, nurse attrition, and decreased nurse productivity, satisfaction, and morale.

In light of this, it is vital that the nursing profession take an active step in preventing incivility in our nursing programs and places of employment. The American Nurses Association (2012) has taken such action by developing a booklet, *Bullying in the Workplace: Reversing a Culture*, to help nurses understand and deal with bullying in the work environment. In addition, the Institute of Medicine Report *The Future of Nursing: Leading Change* (IOM, 2010) includes recommendations that call for healthcare professionals to establish civil and respectful relationships and interactions.

■ Violence in the Workplace

The **violence** in our society is evident and appears to be increasing in frequency and severity. What is more alarming is our desensitization to the constant exposure by Internet, radio, and television. As nurses, we can easily put a face on violence. We see the man in the emergency department with a gunshot wound to the chest. Only 30 minutes before, he was leaving work for a weekend with family when someone decided that they needed his car more than this man needed his life. We see violence at the women's shelter when we rotate through that clinical site in community health nursing. We also see troubled individuals who take out their frustration on colleagues and supervisors by going on a shooting rampage, leaving a path of death and destruction. All of these examples affect nurses because we are caring for the ones who are injured and also providing care to the injurer. Although some nursing education programs might include this topic in the curriculum, nursing academia should take an active stance in making sure nursing graduates are prepared to care for individuals who are directly and indirectly affected by violence. This same effort should be made in healthcare facilities to ensure nurses are knowledgeable of how to act and provide competent care when violent incidents occur.

Registered nurses can assume additional roles when addressing violence. The role of the nurse is not limited to providing care in the hospital or emergency department. To work aggressively to address violence, nurses can function in the role of a sexual assault nurse examiner (SANE), legal nurse consultant, or forensic nurse (Littel, 2001).

To be a sexual assault nurse examiner (SANE), a registered nurse must have advanced education and preparation in forensic examination of sexual assault victims. The Office for Victims of Crime of the U.S. Department of Justice has led the development of SANE programs across the country and provides materials and resources to encourage new programs. As a result of the SANE programs, victims of sexual assault consistently receive attention and compassion without delay (Littel, 2001).

Legal nurse consultants (LNCs) are registered nurses with specialized clinical expertise and education who interpret, research, analyze, and provide expert testimony or opinion on medical-related legal cases. These cases can be related to faulty equipment, malpractice, or side effects of medications (Grutkowski, 2012). Forensic nurses are trained to recognize and collect evidence related to criminal acts of trauma or death (Santiago, 2012). Even though a registered nurse can work in all three areas, each one has its specific responsibilities and duties to be performed.

Nurses must become socially aware and politically involved in preventing violence. We have to support legislation that proactively addresses violence and lobby for funding that provides nursing research into violence prevention and treatment. In every potential case, nurses have to use keen assessment skills to identify people at risk and to promote reporting, treatment, and rehabilitation. The national initiative to increase health for all U.S. citizens, Healthy People 2020, outlines objectives for violence and abuse prevention (Table 5-1).

■ Mental Health Needs

As professional nurses experience the stresses that come with today's healthcare environment, we are obliged to assess our own mental health needs. Consider the registered nurse who has worked for 20 years with the same agency. During this time, he learns the practices of his department and agency. In fact, he becomes highly specialized in his area of nursing expertise. Economic changes require workforce reductions, and he becomes a victim, released from employment as a result of downsizing. With the high demand for professional nurses, you might think securing employment would be an easy task. However, because of his specialization, he is forced to take a job outside his area to maintain an income. In addition to the stress of losing a position after a two-decade investment, he finds himself challenged with some of the fundamental aspects of nursing care. Yet, they are not fundamental to him, and there is no one to help him. People try, but after all, they are very

TABLE 5-1 Healthy People 2020 Violence and Abuse Prevention Objectives

Prevention Objectives	Target by 2020	Baseline Data (2008 & 2009)
Homicides	5.5 per 100,000	6.1 per 100,000
Firearm-related deaths	9.2 per 100,000	10.2 per 100,000
Maltreatment of children 17 years and younger	8.5 per 1,000	9.4 per 1,000
Fatalities caused by maltreatment, 17 years and younger	2.2 per 100,000	2.4 per 100,000
Physical assaults, persons aged 12 years and older	14.7 per 1,000	16.3 per 1,000
Reduce children's exposure to violence	54.5%	60.6%
Physical fighting among adolescents on school property in grades 9 through 12	28.4%	31.5%
Weapon carrying by adolescents on school property in grades 9 through 12	4.6%	5.6%
Reduce bullying among adolescents	17.9%	19.9%

Source: Healthy People 2020 (2012).

busy fulfilling their own roles. He becomes depressed, unfulfilled and wonders what his future holds.

Following the many national crises of the last several years, we have witnessed an increase in the mental health needs of our society. Professional nurses are not immune to this reality. Historically, mental health concerns have taken a backseat to other concerns, such as cancer and heart disease. True, these conditions require our resources, but so do the less glamorous conditions that affect emotional, spiritual, and **mental health**. Later in this text, the authors examine care of the professional self and address key concepts pertinent to this discussion.

▪ Global Aging

The Year of the Older Person—this is what the United Nations called the year 1999 to recognize and reaffirm **global aging**, the fact that our global population is aging at an unprecedented rate (U.S. Census Bureau, 2001). In 2010, adults 62 years of age and older comprised 16.2% (49.9 million) of the U.S.

population compared to 14.7% (41.2 million) in the year 2000. By 2030, it is estimated that the population of older adults will rise to 71 million (Howden & Meyer, 2011).

After World War II, fertility increased, and death rates of all ages decreased. Not only are people in developed countries living longer and healthier but so are those in the developing world. In the 1990s, developed countries had equal numbers of young (people 15 years and younger) and old (people 55 years and older) with approximately 22% of the population in each category. On the other hand, 35% of the people in developing countries were children compared with 10% who were older. Still, absolute numbers of older persons are large and growing. In the year 2000, more than half of the world's older people (59%, or 249 million people) lived in developing nations.

In the United States, a decrease in fertility, an increase in urbanization, better education, and improved health care all contribute to this social phenomenon. In addition, the older baby boomers who turned 65 years of age have started to affect health care significantly with increasing numbers receiving Medicare benefits. The impact this will have on our healthcare system is daunting. With the growing numbers of older adults will come a domino effect of more chronic conditions to treat and increased government funding (e.g., Medicare) to pay for treatment of these medical conditions. According to the USDHHS (2012), more than 60% of older adults will manage more than one chronic medical condition, such as diabetes, arthritis, heart failure, and dementia.

There is a need for clear health policy at a national level if we are to be prepared to care for our aging citizens. Approaches used in the past are inadequate. Because this is a new challenge for us, the correct actions are not clearly defined. Still, the responsibility is ours as a society. Nursing professionals should be knowledgeable of our roles and responsibility in obtaining factual information regarding health policy and take an active role in ensuring that quality health care is available and provided.

Preventive health services for older adults are delineated as provisions made in the Affordable Care Act of 2010. Healthy People 2020 established objectives specifically for older adults that should be used by healthcare professionals, including nurses, to promote healthy outcomes for this population. These are just two examples of health policy initiatives that nurses should be aware of and use when planning care for the older adult.

In the last several years, schools of nursing have incorporated a greater number of gerontology courses and concepts into the curriculum. Some nursing programs have increased the amount of gerontology content from a few hours to a required course in the curriculum. Geriatric Nurse Practitioner programs have grown in number, and some schools offer dual-track Adult/Geri Nurse Practitioner and Gero-Psychiatric Mental Health Nurse Practitioner programs in graduate programs. Clinical experiences in adult health settings are heavily saturated with older persons. Still, we lack an organized plan to make certain that healthcare needs will be met—not just for the aging, but also for those who come after them. Recent federal and local legislation calls for improvements in medication coverage, insurance reimbursements, and reform in malpractice law. Thus far, these attempts have been inadequate to provide the comprehensive care that will be vital if we are to make the right to health care real for everyone.

Other entities have made additional efforts to address the issues and challenges of preparing nurses to provide competent and specialized care to the older adult. The Hartford Institute for Geriatric Nursing (2012) provides a wealth of geriatric tools, continuing education offerings and workshops, and individualized training for nurses and nursing faculty in the care of the older adult and incorporating more geriatric content in the curriculum.

■ Nursing Supply and Demand

Few topics regarding nurses have garnered the level of publicity that the current **nursing shortage** has attracted in recent years. As our general population ages, so does our nursing population. As a result, the number of nurses and nurse faculty is shrinking (Peterson, 2001). The average age of RNs in the United States is 45 years and a large number of nurses will retire in the next 10 to 15 years (USDHHS, 2010). This presents a conundrum because as nurses retire, the population of older adults will steadily increase. This is significant because there will be fewer nurses to care for all patients and even fewer to care for the older adult. It is projected that there will be a shortage of 1.2 million nurses by the year 2014.

So, how will this deficit be addressed? In reality, to meet this need, we would need to graduate double the number of current nurse graduates. Although this might seem attainable, there are other challenges to meeting this goal. First, nursing faculty are aging and will be retiring in the near future. This presents a nursing faculty shortage compounded by the fact that fewer nurses pursue academia as a career choice mainly because of lower salaries compared to that of the clinical nurse. Second, nursing programs might not have the infrastructure or facilities to accommodate an increase in enrollment. These challenges can be quite discouraging and that is why this is a major issue that needs to be addressed sooner rather than later. The major concern is related to the topic discussed in the previous section: Who will care for the old? As people age and experience health problems, their needs are often more complex and acute, thereby demanding an even more highly skilled nursing force.

With the downturn in the nation's economy, healthcare systems tried to cut costs to stay in business. Unfortunately, nursing care was not exempt from the cutbacks. In the mid-1990s, nurses were asked to do more with less, and that expectation continues today. Patients are sicker because they are living

---

KEY COMPETENCY 5-3

Examples of Applicable *Nurse of the Future: Nursing Core Competencies*

Systems-Based Practice:

Knowledge (K6) Is aware of global aspects of health care

Attitudes/Behaviors (A6a) Appreciates the potential of the global environment to influence patient health; (A6b) Appreciates the potential of the global environment to influence nursing practice

Source: Massachusetts Department of Higher Education (2010, p. 21).

longer, resulting in a nurse-to-patient ratio that for the nurse is often stressful, seemingly unbearable, and that leads to burnout.

According to Maslach and Jackson (1986), job-related burnout is a syndrome of emotional exhaustion, depersonalization, and decreased personal accomplishment. Emotional exhaustion is feeling overextended and exhausted, depersonalization is an impersonal response to the recipient of one's care, and decreased personal accomplishment is a feeling of incompetence and lack of achievement. A study by Vahey, Aiken, Sloane, Clarke, and Vargas (2004) found that an improvement in the work environment reduced levels of burnout and improved patient outcomes. It is documented that burnout in nurses has a direct effect on patient care and resulting outcomes. Nurse burnout is all too common and pervasive (Weinberg, 2003). As a result, nurses are leaving the profession (Bingham, 2002). For female nurses, 4.1% left the profession in 2000 compared with 2.7% in 1992. Male nurses left at a rate of 7.5% in 2000, up from 2% in 1992 (Nelson, 2002). According to the U.S. Department of Health and Human Services (2010), nearly 77,000 registered nurses intended to leave the profession in 3 years, and of that number, 54,000 were not sure if they would remain in nursing. Nursing burnout might play a significant role in their decision.

In September 2002, the nursing shortage in the United States was labeled a national security concern (Nelson, 2002). Although the historical picture of nursing supply and demand has fluctuated, other variables influence the current shortage. In 2000, 9% of nurses were younger than 30 years old and more than 330,000 registered nurses were expected to retire by 2008. Although the rate of retirement has slowed as a result of economic conditions between 2008 and 2012, the combination of the growing number of older people requiring care with the number of nurses expected to retire when the U.S. economy recovers means that by 2020 the national nursing shortage is predicted to reach a 20% deficit (Nelson, 2002).

The majority of registered nurses work in hospitals; therefore, those facilities are responsible for discovering innovative and alternative ways of recruiting and retaining professional staff. Cooper (2003) presents some strategies for nursing managers, staff, and faculty to negotiate through this crisis:

- To retain older nurses, reconstruct the patient care environment to make it more ergonomically sensitive, supportive, and tailored to the physical limitations of an aging workforce.
- Provide for and encourage educational pursuits.
- Evaluate and modify work schedules to complement circadian rhythms.
- Provide auxiliary staff around the clock.
- Attend to special needs of the nighttime workers; for example, provide fresh foods and healthy snacks.
- Provide a "resting room" for sleep breaks, especially if employees have a distance to drive home.

Despite the disheartening statistics about the nursing shortage, some great strides have been made in devising innovative, creative, and alternative approaches to increasing the pool of registered nurses. According to the Robert Wood Johnson Foundation (2007), several partnerships among nursing programs, hospitals, and government entities have emerged. Some of the initiatives involve "fast tracks" to prepare nursing faculty, special state fund allocation for nursing education, and hospital loan programs. Still, on the supply side of the equation, nursing faculty are also aging. Assistant and associate professors are an average of 52.1 and 48.5 years old, respectively (Cooper, 2003). The shortage of doctoral-prepared faculty is even more severe. On average, nurses receiving new doctorates are 45 years old (Cooper, 2003). This dilemma presents us with the question: Who will teach our future nurses?

Wieck (2003) points out that people are not choosing nursing as a profession. The younger generation is not attracted to the nursing career option. Some reasons can be related to issues currently discussed in the literature— inflexible work environments, low compensation, poor recognition, high stress, and so on. Another possibility is the tendency for nursing education to resist change to meet the expectations of college-degree-seeking students. Nursing education programs must be aware of what this new generation desires in a learning experience and be prepared to reconfigure and create new ways of instruction: offering courses online; providing personal, frequent feedback; and focusing on outcomes and not just the process (Wieck, 2003). The emerging workforce cannot be convinced to enter nursing for the same reasons that once attracted people to the profession. If we are to draw from the rich pool of young people, we have to find out what they need and find ways to provide it.

■ Consumerism

Since the American Hospital Association's development of "A Patient's Bill of Rights" in 1973, consumers have assumed more control of their healthcare experiences; this shift is called **consumerism**. The 1992 version of the document was replaced by the brochure *The Patient Care Partnership: Understanding Expectations, Rights, and Responsibilities* (American Hospital Association, 2003) and various hospitals have adapted the document specifically for their patient population (such as the Pilgrim Medical Center in Montclair, New Jersey, and St. Anthony's Medical Center in Carroll, Iowa). A summary of the original document is presented in Box 5-1. Gone are the days when patients blindly follow the instructions of their physicians. In part, this is cause for celebration in the nursing arena. Professional nursing has long sought to empower patients to take responsibility for their own health. Although pockets of medical paternalism continue, the general shift is to hold healthcare providers to a higher standard than ever before.

BOX 5-1 THE PATIENT CARE PARTNERSHIP

What to expect during your hospital stay:
1. High-quality patient care
2. A clean and safe environment
3. Involvement in your care
   a. Discussing your medical condition and information about medically appropriate treatment choices
   b. Discussing your treatment plan
   c. Getting information from you
   d. Understanding your healthcare goals and values
   e. Understanding who should make decisions when you cannot
4. Protection of your privacy
5. Preparing you and your family for when you leave the hospital
6. Help with your bill and filing insurance claims

O'Neil and the Pew Health Professions Commission (1998) provide another example of attempts to respond to the changing needs of the American healthcare system. From 1989 to 1999, with a grant from the Pew Charitable Trusts, a commission was established to focus on the healthcare workforce. To improve health care of the American people, professionals in the healthcare delivery system needed guidelines to respond to trends and developments. In 1998, the commission presented its report *Twenty-One Competencies for the Twenty-First Century*. These competencies are presented in Box 5-2. Although this document was developed more than a decade ago, the competencies are still applicable today.

BOX 5-2 TWENTY-ONE COMPETENCIES FOR THE TWENTY-FIRST CENTURY

1. Embrace a personal ethic of social responsibility and service.
2. Exhibit ethical behavior in all professional activities.
3. Provide evidence-based, clinically competent care.
4. Incorporate the multiple determinants of health in clinical care.
5. Apply knowledge of the new sciences.
6. Demonstrate critical thinking, reflection, and problem-solving skills.
7. Understand the role of primary care.
8. Rigorously practice preventive health care.
9. Integrate population-based care and services into practice.
10. Improve access to health care for those with unmet health needs.
11. Practice relationship-centered care with individuals and families.
12. Provide culturally sensitive care to a diverse society.

13. Partner with communities in healthcare decisions.
14. Use communication and information technology effectively and appropriately.
15. Work in interdisciplinary teams.
16. Ensure care that balances individual, professional, system, and societal needs.
17. Practice leadership.
18. Take responsibility for quality of care and health outcomes at all levels.
19. Contribute to continuous improvement of the healthcare system.
20. Advocate for public policy that promotes and protects the health of the public.
21. Continue to learn and help others learn.

Source: O'Neil and the Pew Health Professions Commission (1998).

Bulger (2002) states that four major points must be kept in mind when considering the healthcare system of the future. First, technology and science will have a major impact. Although research and experimentation have made the United States a global leader in informatics, robotics, and genetics, we are cautioned to pause and consider the full potential of such a revolution. Second, multiprofessional collaboration will determine the efficiency and effectiveness with which we respond to the demands in health care. It is not feasible for nursing professionals to work solely with other nurses to solve problems and address issues. In a society with a continually changing healthcare system, it is essential for nurses to collaborate and partner with other healthcare professionals and entities that do not have a health-related focus (e.g., those in business, economics, government). Third, we must educate ourselves as healthcare providers and the public as consumers of health care. Finally, as healthcare professionals, we depend on the research being conducted, which should guide our actions and practice. In the end, nursing professionals have a heavy responsibility to be actively engaged in shaping and determining the future healthcare system.

KEY COMPETENCY 5-4

Examples of Applicable
Nurse of the Future: Nursing Core Competencies

Patient-Centered Care:

Attitudes/Behaviors (A2b)
Respects and encourages the patient's input relative to decisions about health care and services

Source: Massachusetts Department of Higher Education (2010, p. 9).

■ Complementary and Alternative Approaches

As the consumer's perspective grows in influence, and individuals take on greater responsibility in their healthcare decisions, they explore approaches to health care that can actually contrast with Western traditions. Different terminology has been used synonymously to define this growing field, such as *complementary care practices* and *alternative medicine*. According to the National Center for Complementary and Alternative Medicine (2012),

"Complementary and alternative medicine is a group of diverse medical and healthcare systems, practices, and products that are not presently considered to be part of conventional medicine." *Complementary medicine* refers to an approach that combines conventional medicine with less conventional options, whereas *alternative medicine* is an approach used instead of conventional medicine. Major types of **complementary and alternative medicine** include the following:

- Alternative medical systems (built on complete systems of practice such as homeopathic medicine or naturopathic medicine)
- Mind–body interventions (techniques designed to enhance the mind's capacity to affect bodily function such as meditation, prayer, music, and support groups)
- Biologically based therapies (use of substances found in nature such as herbs, foods, and vitamins)
- Manipulative and body-based methods (based on manipulation or movement of one or more parts of the body such as chiropractic manipulation or massage)
- Energy therapies (involves the use of energy fields through either biofield therapies such as therapeutic touch, qi gong, or Reiki; or bioelectromagnetic-based therapies such as magnetic therapy)

Alternative and complementary therapies affect the selection of traditional choices for treatment, and ignoring that they exist is not an option. People persist in the use of alternative and complementary therapies for obvious reasons: (1) the therapies have been found valuable, and (2) Western medicine has limited options. A duty of the professional nurse is to secure an accurate assessment of the patient's needs and circumstances. Therefore, it is imperative that nurses be educated on treatment choices the patient has selected. Nurses should provide a safe, trusting atmosphere where patients feel free to discuss their healthcare routines and preferences. Additionally, nursing educational programs should incorporate more information about the research in this growing field.

■ Technological Changes

Although technology influences in professional nursing are presented in detail later in this text, mention of those changes here is warranted. Undeniably, technologic advances have affected professional nursing practice in ways never imagined. The dream of connecting with patients in their homes by remote video and satellite is now commonplace. Digital, point-of-care documentation systems are the upcoming standard for patient records. Moreover, the equipment used in treatment plans changes at an exponential rate.

Although technology presents new challenges—higher costs, greater educational demands, threats to bedside care—nurses can respond proactively.

KEY COMPETENCY 5-5

Examples of Applicable *Nurse of the Future: Nursing Core Competencies*

Safety:

Attitudes /Behaviors (A3) Recognizes that both individuals and systems are accountable for a safety culture

Source: Massachusetts Department of Higher Education (2010, p. 34).

Ways of caring through technology exist that can actually enhance patient safety through more effective systems and the reduction of human error, which is congruent with Institute of Medicine (2000) recommendations. One example is the adoption of electronic patient records, which provide clearer communication lines among members of the multidisciplinary team. Also, documentation can be recorded in real time, thereby allowing the nurse to spend time with the patient. Patient safety is not compromised with poor handwriting and delayed orders (Meadows, 2003). Another example is the use of telehealth approaches to improve healthcare service in rural and underserved communities (Buckwalter, Davis, Wakefield, Kienzle, & Murray, 2002).

Information technology has given patients and care providers an enormous resource for gaining knowledge about diseases, medications, treatment options, and support groups. A basic part of any nursing plan of care should include providing reputable and evidence-based resources for the patient that can be accessed over the Internet. In today's healthcare environment, people search for answers to their healthcare questions. Who better to guide them to good information than a professional registered nurse?

■ Disaster Preparedness

Prior to the turn of this century, **disaster preparedness** was not a major topic of discussion in programs of nursing. Further, the key roles that professional nurses now play in preparing and responding to disasters were unexplored until recently. The World Trade Center attack in 2001 and the shock of Hurricane Katrina in 2005 opened the nation's eyes to our vulnerabilities and our strengths. As a result, disaster management has become common language in our schools, agencies, and communities.

Disaster management, plans designating responses during an emergency, is coordinated by local, state, and federal groups. Firefighters, police officers, and healthcare professionals are part of response teams. Disaster training is also available to other volunteers. We have learned that caring for large groups affected by disaster requires an organized, thoughtful, unbiased approach by our leaders.

> **Disaster management has become common language in our schools, agencies, and communities.**

Professional nurses carry the burden of being knowledgeable about potential disasters, such as Avian influenza, educating the public about the risks, and responding when persons are affected. The ANA makes available policies, resources, and educational opportunities on disaster preparedness for nurses. In addition, the Institute of Medicine (2009) prepared a document that provides guidance for entities establishing standards of care for disaster preparedness. The Centers for Disease Control and Prevention (CDC) Clinician Outreach and Communication Activity program formed in 2011 in response to the anthrax attacks in the United States with the mission to help healthcare professionals provide optimal care by facilitating communication between clinicians and CDC about emerging health threats, identifying clinical issues during emergencies to help inform outreach strategies, and disseminating evidence-based health information and public health emergency messages (CDC, 2012).

■ Research Needs

Addressing the context of professional nursing in today's world raises important research questions. Key variables are the changes in patient acuity and the effect on nurse staffing (Robert Wood Johnson Foundation, 2007). Models of nurse staffing, including fixed minimum ratios and pay-for-performance, are being tested. Although not independently, staffing ratios offer promise to improve nursing work environments. Research regarding the future of nursing must center on efforts aimed at creating practice environments that increase nurse satisfaction and improve productivity. Specific areas identified by the Robert Wood Johnson Foundation (2007) include increasing nurses' authority, increasing trust between nurses and management, reorganizing nurses' work, and prohibiting mandatory overtime. As nursing specialties develop standards of care, it is also vital that the standards have an evidenced-based foundation. As a profession, nursing needs to base practice on research and primarily on experiential successes.

> Research regarding the future of nursing must center on efforts aimed at creating practice environments that increase nurse satisfaction and improve productivity.

Conclusion

Now, when you hear the word *nursing*, what image comes to mind? If the picture is blurry or confused by the expanding social context presented in this chapter—good! The cloudiness indicates that the tradition continues to be questioned. We have looked at some of the social phenomena that help define nursing. Because those experiences change constantly, what we envision now will also be transformed. Nevertheless, we have to question the image and explore the factors that influence it. We are challenged to do this on a regular basis. Only then can we evolve in meaningful ways to better meet the nursing needs of our society.

Web Resources

American Assembly for Men in Nursing: www.aamn.org
American Association of Colleges of Nursing: www.aacn.nche.edu
American Hospital Association: www.aha.org
American Nurses Association: www.nursingworld.org

Campaign for Nursing's Future: www.discovernursing.com
Diversity Nursing: www.diversitynursing.com
Healthy People 2020: www.healthypeople.gov
Minority Nurse: www.minoritynurse.com
National Association of Hispanic Nurses: www.thehispanicnurses.org
National Black Nurses Association: www.nbna.org
National Center for Complementary and Alternative Medicine: www.nccam.nih.gov
National League for Nursing: www.nln.org
National Student Nurses Association: www.nsna.org
Office for Victims of Crime, U.S. Department of Justice: www.ojp.usdoj.gov/ovc
Pew Health Professions Commission: http://futurehealth.ucsf.edu/Public/Center-Home.aspx
Sexual Assault Nurse Examiners: www.sane-sart.com
Transcultural Nursing Society: www.tcns.org
TRICARE: www.tricare.mil
U.S. Bureau of the Census: www.census.gov
U.S. Department of Labor: www.stats.bls.gov

References

Agency for Healthcare Research and Quality. (2010). National healthcare disparities reports 2010. Retrieved from www.ahrq.gov/qual/qrdr10.htm

American Hospital Association. (2003). The patient care partnership: Understanding expectations, rights, and responsibilities. Retrieved from http://www.aha.org/aha/issues/Communicating-With-Patients/pt-care-partnership.html

American Nurses Association. (2007). American Nurses Association recognizes the contributions of men in nursing with the (ANA) Luther Christman Award. *Wyoming Nurse, 20*(2), 13.

American Nurses Association. (2012). *Bullying in the workplace: Reversing a culture*. Silver Spring, MD: Author.

American Society of Registered Nurses. (2008). Men in nursing. Retrieved from http://www.asrn.org/journal-nursing/374-men-in-nursing.html

Armstrong, F. (2002). Not just women's business: Men in nursing. *Australian Nursing Journal, 9*(11), 24–26.

Berlin, L. E., Stennett, J., & Bednash, G. D. (2003). *2002–2003 enrollment and graduations in baccalaureate and graduate programs in nursing*. Washington, DC: American Association of Colleges of Nursing.

Berlin, L. E., Stennett, J., & Bednash, G. D. (2004). *2003–2004 enrollment and graduations in baccalaureate and graduate programs in nursing*. Washington, DC: American Association of Colleges of Nursing.

Bingham, R. (2002). Leaving nursing [Electronic version]. *Health Affairs, 21*, 211–218.

Blais, K., Hayes, J. S., Kozier, B., & Erb, G. (2001). *Professional nursing practice: Concepts and perspectives* (4th ed.). Upper Saddle River, NJ: Pearson.

Brady, M. S., & Sherrod, D. R. (2003). Retaining men in nursing programs designed for women [Electronic version]. *Journal of Nursing Education, 42*, 159–163.

Buckwalter, K. C., Davis, L. L., Wakefield, B. J., Kienzle, M. G., & Murray, M. A. (2002). Telehealth for elders and their caregivers in rural communities. *Family and Community Health, 25*(3), 31–40.

Bulger, R. J. (2002). What will health care look like in the future? In E. J. Sullivan (Ed.), *Creating nursing's future: Issues, opportunities and challenges* (pp. 14–31). St. Louis, MO: Mosby.

Buresh, B., & Gordon, S. (2000). *From silence to voice: What nurses know and must communicate to the public.* New York, NY: Cornell University Press.

Buresh, B., & Gordon, S. (2006). *From silence to voice: What nurses know and must communicate to the public.* New York, NY: Cornell University Press.

Cardillo, D. W. (2001). *Your first year as a nurse: Making the transition from total novice to successful professional.* Roseville, CA: Prima.

Centers for Disease Control and Prevention. (2012). Clinical outreach and communication activity. Retrieved from http://www.bt.cdc.gov/coca

Chitty, K., & Campbell, C. (2001). The social context of nursing. In K. K. Chitty (Ed.), *Professional nursing: Concepts and challenges* (pp. 64–100). Philadelphia, PA: Saunders.

Chung, V. (2001). Men in nursing. *Minority Nurse.* Retrieved from http://www.minoritynurse.com/?q=men-nursing/men-nursing

Cooper, E. E. (2003). Pieces of the shortage puzzle: Aging and shift work [Electronic version]. *Nursing Economics, 21*(2), 75–80.

Gibbs, D. M., & Waugaman, W. R. (2004). Diversity behind the mask: Ethnicity, gender, and past career experience in a nurse anesthesiology program [Electronic version]. *Journal of Multicultural Nursing & Health, 10*, 77–82.

Gordon, S. (2005). *Nursing against the odds: How health care cost cutting, media stereotypes, and medical hubris undermine nurses and patient care.* Ithaca, NY: Cornell University Press.

Gordon, S. (2010). *When chicken soup isn't enough: Stories of nurses standing up for themselves, their patients, and their profession.* Ithaca, NY: Cornell University Press.

Gordon, S., Buchanan, J., & Bretherton, T. (2008). *Safety in numbers: Nurse-to-patient ratios and the future of health care.* Ithaca, NY: Cornell University Press.

Grant, L. F., & Letzring, T. D. (2003). Status of cultural competence in nursing education: A literature review [Electronic version]. *Journal of Multicultural Nursing & Health, 9*(2), 6–13.

Grutkowski, L. L. (2012). Top 5 legal nurse consulting responsibilities. Retrieved from http://www.allnursingschools.com/nursing-careers/career/lnc

Hartford Institute for Geriatric Nursing. (2012). Home page. Retrieved from http://www.hartfordign.org

Health Careers Center. (2012). 2005 Mississippi men in nursing calendar. Retrieved from http://www.mshealthcareers.com/media/2005meninnursing_pressrelease.htm

Howden, L. M., & Meyer, J. A. (2011). *Age and sex composition: 2010.* Washington, DC: U.S. Census Bureau. Retrieved from http://www.census.gov/prod/cen2010/briefs/c2010br-03.pdf

Institute of Medicine. (2000). *To err is human: Building a safer health system.* Washington, DC: National Academy Press.

Institute of Medicine. (2009). Guidance for establishing standards of care for use in disaster situations. Retrieved from http://www.iom.edu/Activities/PublicHealth/DisasterCareStandards.aspx

Institute of Medicine. (2010). *The future of nursing: Leading change, Advancing health*. Retrieved from http://books.nap.edu/openbook.php?record_id=12956

Jacob, S. R., & Carnegie, M. E. (2002). Cultural competency and social issues in nursing and health care. In B. Cherry (Ed.), *Contemporary nursing: Issues, trends, & management* (pp. 239–262). St. Louis, MO: Mosby.

Jones, J. M. (2012). Record 64% rate honesty, ethics of members of Congress low: Ratings of nurses, pharmacists, and, medical doctors most positive. Retrieved from http://www.gallup.com/poll/151460/record-rate-honesty-ethics-members-congress-low.aspx

Kavanagh, K. H. (2001). Social and cultural dimensions of health and health care. In J. L. Creasia & B. Parker (Eds.), *Conceptual foundations: The bridge to professional nursing practice* (pp. 294–314). St. Louis, MO: Mosby.

Keogh, B., & O'Lynn, C. (2007). Male nurses' experiences of gender barriers: Irish and American perspectives. *Nurse Educator, 32*(6), 256–259.

Leininger, M. M. (1991). *Culture care diversity and universality*. New York, NY: National League for Nursing Press.

Levine, K. (2012). When speaking the same language means speaking different languages. Retrieved from http://www.minoritynurse.com/when-speaking-same-language-means-speaking-different-languages

Littel, K. (2001). Sexual assault nurse examiner (SANE) programs: Improving the community response to sexual assault victims. Retrieved from http://new.vawnet.org/Assoc_Files_VAWnet/OVC_SANE0401-186366.pdf

Maslach, C., & Jackson, S. (1986). *Maslach burnout inventory manual*. Palo Alto, CA: Consulting Psychologists Press.

Massachusetts Department of Higher Education. (2010). *Nurse of the future: Nursing core competencies*. Retrieved from http://www.mass.edu/currentinit/documents/NursingCoreCompetencies.pdf

Meadows, G. (2003). Improving the patient experience with information technology [Electronic version]. *Nursing Economics, 21*, 300–302.

Meyers, S. (2003). Real men chose nursing [Electronic version]. *Hospitals & Health Networks, 77*(6), 72–74.

Minority Nurse. (2012). The TAKE PRIDE campaign. Retrieved from http://www.minoritynurse.com/print/80841

National Advisory Council on Nurse Education and Practice. (2003). *Third report to the secretary of Health and Human Services and Congress*. Retrieved from http://www.hrsa.gov/advisorycommittees/bhpradvisory/nacnep/Reports/thirdreport.pdf

National Center for Complementary and Alternative Medicine. (2012). What is complementary and alternative medicine (CAM)? Retrieved from http://nccam.nih.gov/health/whatiscam

National League for Nursing. (2012). Annual survey of schools of nursing. Retrieved from http://www.nln.org/aboutnln/research_survey.htm

Nelson, R. (2002). US nursing shortage a "national security concern" [Electronic version]. *Lancet, 360*, 855–857.

O'Neil, E. H., & the Pew Health Professions Commission. (1998). *Twenty-one competencies for the twenty-first century*. San Francisco, CA: Pew Health Professions Commission.

Oregon Center for Nursing. (2003). Are you man enough … to be a nurse? Retrieved from http://www.oregoncenterfornursing.org/index.php?mode=postersandmore

Otto, L. A., & Gurney, C. (2006, Fall/Winter). Ethnic diversity in the nurse workforce: A literature review. *Journal of the New York State Nurses Association, 16–21.*

Peterson, C. (2001). Issues update. In short supply: Around the world, the need for nurses grows. *American Journal of Nursing, 101*(9), 61–64.

Robert Wood Johnson Foundation. (2007). *Charting nursing's future: Reports on policies that can transform patient care.* Princeton, NJ: Author.

Rocker, C. F. (2008). Addressing nurse-to-nurse bullying to promote nurse retention. *Journal of Issues in Nursing, 13*(3).

Santiago, A. (2012). Forensic nursing careers. Retrieved from http://healthcareers.about.com/od/nursingcareers/a/ForensicNursing.htm

Sigma Theta Tau International. (1998). *The Woodhull study on nursing and the media: Health care's invisible partner.* Indianapolis, IN: STTI Center Nursing Press.

Trossman, S. (2003). Caring knows no gender: Break the stereotype and boost the number of men in nursing. *American Journal of Nursing, 103,* 65–68.

Turkeltaub, M. (2004). Nurse-managed centers: Increasing access to health care [Electronic version]. *Journal of Nursing Education, 43*(2), 53–54.

U.S. Census Bureau. (2001). *An aging world: 2001.* Retrieved from http://www.census.gov/prod/2001pubs/p95-01-1.pdf

U.S. Department of Health and Human Services. (2010). *The registered nurse population: Initial findings from the 2008 national sample survey of registered nurses.* Retrieved from http://bhpr.hrsa.gov/healthworkforce/rnsurvey

U.S. Department of Health and Human Services. (2012). *Healthy people 2020: Injury and violence prevention.* Retrieved from http://www.healthypeople.gov/2020/topicsobjectives2020/overview.aspx?topicid=24

Vahey, D., Aiken, L. H., Sloane, D. M., Clarke, S. P., & Vargas, D. (2004). Nurse burnout and patient satisfaction. *Med Care, 42*(2), 1157–1166.

Waters, V. L. (2004). Cultivate corporate culture and diversity [Electronic version]. *Nursing Management, 35,* 36–40.

Weinberg, D. B. (2003). *Code green.* Ithaca, NY: Cornell University Press.

White House. (2012). Joining forces. Retrieved from http://www.whitehouse.gov/joiningforces

Wieck, K. L. (2003). Faculty for the millennium: Changes needed to attract the emerging workforce into nursing. *Journal of Nursing Education, 42,* 151–159.

Education and Socialization to the Professional Nursing Role

Melanie Gilmore

6

Key Terms and Concepts

» **Socialization**
» Formation
» Professional values
» Novice
» Advanced beginner
» Competent
» Proficient
» Expert
» Role transition

Socialization to professional nursing is the process of acquiring the knowledge, skills, and sense of identity that are characteristic of the profession. It is a process by which a student internalizes the attitudes, beliefs, norms, values, and standards of the profession into his or her own behavior pattern (Cohen, 1981). Professional socialization has four goals: (1) to learn the technology of the profession—the facts, skills, and theory, (2) to learn to internalize the professional culture, (3) to find a personally and professionally acceptable version of the role, and (4) to integrate this professional role into all of the other life roles (Hentz, 2009).

Recently, Benner, Sutphen, Leonard, and Day (2010) made the case for using the term **formation** to describe this process that occurs over time because it better denotes "the development of perceptual abilities, the ability to draw on knowledge and skilled know-how, and a way of being and acting in practice and in the world" (p. 166).

Whatever terminology is chosen, the process described in this chapter refers to the transformation of the layperson into a skilled nurse who is prepared to respond skillfully and respectfully to persons in need of nursing care or, as described by Benner et al. (2010) in their discussion of formation, "the lay student moves from *acting* like a nurse to *being* a nurse" (p. 177). This development of professional identity occurs initially through the formal educational process and culminates in the practice setting.

Learning Objectives

After completing this chapter, the student should be able to:

1. Discuss professionalism and nursing.
2. Describe socialization to professional nursing.
3. Describe how nursing education affects the socialization of nurses.
4. Describe the stages of skill and knowledge acquisition as defined by Benner.
5. Identify factors that facilitate professional role development.

Professional nursing continues to evolve into a profession with a distinct body of knowledge, specialized practice, standards of practice, and social contract. The professional nurse is responsible for practice that incorporates this specialized body of knowledge and standards of practice.

Professional Nursing Values

Professional values are beliefs or ideals that guide interactions with patients, colleagues, other professionals, and the public. Professional values are considered a component of excellence, and the existence of a code is considered a hallmark of professionalism. The development of professional values begins with professional education in nursing and continues along a continuum throughout the years of nursing practice. Professional values associated with nursing are outlined in the American Nurses Association *Code of Ethics* (ANA, 2001). The values of (1) commitment to public service, (2) autonomy, (3) commitment to lifelong learning and education, and (4) a belief in the dignity and worth of each person epitomize the caring, professional nurse.

> **Professional values are beliefs or ideals that guide interactions with patients, colleagues, other professionals, and the public.**

Nursing is a helping profession directed toward health promotion and disease prevention of individuals, families, and communities. Caring is a concept central to the profession of nursing. Inherent in this value is a strong commitment to public service. The role of the nurse is focused on assessing and promoting the health and well-being of all humans. Registered nurses remain in nursing to promote, advocate, and strive to protect the health and safety of patients, families, and communities (ANA, 2004).

Autonomy is the right to self-determination as a profession. The role of the professional nurse is to honor and assist individuals and families to make informed decisions about health care and provide information so that they can make informed choices. The professional nurse respects patients' rights to make decisions about their health care.

Commitment to lifelong learning and education is necessary in the dynamic healthcare arena that surrounds nursing practice in this century. Nurses need continuous education to maintain a safe level of practice and expand their level of competence as professionals. With new technologies and the rapid expansion of medical and nursing knowledge, the nurse must continuously seek to expand the body of professional knowledge. Professional nursing involves a commitment to be resourceful, to respond to the dynamic challenges of delivering health care, to incorporate technology into their art and caring, and to remain visionaries as the future unfolds (ANA, 2004).

KEY COMPETENCY 6-1

Examples of Applicable *Nurse of the Future: Nursing Core Competencies*

Professionalism:

Knowledge (K4a) Describes factors essential to the promotion of professional development

Skills (S4a) Participates in life-long learning

Attitudes/Behaviors (A4a) Committed to life-long learning

Source: Massachusetts Department of Higher Education (2010), p. 13.

Human dignity is respect for the inherent worth and uniqueness of individuals and communities. According to the International Council of Nurses' (ICN's) *Code of Ethics for Nurses* (ICN, 2006), "inherent in nursing is respect for human rights, including cultural rights, the right to life and choice, to dignity and to be treated with respect. Nursing care is respectful of and unrestricted by considerations of age, color, creed, culture, disability or illness, gender, sexual orientation, nationality, politics, race or social status" (p. 1).

> **www] CRITICAL THINKING QUESTIONS ✳**
>
> As a nursing student, do you share the values of commitment to public service, autonomy, commitment to lifelong learning and education, and the belief in the dignity and worth of each person? Do nurses with whom you have interacted demonstrate these values? ✳

Socialization Process

■ Educational Socialization

Socialization into a profession is a process of adapting to and becoming a part of a culture (Ousey, 2009). Part of socialization is about individuals learning what it means to be a professional. Students new to the nursing profession learn the role in the educational setting. Cohen (1981) uses the theories of cognitive development to develop a model of professional nursing socialization through education. The model describes four stages students must experience as they begin to internalize the roles of a profession. In stage 1, Unilateral Dependence, the individual places complete reliance on external controls and searches for the one right answer (Cohen, 1981, p. 16). In essence, the student looks to the instructor for the right answers and is unlikely to question the authority. As the student gains foundational knowledge and skill, there begins the process of questioning the authority.

During stage 2, Negative/Independence, the student begins to pull away from external controls and is characterized by cognitive rebellion. The student begins to think critically and begins to question the instructor and relies more on his or her own judgments. Stage 3, Dependence/Mutuality, marks the beginning of empathy and commitment to others (Cohen, 1981, p. 18). In this stage, the student begins to apply knowledge to practice and the student tests information and facts. "Students have a knowledge base upon which to anchor critical thought and can relate new material to their previous knowledge base" (Cohen, 1981, p. 18). In this stage, the student is actively engaged in the learning, thinking through problems. For this stage to emerge, the learning environment must support and value risk taking. The role of the teacher is that of coach, mentor, and senior learner. The mentor helps the student link theory to practice while in the clinical areas, thus helping the student to learn from experiences and to improve practices to support professional socialization.

Stage 4, Interdependence, occurs when neither mutuality nor autonomy is dominant. Learning from others and the ability to solve problems independently are evident. This is the stage of the professional lifelong learner who demonstrates reflection in practice and is responsible for continued learning. Professional socialization toward the stage of interdependence requires a supportive educational climate that values autonomy, independent thinking, and authenticity. Students become professionals.

■ Professional Socialization

Several models in the literature describe professional socialization. Regardless of the model embraced, socialization into the nursing profession must include new competencies for the 21st century. The Institute of Medicine (IOM, 2011) reported that nurses need requisite competencies including leadership, health policy, system improvement, research and evidence-based practice, and teamwork and collaboration to meet the needs of the current dynamic healthcare environment. Nursing educators must give students the requisite skills and practice opportunities that equip them for the profession and instill in them the desire to become lifelong learners. Nurses need continuous education to maintain a safe level of practice and expand their level of competence as professionals. With new technologies and the rapid expansion of medical and nursing knowledge, the nurse must continuously seek to expand the body of professional knowledge. Professional nursing involves a commitment to be resourceful, to respond to the dynamic challenges of delivering health care, to incorporate technology into their art and caring, and to remain visionaries as the future unfolds (ANA, 2004).

■ Model of Professional Socialization: From Novice to Expert

Benner (1984) describes the development of professional clinical practice of nurses. Benner's model identifies the stages of novice, advanced beginner, competent, proficient, and expert that are based on the nurse's experience in practice. With an understanding of this progression of knowledge and skills, educational programs have developed supportive curricula using a continuum of experiences to enhance skill and knowledge development. Healthcare environments have also incorporated this model to facilitate the nurse's professional practice by assessing the nurse's stage of development. This model is not limited to the student experience or to that of the new graduate nurse. Experienced nurses too can benefit from experiences designed to move toward expert.

> Benner's model identifies the stages of novice, advanced beginner, competent, proficient, and expert that are based on the nurse's experience in practice.

The first stage, **novice**, is characterized by a lack of knowledge and experience. In this stage, the facts, rules, and guidelines for practice are the focus. Rules for practice are context free, and the student task is to acquire the knowledge and skills. The stage of novice is not related to the age of the student but rather to the knowledge and skill in the area of study. For example, learning how to give injections would be presented with the procedural guidelines, and the novice would then practice the skill. At this stage, much of the student's energy and attention is aimed at remembering the rules.

In the next stage, **advanced beginner**, the student can formulate principles that dictate action (Benner, 1984). For example, the advanced beginner grasps the rationale behind why different medications require different injection techniques. However, advanced beginners still lack the experience to know how to prioritize in more complex situations and might feel at a loss in terms of what they can safely leave out. They emphasize the rules and do not have the experience to adjust or adapt the rules to the situation. Both the advanced beginner and the novice stages require guidance. These stages parallel Cohen's professional development stage of dependence. Given the complexity of nursing practice and the range of clinical experiences, many new graduates can be described as advanced beginners.

Benner's stage 3, **competent**, is characterized by the ability to analyze problems and prioritize. The nurse has a solid grasp of the rules and principles. Movement from one stage to the next does not cross distinct boundaries. The nurse at this stage has had experience in a variety of clinical situations and can draw on prior knowledge and experience. The nurse has the ability to plan as well as to alter plans as necessary. Students who have the opportunity to have extended internships in a specialty area during their education can graduate entering this stage. Cohen's stage of dependence/mutuality corresponds to this stage.

Stage 4, **proficient**, refers to the professional who can grasp the situation contextually and as a whole. This nurse has a solid grasp of the norms as well as solid experiences that shed light on the variations from the norm. Incorporated into practice is the ability to test knowledge against situations that might not fit and to solve problems with alternative approaches. In this stage, the professional tests the rules and theories and looks at cases that can lead to developing alternative rules and theories. One might say that this is the stage when the professional begins to "break the rules" because he or she sees that the rules do not always apply.

Benner's final stage, **expert**, means the nurse has moved beyond a fixed set of rules. The expert has an internalized understanding grounded in a wealth of experience as well as depth of knowledge. The expert is always learning and always questioning using subjective and objective knowing. Benner (1984) proposes that not all nurses can obtain this stage.

Reality Shock

Professional socialization requires that the student learn the technology of the profession, learn to internalize the professional culture, find a personally and professionally acceptable version of the role, and integrate this professional role into all the other life roles (Cohen, 1981). Students are taught an ideal, theoretical, research-based practice that shelters them from the realities of the world where nursing practice consists not only of the theory and research but human emotion and response, along with policies and procedures of the particular working environment. This concept of idealism is important to the profession because it contributes to a high standard of professional practice. The perceived disconnect between education and practice is known as role discrepancy. Therefore, when students enter the real world, the culture of the classroom and the culture of clinical practice can seem worlds apart. The transition from nursing student to registered nurse is referred to as reality shock (Kramer, 1974).

Reality shock occurs when the perceived role (how an individual believes he or she should perform in a role) comes into conflict with the performed role (Catalano, 2009). Many new graduates experience this reality shock of knowing what to do and how to do it but encountering circumstances that prevent them from performing the role in that way (Blais, Hayes, Kozier, & Erb, 2005, p. 21). Role transition shock is the experience of moving from the known role of student to the role of practicing professional (Duchscher, 2009). Role conflict exists when a nurse cannot integrate the ideal, the perceived, and the actual performed role into one professional role. For many nursing students, role conflict occurs when they transition from the role of student to that of registered nurse (Pellico, Brewer, & Kovner, 2009). The new graduate moves from a perceived role of what the professional nurse is and does to the actual performed role where his or her actions and beliefs might be challenged.

The reality shock, or role transition shock, new graduates experience can be reduced to some extent. Schools of nursing have implemented opportunities for externships or prolonged preceptor clinical experiences with a professional nurse prior to graduation. Research (Ruth-Sahd, Beck, & McCall, 2010) shows how participation in extern programs eases the gap between education and practice. One goal of this experience is to help the student assimilate the role of the professional nurse just prior to graduation. The student can experience a more realistic view of clinical practice in the real world. As one student reported, "All the lectures and assignments in nursing school cannot compare with the application of

www CRITICAL THINKING QUESTIONS *

What do you think are the barriers to the process of professional socialization or formation? Do you think different environments might foster or hinder the process of professional socialization or formation? Do you think that personal characteristics of nurses might influence the process of professional socialization or formation? *

theory that this externship offered" (Ruth-Sahd et al., 2010, p. 83). Externships and preceptor clinical experiences can help nursing students begin the **role transition** from perceived role expectations to actual role expectations, thus easing the transition from student nurse to practicing professional.

Facilitating the Transition to Professional Practice

The American Association of Colleges of Nursing (AACN, 2008) lists the roles of the professional nurse as provider of care, designer/manager/coordinator of care, and member of a profession to facilitate the development of professional nursing values. The concepts of patient-centered care, interprofessional teams, evidence-based practice, quality improvement, patient safety, informatics, clinical reasoning/critical thinking, genetics and genomics, cultural sensitivity, professionalism, and practice across the life span in an ever-changing and complex healthcare environment are emphasized as the essentials of professional nursing education.

Professional socialization of nurses toward a profession that fully embraces caring for self and others reflects the internalization of what Roach (1991) refers to as "the five C's: compassion, competence, confidence, conscience, and commitment" (p. 132), representing a framework for human response from which professional caring is expressed. Caring as a core value of nursing represents the essence of the history of nursing and the foundation for the future (Watson, 1988).

The goal in the socialization of nurses today and for the future is to achieve caring with autonomy. To facilitate the socialization into the profession, hospitals offer formalized graduate nurse programs or internships that provide graduates with rotations through a number of clinical areas that include preceptor support. After the completion of such programs, new nurses gain a sense of belonging and can complete their socialization into the clinical workplace (McKenna & Newton, 2009). In addition to formal education, preceptors can assist students to develop skills of assertion, reflection, and critical thinking, which are needed to provide holistic, evidence-based care (Mooney, 2007). The challenge for the profession is capitalizing on the strengths of everyone and finding a means of accommodating all individuals as a way of maintaining the viability of the profession (Leduc & Kotzer, 2009). To meet this challenge, it is imperative that educators, students, and practitioners recognize and integrate the ANA *Code of Ethics* in both education and practice. The result will be a more adaptable work environment that nurtures each individual while achieving harmony and balance within the profession.

Conclusions: Reflective Professional Practice

Nursing education should be humanistic and caring, with caring experts as role models who contribute to the socialization of future generations of nurses and help them become caring experts in nursing practice. Through their research, Condon and Sharts-Hopko (2010) report that reflection can be an effective means of understanding human emotion and responses. One student stated, "I think the most important time is after the clinical training when I go home. I think about the information I get from the patient. What does it mean? What does it mean for the patient? I should connect to it" (Condon & Sharts-Hopko, 2010, p. 169). Regarding role development and socialization, it is important to remember that we learn what we live (Becker-Hentz, 2004).

Classroom Activity

Incorporate actual quotes from the nurses who were interviewed in Benner's book *From Novice to Expert* (1984) in class discussions to illustrate the differences between each of the stages: novice, advanced beginner, competent, proficient, and expert. This activity is simple but enlightening to students. www

References

American Association of Colleges of Nursing. (2008). *The Essentials of baccalaureate education for professional nursing practice*. Washington, DC: Author.

American Nurses Association. (2001). *Code of ethics for nurses with interpretive statements*. Washington, DC: Author.

American Nurses Association. (2004). *Scope and standards of practice*. Washington, DC: Author.

Becker-Hentz, P. (2004). *Understanding relationships: Learning what we live*. Unpublished manuscript.

Benner, P. (1984). *From novice to expert*. Menlo-Park, CA: Addison-Wesley.

Benner, P., Sutphen, M., Leonard, V., & Day, L. (2010). *Educating nurses: A call for radical transformation*. San Francisco, CA: Jossey-Bass.

Blais, K. K., Hayes, J. S., Kozier, B., & Erb, G. (2005). Socialization to professional nursing roles. In K. K. Blais, J. S. Hayes, B. Kozier, & G. Erb (Eds.), *Professional nursing practice: Concepts and perspectives* (4th ed.). Upper Saddle River, NJ: Prentice Hall.

Catalano, J. (2009). *Nursing now!* (5th ed.). Philadelphia, PA: F. A. Davis.

Cohen, H. A. (1981). *The nurse's quest for a professional identity*. Menlo-Park, CA: Addison-Wesley.

Condon, E., & Sharts-Hopko, N. (2010). Socialization of Japanese nursing students. *Nursing Education Perspectives, 31*(3), 167–169.

Duchscher, J. E. B. (2009). Transition shock: The initial stage of role adaptation for newly graduated registered nurses. *Journal of Advanced Nursing, 65*(5), 1103–1113. doi:10.1111/j.1365-2648.2008.04898.x

Hentz, P. B. (2009). Socialization of nurses: A historical view. In *Role development in professional nursing practice* (2nd ed.). Sudbury, MA: Jones and Bartlett.

Institute of Medicine. (2011). *The future of nursing: Leading change, advancing health*. Washington. DC: National Academies Press.

International Council of Nurses. (2006). *Code of ethics for nurses*. Retrieved from http://www.icn.ch/about-icn/code-of-ethics-for-nurses

Kramer, M. (1974). *Reality shock, why nurses leave nursing*. St. Louis, MO: Mosby.

Leduc, K., & Kotzer, M. (2009). Bridging the gap: A comparison of the professional nursing values of students, new graduates and seasoned professionals. *Nursing Education Perspectives, 30*(5), 279–284.

Massachusetts Department of Higher Education. (2010). *Nurse of the future: Nursing core competencies*. Retrieved from http://www.mass.edu/currentinit/documents/NursingCoreCompetencies.pdf

McKenna, L., & Newton, J. M. (2009). After the graduate year: A phenomenological exploration of how new nurses develop their knowledge and skill over the first 18 months following graduation. *Contemporary Nurse: A Journal for the Australian Nursing Profession, 31*(2), 153–162.

Mooney, M. (2007). Professional socialization: The key to survival as a newly qualified nurse. *International Journal of Nursing Practice, 30*, 75–80.

Ousey, K. (2009). Socialization of student nurses—the role of the mentor. *Learning in Health and Social Care, 8*(3), 175–184.

Pellico, L. H., Brewer, C. S., & Kovner, C. T. (2009). What newly licensed registered nurses have to say about their first experiences. *Nursing Outlook, 57*, 194–203.

Roach, M. S. (1991). Creating communities of caring. In National League for Nursing (Eds.), *Curriculum revolution: Community building and activism* (pp. 123–138). New York, NY: National League for Nursing Press.

Ruth-Sahd, L. A., Beck, J., & McCall, C. (2010). Transformative learning during a nursing externship program: The reflections of senior nursing students. *Nursing Education Perspectives, 31*(2), 78–83.

Watson, J. (1988). *Nursing: Human science and human care*. New York, NY: National League for Nursing Press.

Career Management and Care of the Professional Self

7

Luann M. Daggett

Sharon is a 23-year-old registered nurse (RN) who graduated from an associate's degree nursing program 3 years ago. Since graduation, she has worked at a large university-based hospital in a major metropolitan area. Her first assignment was in an oncology unit where she worked as a staff nurse for a year before transferring to the cardiovascular recovery unit. Sharon is an outstanding staff nurse, providing excellent care to her patients and working well as a member of the healthcare team. Her performance appraisals have been positive. Although Sharon would like to return to school for her baccalaureate degree, working rotating shifts with varying schedules has prevented her from taking classes.

Recently, there was an opening on her unit for an assistant nurse manager. Sharon hoped to be considered for the position and was disappointed when another nurse whom she considered less qualified got the position. Discussing the decision with her supervisor, Sharon asked why she had not been given the job. To her surprise, the supervisor replied, "Why, Sharon, I had no idea you were interested!" Sharon left the meeting feeling hurt, angry, frustrated, and devalued. She could not understand why all of her hard work had gone unnoticed (and unrewarded) by her supervisor. Although inconvenient, Sharon is thinking about changing jobs and moving to a new hospital in a different part of the city.

Key Terms and Concepts

- » **Career management**
- » Journaling
- » Core values
- » Mission statement
- » Success
- » Objectives
- » 5-year plan
- » Public speaking
- » Networking
- » Mentoring
- » Feedback
- » Lifelong learning
- » Burnout
- » Self-care
- » Life management

Learning Objectives

After completing this chapter, the student should be able to:

1. Describe the difference between an occupation and a career.
2. Articulate the importance of assuming a proactive role in managing your nursing career.
3. Set career goals and formulate objectives designed to meet the goals.
4. Describe specific strategies for increasing personal visibility within an organization.
5. Explain methods for obtaining feedback on personal performance.
6. Describe the effects of work-related stress on health and career longevity.
7. Articulate the importance of life management for optimal personal and professional health.

Sharon's story, unfortunately, is typical of the way many nurses approach their jobs. Career management is not a concept that is familiar to them. For many, nursing is still viewed as a calling or vocation rather than as a career that needs managing. Despite the increasing number of men entering nursing in the past few years, nursing is still a female-dominated profession, and women see career management as self-promotion. They are uncomfortable calling attention to their accomplishments, asking for recognition, or negotiating raises and promotions. As a result, many nurses do not receive the positive feedback, recognition, and career advancement opportunities that they deserve. Feeling chronically undervalued and unappreciated, nurses become burned out, change jobs, or leave the profession altogether.

Occupation vs. Career

Nursing as a career is as much a philosophical approach as it is a professional choice. The difference is whether one considers nursing an occupation or a career. Occupation is defined as (1) an activity that keeps a person busy or (2) one's job or employment (Oxford University Press, 1996). In comparison, a career is a course of professional life or employment that affords the individual opportunities for personal advancement, progress, or achievement (Miller, 2003). Some people view nursing as a job or an occupation, whereas others take the approach that nursing is a profession requiring a lifelong commitment. Table 7-1 compares attitudes toward nursing as either an occupation or a career. If you choose to view nursing as a professional career, you will behave differently than if you consider it as merely a job that is most likely temporary or a means to an end.

> **Whether one considers nursing a vocation, an occupation, or a career, it remains only one aspect of an individual's life and must not become all-consuming.**

A career is not something that is automatically conferred along with a college degree; it is a life choice that must be actively planned and pursued. A degree and a nursing license might be the ticket that gets you started on the journey, but without a destination, an itinerary, and a map, you will not travel very far. Like any important journey, a career requires research and planning; otherwise, you risk missing opportunities and critical milestones along the way. One should always assess the current location before planning future directions. Just as you track progress with a map while on a road trip, you should have a plan for managing your career, lest you find yourself wandering in the wilderness without making any true progress toward your career goals. **Career management** can be defined as a planned logical progression of one's professional life that includes clearly defined goals and objectives and a plan for achievement. Joel (2003) advises building a nursing

www. CRITICAL THINKING QUESTIONS ✳

Do you view nursing as a career or a job? What are your goals related to nursing? ✳

TABLE 7-1 Comparison of Attitudes: Occupation vs. Career		
Factor	**Occupation**	**Career**
Longevity	Temporary, a means to an end	Lifelong vocation
Educational Preparation	Minimal training that is required, usually associate degree	University professional degree program based on a foundation of core liberal arts
Continuing Education	Only what is required for the job or to get a raise/promotion	Lifelong learning, continuous efforts to gain new knowledge, skills, and abilities
Level of Commitment	Short-term, as long as job meets personal needs	Long-term commitment to organization and profession
Expectations	Reasonable work for reasonable pay; responsibility ends with shift	Will assume additional responsibilities, volunteer for organizational activities and community-based events

career cautiously and deliberately, laying each brick in a predetermined pattern. This requires careful consideration of what it is you like to do, what you are good at, where you would eventually like to be professionally, and what skills and education you will need to get there.

Common Myths and Misconceptions

Table 7-2 lists a number of common myths and misconceptions that many nurses hold. The attitude that one's supervisor is responsible for taking care of you is a common example of an employee's flawed thinking. Good works do not speak for themselves—mistakes speak for themselves, and they speak loudly and clearly. Quality patient care is an expectation of the nurse's job and generally goes unnoticed until either a mistake is made or a complaint is received. Your supervisor has many role responsibilities—looking out for your career is not them.

> **Your supervisor has many role responsibilities—looking out for your career is not one of them.**

Many nurses believe that because of the nursing shortage they will be guaranteed a job. In fact, a large number of students enter nursing programs thinking that they will always have job security. Although graduates of nursing programs generally have highly marketable skills, nursing positions are as

> ### TABLE 7-2   Common Myths and Misconceptions
>
> - If I work hard, I will be rewarded.
> - Good works speak for themselves.
> - It is my boss's job to recommend me for special assignments or promotion.
> - As a registered nurse, I will always have a job.
> - My hospital will look out for me.

susceptible to economic fluctuations as those in any other field. The nursing shortage does not mean job security; a nursing shortage usually leads to a proliferation of unlicensed assistive personnel that actually erodes the role of professional nurses. The notion that hospitals and healthcare agencies look out for the concerns of nurses is unrealistic. Whether operated for profit or not, healthcare facilities are businesses that are concerned with providing services to customers for a fee. If production costs exceed profits, adjustments must be made or the business will fold. Nursing care is expensive to provide, and thus, it is often targeted for cost reduction. Healthcare agencies operate in their own best interests, which might not coincide with the interests of the nursing staff.

It is our responsibility to manage our own careers. Your boss has other things to do than to follow your career. It is your responsibility to get the level of recognition that you need and to seek opportunities that will advance your own career. Passive, obedient behavior does not get you far in the real world and neither does sitting back waiting for others to look out for you. In the real world, you cannot afford to wait your turn for good things to happen—you have to make them happen.

Setting Personal Goals

The first step in career management is to know where you want to go professionally. Unless you have a clear understanding of the final destination, it is impossible to select the best route to follow to get there. If you set out on a trip without knowing your final destination, how can you possibly choose the best road to take to get there? This is probably the most difficult part of career management. A reasonable approach would be to consider which aspects of nursing are most appealing to you. Do you like the interaction of direct patient care, or do you prefer to direct others in providing care? Are you more comfortable in an acute care setting, or do you favor the stability of long-term care or rehabilitation settings? Do you like to teach others? Are you more at ease leading or following? Because professional activities always take place within the context of personal needs and responsibilities, it is important to consider what those might be as well.

For many of us, goal setting and visualizing a desired future are difficult tasks. At some point in our early education, we made the decision to become a nurse and set our sights on preparing for entrance into a nursing program. Then we focused on surviving the rigorous course of study and graduating. After graduation came the challenge of finding and adjusting to our first nursing position. Long-range goals were not something we gave much thought to until reaching a point where being a staff nurse was no longer exciting or challenging. At this point, many nurses decide to return to school to seek an advanced degree in nursing with little thought as to what exactly they wish to study or what they ultimately plan to do with an additional degree. They choose programs that are convenient or accessible, rather than searching for the right educational program to meet specific learning needs. Often they decide to apply to school because friends or colleagues are doing so, and they do not want to feel left behind.

The decision to return to school or make a major career change should never be made hastily; rather, it should occur after a period of careful introspection and discernment. Consideration should be given to issues such as the following:

- Personal values
- Professional values
- Family issues and responsibilities
- Lifestyle choices
- Economic factors
- Community and recreational involvement

Educational programs are demanding and costly—financially, psychologically, and socially. Returning to school requires commitment, not just from the individual who will be studying, but also from family members, friends, employers, and other people in one's social network. Likewise, job or career changes are stressful and have long-term effects on finances, personal happiness, and interpersonal relationships. These decisions should never be made casually or impetuously.

■ Journaling Techniques, Writing Objectives

Various exercises and books on values clarification are available in bookstores or on the Internet; however, one of the most effective means of introspection is journaling. **Journaling** is the process by which one sits down quietly on a daily or regular basis to think and record one's thoughts and ideas in a notebook. There are many suggested techniques for journaling; one useful method is to record three things—events, ideas, or thoughts—that were important to you that day. These can include things that happened at work or in your personal life. As you record your thoughts, be sure to include any particular insights that occur to you. It is important that you do this on a daily basis or at least five to six times a week. At the end of the week, review your journal entries, looking for themes or patterns in your writing. Be sure to write these observations. Once a month look back through your journal to assess the issues, ideas, or events that were important to you that month. Record your insights.

As you write, the emphasis should be on recording your thoughts as they occur to you. Grammar, spelling, sentence structure, and handwriting are not important. This journal is for your eyes only, and substance is more important than form. Some people are more comfortable writing fragments of sentences or making lists of their ideas, whereas others prefer the catharsis of writing pages of text. Either style is effective, whichever works best for you. The important thing is regularity. One's daily activities are like the fine stitches of a tapestry; examined close-up they are interesting but limited. By stepping back and looking at the details of one's life over a period of time, you see a more complete picture and gain a sense of the core values that give depth and meaning to life. **Core values** are those values that are most important to us, the values that define who we are as human beings. There must be congruence between what it is you value and what it is you do before satisfaction can be derived from one's work.

CRITICAL THINKING QUESTIONS ✳

What are your core values? Do you see congruence between what you value and your career? ✳

Once you have an appreciation of what is truly important to you, Covey (1989) recommends developing a personal mission statement that includes all of your life roles and the values that you attach to or express in those roles. A **mission statement** is a clear, concise statement of who you are and what you are about in life. It can be a powerful tool for helping you find meaning and give direction to your life. Until one understands what is truly important and essential to one's happiness in both the professional and personal arenas, it is impossible to plan a future or manage a career effectively. Understanding your values and life mission allows you to discern which professional activities provide you with a sense of accomplishment and reward. As you feel the need to grow professionally, it is important that you set goals and make choices based on core values instead of circumstance or whim. **Success** in life can be defined as doing what you want, where you want, and with the people you want to do it with. This implies balance within the various arenas of your life—professional, personal, social, and spiritual.

When you have decided on a direction for your professional career, it is essential that you can visualize clearly the outcome you desire. Covey (1989) believes that visualizing something organizes one's ability to accomplish it; one must begin with the end in mind. The more precisely you are able to visualize exactly what it is you desire, the more clearly you will be able to distinguish the steps it will take for you to achieve your goal. **Objectives** are specific measures that you will take in achievement of your goal. Writing objectives provides you with a plan on how you are going to get from where

TABLE 7-3 Career Goal: Family Nurse Practitioner

Goal: To become a certified Family Nurse Practitioner
Objectives:
- Contact university for program information and application materials.
- Schedule the Graduate Record Examination.
- Purchase the Graduate Record Examination study guide and review one chapter per week.
- Contact three professional sources for reference letters.
- Complete health information forms and schedule physical examination.
- Submit application materials before the fall deadline.
- Apply for financial aid.
- Make appointment with academic advisor to plan program of study.
- Register for classes.

you are to your desired future. Objectives should be specific and measurable, serving as milestones that mark your progress. Objectives must include a time frame for their accomplishment. Table 7-3 shows an example of a goal and its concomitant objectives for a nurse who wants to become a family nurse practitioner. It is clear from this example that one could realistically attain this goal by following the objectives in this plan. The more detailed and specific your objectives, the easier it will be to follow the steps required to reach your goal. The difference between people who are successful in life and those who only dream of success is the ability to visualize their dreams and complete the steps that connect their present with their future.

Although it is highly desirable to know one's ultimate professional goals, for many of us, it might be unrealistic to look that far into the future. That does not mean your career should proceed without a plan; rather, your plans may be more short term. Developing short-range goals such as where you would like to be in 5 years might be a more reasonable approach for you. Defining a **5-year plan** enables you to set clear objectives and follow specific steps on how to meet those objectives while allowing for flexibility in adjusting to changing life circumstances.

Career Management Strategies

Assessing your current position is a good place to begin managing your career. Are you engaged in work that is socially significant, challenging, rewarding, and fulfilling? Do you generally look forward to going to work and enjoy the time that you spend there? Do you like and respect the people with whom you work? Are the salary and benefits you receive for your work reasonable and sufficient to accommodate your lifestyle? Are there opportunities for advancement within your organization? If you cannot respond positively to these questions, you have two choices: Either stay where you are and work to improve the situation, or look for another position. Only you can make this decision, however; if your job situation is not working for you, it is up to you to do something about it.

Once you have decided that a job change is the right move for you, it is important that you set about finding a position that will meet your personal and professional needs. Knowing what you are looking for is vital to your success. A careful analysis of your old job—what you liked and disliked about the job and your role in creating and sustaining the situation—can help you avoid similar pitfalls in your next position. This is where journaling can be very useful in clearly defining your expectations.

If possible, never leave a job until you have a firm commitment from a new employer. Finding the perfect job is labor intensive and time consuming. Trying to do so when you are unemployed and facing financial hardship is almost impossible. The old adage "good jobs are hard to find" is very true. Many people hunt for prospective jobs in newspapers or visit Internet career websites. This strategy might be the best option if you are unfamiliar with the local job market or are relocating to a new area. Keep in mind, however, that most organizations first post position openings in house to allow their employees opportunities for advancement or lateral transfers. Because it can be difficult for outsiders to know about these openings, you might consider beginning your job search within your present organization. Along with contacting the human resources department for a listing of current job openings, it is important for you to begin networking and talking to people within your organization who might be able to help you advance your career goals. Your unit supervisor, other managers, or your nursing service administrator are all potential sources for leads. Even if there is not a current opening in the area you seek, expressing your interest to influential people puts you in mind if something becomes available.

If your job search takes you to unfamiliar territory, modern job hunting can be facilitated by technology. Most healthcare agencies have websites that post current position openings along with a description of the facility, the services it offers, and its mission statement and philosophy. You might also consider posting your résumé with an online health careers database where prospective employers can search for qualified employees. Because there is no control over who has access to your information, use caution in listing personal information in an online résumé. Alternatively, you might want to contact colleagues in a geographical locale by joining local chapters of a professional organization or registering for newsgroups or chat rooms to make professional contacts. Regardless of whether you choose to look internally or externally for job opportunities, creating a positive first impression of you and your work is exceedingly important.

■ First Impressions

First impressions—whether it is by telephone, letter of inquiry, résumé, email, or personal interview—begin with your initial contact with an organization. A favorable first impression creates a halo effect that lasts a long time. Likewise, it is very difficult to alter an initial negative impression, and the more negative the impression, the harder it is to change. You want to present yourself in such a way that people take you seriously and listen to what you have to offer. If your first contact is a written communication, either a letter of inquiry, résumé, or a job application form, be sure your writing conveys a true representation of who you are. Letters should always be typed and written clearly and concisely and be free of spelling, punctuation, and grammatical errors. Likewise, application forms should be typed or printed clearly using black ink. The information must be complete, accurate, and free of errors. If your written communication is sloppy or grammatically incorrect, the reviewer will assume that you are careless or uneducated. This is not the impression you want to convey to a prospective employer. Useful hints for résumé preparation can be found on various websites such as nursinglink.monster.com/benefits/articles/7394-7-best-resume-tips-for-nurses and www.nursing-exams.ca/blog/the-internets-best-resume-preparation-sites.

> **First impressions begin with your initial contact with an organization.**

If your first contact with an organization is a personal interview, you must prepare yourself for the interview and present yourself as a serious prospect. Dress professionally. For men this means a coat and tie and for women a business suit or dress. Regardless of your personal style, the goal is to look like you will belong in this organization; thus, be sure to dress appropriately. Arrive at least 5 minutes before your scheduled appointment time. Do your homework by learning as much as you can about the organization, including its philosophy and mission statement. Keep in mind that you will be interviewing the organizational representatives as much as they will be interviewing you; thus, come prepared with questions. During the interview, you will want to learn as much as possible about the job expectations and convey information about what you have to offer to the organization. Be prepared to discuss your strengths and limitations. It is customary not to inquire about salary or benefits until a job offer has been made. Employers typically interview several prospects before deciding on an individual, and salary is based on education and experience. There is usually a salary range for a given position, and thus, be prepared to negotiate if the initial offer is unacceptable. Even if the employer is unwilling to increase the quoted salary, you will at least learn whether you were offered the maximum allocated to the position for someone with your experience and background.

The better the job, the more competition you will have in applying for it; thus, find positive ways to separate yourself from other applicants. Preparation and a professional appearance are a good start, but you might need to do more to stand out from the crowd. Discuss not only your present qualifications, but share your plans for future professional growth or aspirations. The more you align yourself with the mission and goals of the organization, the more acceptable you will be to an employer. Follow an interview immediately with a written letter thanking the interviewer for his or her time and consideration of your application. This crucial step is often overlooked by applicants and can tip the balance in your favor.

Before concluding the interview, ask about the time frame for decision making about the position. If you know when the employer expects to choose a candidate and you have not been notified of your selection, you can follow up with a telephone call at the appropriate time. Even if you are not selected for this position, maintain your positive first impression by thanking the employer for interviewing you and asking to have your application kept on file so that you might be considered for future positions.

As stated previously, the interview is also a time for you to find out more about the organization. The American Association of Colleges of Nursing (AACN) has identified eight key characteristics or hallmarks that each nurse should consider when screening potential employers (AACN, 2002). To assess the practice environment of the organization, the AACN suggests that the nurse ask questions during the interview that relate to the following eight key organizational characteristics:

1. Does the potential employer manifest a philosophy of clinical care emphasizing quality, safety, interdisciplinary collaboration, continuity of care, and professional accountability?
2. Does the potential employer recognize the value of nurses' expertise on clinical care quality and patient outcomes?
3. Does the potential employer promote executive-level nursing leadership?
4. Does the potential employer empower nurses' participation in clinical decision making and organization of clinical care systems?
5. Does the potential employer demonstrate professional development support for nurses?
6. Does the potential employer maintain clinical advancement programs based on education, certification, and advanced preparation?
7. Does the potential employer create collaborative relationships among members of the healthcare team?
8. Does the potential employer utilize technological advances in clinical care and information systems?

Other information about the organization that might be of interest to the potential nurse employee during the interview is the RN vacancy and turnover rate, patient satisfaction scores, educational mix of nursing staff, average tenure of nursing staff, employee satisfaction scores, percentage of travel nurses utilized, key human resource policies, whether the nurses are unionized (if so, a copy of the contract), and the most recent Joint Commission report on the organization (AACN, 2002). The full white paper and summary brochure are available online.

Knowing the characteristics of the practice environment before you accept a position assists you in making the best decision possible. Making an informed decision about where to practice nursing, whether you are a new graduate or an experienced nurse, contributes to your long-term success and job satisfaction as a nurse.

> **www CRITICAL THINKING QUESTION ✶**
>
> What kind of first impression do you make when searching for a new position? ✶

Maximizing Your Visibility

Developing and managing a career is very different from merely showing up and doing your job. A career involves a commitment not just to the work of an employee but to the well-being of the entire organization. This means that your efforts extend beyond the care of your patients on your assigned nursing unit to assume responsibilities beyond those for which you were hired. Administering high-quality patient care is an important part of the nurse's role; however, this is only one aspect of the professional nursing role. If you wish to advance your career in a given institution, you must be seen as a committed member of that organization. To do this, you must be visible within the organization.

> **If you wish to advance your career in a given institution, you must be seen as a committed member of that organization.**

Remember the myth that good works speak for themselves. Nurses who show up on time, do their jobs well, and go home rarely come to the attention of influential people within the organization unless a problem occurs. Then, the nurses receive a lot of negative attention. Nurses and other employees who work the night shift are rarely if ever seen by hospital administrators and risk being invisible within the organization unless they purposely engage in activities that take place during normal business hours. Thus, how does one increase his or her visibility in a positive way?

Most hospitals and healthcare agencies provide some degree of self-governance within the organizational structure. Committees composed of physicians, nurses, and administrators assume important functions of governance such as ethics committees, research protocol review committees, patient care review committees (quality assurance), and others. Volunteering to serve on self-governance committees not only contributes to nurses' professional autonomy but also affords opportunities for you to be seen in a different light by people who can be helpful to you in your career. Similarly, most healthcare institutions are committed to supporting health-related community activities such as blood drives, fund-raising walks, and health fairs. These also provide opportunities for nurses to contribute to their community while getting to know people in other areas of their organization.

As a professional nurse, you represent your organization both in and out of the workplace. Volunteering to be a spokesperson for the organization can increase your visibility dramatically. **Public speaking** is a daunting task for many nurses who are otherwise fearless in their other professional activities. Most nurses would rather work double shifts, manage disasters, or care for multiple acutely ill unstable patients simultaneously than stand up in front of a group and deliver a speech. Unfortunately, it is hard to be a spokesperson for an organization without engaging in some public speaking. The higher in an organization you rise, the more you are going to be called on to speak in public. If you are comfortable speaking in front of others, it will be much easier for you to establish your authority and credibility with a group. The good news is that it is not only possible to become a skilled speaker but to enjoy that aspect of your professional nursing role. The bad news is that the only way to become comfortable being a public speaker is to speak in public.

If you are inexperienced or uncomfortable speaking before a group, start slowly. Begin by speaking out in a staff meeting or volunteering to do an in-service presentation for the staff on your nursing unit. Agree to chair a hospital committee, accept a leadership position in your professional nursing organization, or travel to local schools or colleges to recruit nurses for your institution. Soon you will be making presentations to community organizations, church groups, or schools. Developing this important skill will increase your poise and self-confidence, ensuring that your ideas will be heard.

Writing letters is a powerful tool to support others while increasing your own visibility within the organization. Writing letters to individuals who have done a good job or gone out of their way to help you, thanking them for their efforts, not only supports your colleagues but also ensures that you will receive similar high levels of cooperation in the future. By directing the letter to the supervisor while sending a copy to the individual, a powerful message is sent that has the secondary benefit of marking you as a team player. This strategy may seem manipulative and self-serving; however, members of an organization have an obligation to support each other. We must reframe our thinking to understand that by advancing the careers of our colleagues and ourselves we are in fact strengthening the organization.

Likewise, it is important to get letters of support for ourselves. Think of all of the times patients and family members have complimented you on the care they have received from you. Although it is always nice to know that your efforts are appreciated, would it not be nice if your supervisors were able to hear those comments? The next time you receive a verbal compliment, ask the person to put it in writing. Good work counts when someone sees it or knows about it. Try saying, "Thank you. I really appreciate you telling me that. I wish my boss could hear it. Would you mind putting that in writing?"

Most people respond positively and wonder why they had not thought to do it themselves.

Letters document your skills and validate your abilities. Save these letters and use them to get new jobs or promotions. Letters can be presented as samples of your work. Never leave a job without getting at least three letters of reference from supervisors and colleagues. If you are not immediately moving to another position, have the references addressed to "To Whom It May Concern." Often, if there is a gap in your employment, when you go to apply for a new position, the people who knew you before and who could attest to your work have retired or moved to other institutions themselves. These letters of reference are just as valid as those written currently by specific individuals.

Networking

The more people who know you and who know the quality of your work and what you have to offer, the more doors will be open to you and greater opportunities will come your way. **Networking** is the process by which you get to know people within your organization and within your profession. Networking is important because it allows people to know one another on a personal level, forging relationships that enhance communication and increase productivity. Networking creates a sense of belonging among members of an organization or professional group.

> The more people who know you and who know the quality of your work and what you have to offer, the more doors will be open to you and greater opportunities will come your way.

One of the best ways to network with other nurses is to join or become more active in your professional organization. By attending meetings, working on a committee, contributing to the newsletter, or speaking at an organizational function, you increase your professional contacts and enhance your reputation in your field. Attend regional or national conventions, join a panel discussion, or make a presentation. Be sure to send a copy of your speech to your supervisor and nursing service administrator so that they know that you are representing your organization well.

If you tend to shy away from meetings because you are uncomfortable in social situations where you might not know people, keep in mind that others probably feel the same way. Assume that you are going to be welcomed and accepted. Take on the role of welcoming other people and putting them at ease. Come prepared with small talk—topics that you can share comfortably with others. Keep abreast of developments in your field, controversial legislative proposals, news items, or amusing anecdotes. If you arrive at the meeting with ideas to share, it is much easier to strike up conversations with relative strangers. Occasionally, you might find that it is difficult to detach

TABLE 7-4 Getting the Most out of Meetings	
• Attend three meetings before deciding about a group: once to overcome your fear, once to learn about it, and once to decide if you like it. • Introduce yourself by giving your first and last name and telling something about yourself to get the conversation going. • Say your first and last name as you meet people. Even people who know you well or have met you before can have temporary amnesia for names.	• Wear your name tag on the right side so that people can see it when you shake hands. • Wear comfortable shoes and clothing; you might be standing for a while. • Plan your conversation ahead of time. Come prepared with small talk. • Keep your business cards handy; use them to leave a tangible reminder of who you are. • Relax and try to enjoy yourself. If you are uncomfortable, find someone who looks nervous and try to set that person at ease.

yourself from someone with whom you have started a conversation. If this is a concern, stand by the door and greet people as they arrive. Speak to them briefly before directing them to others or the refreshments. You will find you get to meet a lot of people for a short time and you will not have to worry about disengaging. Table 7-4 offers further hints on getting the most out of meetings. If you are still uncomfortable, give yourself an assignment: Stay for 1 hour, and speak to five people; then you can leave. You might find that you remain for the entire meeting and enjoy doing so. After one or two meetings, you'll arrive to a meeting of friends and colleagues rather than strangers. The informal conversations that take place at professional meetings can be more valuable to you and your career than the formal business of the group.

Mentoring

Just as we are responsible for developing and managing our own careers, we are obliged to encourage others to develop professionally as well. Too often nurses compete to maintain the status quo rather than supporting the advancement of colleagues. Nurses who choose to further their careers by returning to school for advanced degrees or seeking promotions are somehow perceived as a threat and are frequently discouraged or even sabotaged in subtle ways by their colleagues. There is a scarcity mentality in which another's progress is perceived as a loss in one's own status. This phenomenon has a detrimental effect on the profession as a whole.

Experienced nurses can usually recall other nurses who served as role models or mentors, providing leadership and guidance to them as they began their nursing careers or faced professional challenges. The relationships between new and experienced nurses take many forms and vary from friend and informal advisor to that of a formal contractual mentor. **Mentoring** has been defined as a developmental, empowering, and nurturing relationship that extends over time and in which mutual sharing, learning, and growth occur in an atmosphere of respect, collegiality, and affirmation (Vance & Olson, 1998). Ideally, all graduate nurses should be assigned mentors who work closely with them during the difficult transition between the student and staff nurse roles. A true mentor, however, is someone who is willing to maintain a long-term relationship, advising and guiding an individual as needed throughout the professional career.

Unfortunately, few organizations are able to provide formal mentors for all new employees. Mentorship, however, is such an important component of successful career management that individuals should actively seek out formal or informal mentors to guide and support them. Mentoring relationships can develop through networking as you meet and interact with colleagues who you respect and admire. When selecting a mentor, it is important to seek someone with whom it is easy to communicate and who has the time and interest to work with you to discuss various professional issues. A mentor is not just someone who offers advice, but someone who challenges your ideas and encourages you to strive for excellence.

> **KEY COMPETENCY 7-2**
>
> Examples of Applicable *Nurse of the Future: Nursing Core Competencies*
>
> Professionalism:
>
> Skills (S8g) Develops personal goals for professional development
>
> Attitudes/Behaviors (A4b) Values the mentoring relationship for professional development
>
> *Source:* Massachusetts Department of Higher Education (2010), pp. 13, 15.

Evaluating Your Performance

What do people really think of you and your work? Aside from asking a trusted colleague how he or she rates your performance professionally, you can either rely on the formal process of the performance appraisal done annually by your supervisor, or you can actively solicit feedback from others. Most people are creatures of habit and will continue behaviors that seem to have been effective in the past until someone informs them otherwise. It is difficult for us to directly observe the effects of our words or actions on another person. We must rely on the social mirror in which we see ourselves reflected through the responses of others. **Feedback** is information that we receive from others about the impact of our behavior on them; it allows us to view ourselves from another's perspective. Soliciting feedback from peers is one way to gain direct information on how people perceive our words, actions, and abilities. Feedback differs from advice in that it describes the effect of another's behavior on us. It does not include advice on changing that behavior; rather, it is up to the individual soliciting feedback to decide if change is warranted (Riley, 2004).

Feedback can be difficult to hear, especially if it is unexpectedly negative. Be sure that you truly want to hear the information you are asking another to give. If you want to receive only positive feedback, forget about asking people to be honest with you. It is risky asking others to jeopardize a relationship by divulging opinions that might not be welcomed. Riley (2004) recommends you take the following steps when you solicit feedback:

- *Get focused:* Ensure that you are not distracted by other issues and can give your full attention to the information you are receiving.
- *Allocate sufficient time:* Schedule enough time so that you can listen and reflect on the information without being rushed.
- *Understand the feedback:* Seek clarification or ask for repetition of information that is unclear.
- *Ask for guidance:* If the feedback indicates the need for a change in behavior, ask for advice or directions for change.
- *Show appreciation:* The person giving feedback has taken a big risk and made an effort to provide you with useful information. Thank him or her for the effort.
- *Think about the feedback:* Evaluate your behavior in light of this new information. Reflect on the implications and consider changes.

Asking for and receiving feedback, especially if it is negative, is a courageous act. Regardless of whether you choose to act on the information, it is important to know how others perceive you.

CRITICAL THINKING QUESTIONS ✳

Do you have the courage to ask for honest feedback? Do you have the courage to give honest feedback to a friend or colleague? How do you respond to negative feedback? ✳

The process of performance appraisal is a more formalized means of obtaining feedback on your professional activities. Performance appraisals are formal evaluations of employees by a superior, usually a manager or supervisor of some kind, comparing the employee's behavior with a set of standards (Tappan, 2001). When done correctly, the performance appraisal process can be a highly effective tool for motivating employees to continue high-level performance and to strive for even greater accomplishments. Too often, however, the process is perfunctory or, at worst, punitive, serving to discourage rather than reward employees. Optimally, a good manager collects data for the employees' annual reviews throughout the reviewing period, which is usually 1 year. Collecting anecdotal notes on incidents of positive performance as well as negative episodes helps to present a balanced picture of an individual's performance. Annual reviews are too often based on an employee's performance during the week or weeks immediately preceding the review, thus creating an artificial halo or horns effect (Table 7-5). To counter this possibility, it is important for you to take a proactive role in the process by providing your supervisor with accurate information about your performance and accomplishments throughout the reporting period.

Most organizations have a set time in the year when performance appraisals are conducted. Commonly, this takes place early in the calendar year and reflects employee performance during the previous 12-month period. Newer employees might be evaluated more frequently. Keeping in mind the

TABLE 7-5 Halo vs. Horns Effect	
Halo Effect: Overrating an employee's total performance based on a single positive event. • Strong social skills and a pleasant personality masking poor performance • Rating based on past positive performance rather than current observations • History of mediocrity punctuated by a single recent stellar performance	• Friendship or shared interests with the manager Horns Effect: Underrating an employee's total performance based on a single negative event. • Positive performance interrupted by a serious error committed recently • Consistent good work but disagrees with manager • Associating with substandard peers • Poor physical appearance in dress, manners, or hygiene

fact that your supervisor has more important things to do than to track your career, you can assist in this process by providing your supervisor with information that you believe should be included in your performance appraisal such as the following:

• Continuing education courses, workshops, seminars, or formal programs of study attended
• Special projects completed, such as preparing teaching materials, in-service educational programs, or developing patient care policies
• Special assignments carried out in other areas of the organization
• Awards, letters of commendation, or recognition received for your professional activities
• Examples of instances when you performed above and beyond what was expected or required
• Plans for further education and/or professional development activities in the next year

Most managers appreciate this type of assistance and welcome having the information at their disposal as they fill out the appraisal forms. If you have made serious errors or committed a recent professional faux pas, this might still show up on your evaluation; however, you are more likely to receive a balanced review.

Once the performance appraisal evaluation form has been completed, most organizations require a conference between the employee and supervisor to discuss the review. If your unit manager does not already do this, request a meeting at a time that is convenient for both of you when you can be relatively free from interruptions. For many of us, these meetings conjure up painful memories of being called to the principal's office in school to be reprimanded for some infraction of the rules—not a pleasant association. Keep in mind, however, that the purpose of the meeting is to discuss the review ratings, identify strengths and limitations, and brainstorm activities that will contribute to your professional growth. Motivation is the goal. Your role in the meeting is to listen carefully to what is being said, whether or not you agree with the findings. If the review is positive, the discussion will be easy for both sides. If the review is disappointing, it is important that you remain neutral and not react negatively, making a difficult situation worse.

Coping with Adversity

We never like to hear negative things about our performance, especially if the comments are unexpected or unwarranted. Responding to a negative performance appraisal with anger or defensiveness is not going to advance your career. Whether or not you agree with the appraisal, the report reflects your supervisor's perceptions of your performance, which might or might not be accurate. Either way, you have a problem. Remember, your role in this meeting is to listen to feedback. Your career is at stake here; thus, you do not have the luxury of getting angry and storming out of the meeting. If you become emotional or feel that you might lose control, ask for time to reflect on the report and schedule another meeting to continue the discussion.

Be careful what you sign and know what your signature implies. Does it mean that you concur with the performance appraisal or only that you have received the report? If your supervisor insists that you sign the report, it is appropriate that you write in what your signature indicates (e.g., "signature reflects receipt of report only, not concurrence with findings" or "see attached response"). It is strongly recommended that you take time to distance yourself and gain perspective about a negative performance appraisal before responding either in person or in writing. You might want to validate the findings with your mentor or trusted colleagues.

If you believe the findings are inaccurate, you need to explore how your supervisor reached those conclusions. This can be accomplished only by having a frank discussion with him or her about your performance and how it varies from the expectations. This discussion should afford you an equal opportunity to describe your point of view. If you are concerned about the emotional level of the meeting, you can request that a disinterested third party attend to mediate. You can do a great deal to diffuse a potentially hostile meeting by acknowledging your role in creating the situation: "Given the information you have, I can see where you might draw that conclusion," or "I see where you might think that." This does not mean that you agree with your supervisor's statements but allows for the possibility that the supervisor's impressions might be accurate given limited or erroneous information. If the appraisal is inaccurate, you should present specific facts that contradict the findings and request that the ratings be changed. It is hoped the outcome of the interview is that you each have a greater appreciation for the other's perspective and expectations.

If your supervisor disagrees or is unwilling to change the ratings, you should then attach a typewritten page of comments to the report stating factually the events from your point of view. Be sure to keep copies of all documents for your personal records. At the end of the meeting, if you are still dissatisfied or believe that you have been treated unfairly, you need to seek redress by following the chain of command in your organization. Consult your employee handbook or policy manual for information on how to appeal an erroneous performance appraisal. As much as it might give temporary relief, if would be a grave mistake to go outside the chain of command and storm the nursing administrator's office. At some point, you will have to decide how far the matter is worth pursuing. If you are unable to resolve your differences with the supervisor, it might be time to look for another position either within the organization or at a different agency.

Given the numbers and types of decisions that nurses are required to make daily, it is practically inevitable that mistakes will be made in the clinical area. Fortunately, most errors can be corrected without patients experiencing adverse effects. Whenever a mistake is made, however, it is important that the nurse notify the patient and family if appropriate, the supervisor, the physician, and any other members of the healthcare team who might be concerned. Every organization has a procedure for documenting errors or events that cause a risk of injury or possible litigation. The manner in which mistakes are handled on a unit is indicative of the relationships among the individuals working there. Errors are generally symptoms of more important problems that must be addressed. Although errors are obviously undesirable, they create opportunities for learning as well as developing policies and procedures for preventing their occurrence in the future. As a professional, you should always be honest and take responsibility for your actions. When an error is made, admit that you did something wrong, apologize, and do whatever is necessary to either correct the error or mitigate the consequences. Take steps to ensure that similar mistakes are prevented. Making excuses or blaming others only makes an adverse situation worse. Hospital administrators and managers would much prefer honest employees who make mistakes and take steps to correct the situation than individuals who lie or attempt to cover up errors that might lead to costly litigation later.

Commitment to the Profession

Nursing is more than just a job; it is a profession and requires serious commitments from its members. One of the characteristics of a profession is a commitment to **lifelong learning**. Undergraduate nursing programs,

> **Nursing is more than just a job; it is a profession and requires serious commitments from its members.**

www **CRITICAL THINKING QUESTIONS** ✳

Do you plan to be a part of a professional organization after graduation? Why or why not? What do you anticipate will be your level of involvement? ✳

KEY COMPETENCY 7-3

Examples of Applicable *Nurse of the Future: Nursing Core Competencies*

Professionalism:

Knowledge (K4b) Describes the role of a professional organization in shaping the practice of nursing; (K8a) Understands the responsibilities inherent in being a member of the nursing profession

Skills (S8i) Assumes professional responsibility through participation in professional nursing organizations

Attitudes/Behaviors (A8a) Recognizes need for personal and professional behaviors that promote the profession of nursing

Source: Massachusetts Department of Higher Education (2010), pp. 13, 15.

regardless of whether they are diploma, associate degree, or baccalaureate degree programs, are designed to prepare individuals to function in entry-level nursing positions under the supervision of more experienced nurses. Successful completion of the NCLEX-RN examination and qualifying for state licensure imply that you have met the minimal requirements to practice safely as an RN. Many nurses say that their real education began not in school, but on their first job. Nursing is one of the most rapidly developing professional disciplines. It is impossible for any educational program to provide nurses with all of the information that they need to know to practice over the course of a lifetime. The best that education can do is to provide the basics while teaching students how to learn and how to access information. It is up to the individual to continue to develop professionally by acquiring new skills and knowledge.

As members of a professional discipline, we have an obligation to support our profession. Our responsibilities do not end at the close of our shift; we are responsible for keeping abreast of developments in the field and ensuring that the care our patients receive is the highest quality and most current treatment available. It is also important for nurses to have a voice in health care and related issues. The public considers nurses to be the most trusted of all healthcare providers, yet few people can describe exactly what nurses do. The media more often portray nurses as sex objects than as competent clinical practitioners. The media rarely view nurses as experts in health-related issues. It is vital that we articulate our role and educate elected officials and the public about the valuable contribution that nurses make. Nurses should take every opportunity to promote their profession.

One important way to do this is by joining professional organizations. Whatever your clinical interests, there is a professional organization that supports them. By joining an organization, you have access to journals, continuing education offerings, professional meetings, and a network of other nurses who share your interests. The American Nurses Association and its state chapters are the recognized voice of nursing in the United States, although only 10% of registered nurses are members. This means that the vast majority of nurses are not heard or consulted when public policies concerning healthcare issues are discussed. Organizations such as the National League for Nursing and the American Association of Colleges of Nursing have an important role in setting educational standards and ensuring that those standards are met. These organizations depend on the contributions of members who volunteer their time, energy, and support to advance the goals of nursing.

Commitment to Ourselves

As nurses, we have the privilege of interacting with people during the most significant moments of their lives—birth, death, and times of illness and injury. In the course of our work, we routinely engage in activities that affect the lives of others at times when they are most vulnerable and in need of caring professionals. Our work matters, our actions count. As a result, the public views nurses very positively. We have the reputation of being honest, caring, reliable, concerned, and approachable. Although we enjoy the status of being members of this prestigious profession, there is a downside to it.

Nurses, unfortunately, are particularly vulnerable to stress and burnout. Nursing is publicly perceived to be not just a profession, but a vocation to which members pledge lifelong commitment. There is an assumption that nurses should be readily available at all times to listen to problems and discuss health issues even when they are not on the job. Nurses are caring and approachable; therefore, people often seek out nurses for advice and treatment where they would never presume to impose on a physician outside of a working situation. Family members frequently assume that nurses will step forward and volunteer to care for sick or elderly relatives simply because they are nurses, regardless of their professional career responsibilities—and we respond as expected. Men and women who are attracted to the nursing profession tend to be "people pleasers" who are generous with their time and resources. They often have trouble saying "no" to requests for assistance. Being needed makes us feel valued and important. Although there is nothing inherently wrong with this trait, it does open us up to abuse and disregard for our personal needs.

■ Stress in the Work Environment

Nursing is demanding work. Nurses work long hours in high-stress environments caring for clients whose conditions are often unstable. The decisions nurses make have serious implications for the health and lives of their patients. Our clients are sick and family members are stressed by the hospitalization, so nurses regularly interact with people who are not at their best. Hospitals are fast-paced, intense work environments where situations change rapidly and nurses must respond quickly and accurately to a multitude of competing demands. The nursing shortage further complicates the situation in that many units are chronically understaffed. There is often a rapid turnover of staff members and a lack of experienced nurses. Many hospitals have implemented 12-hour shifts for nurses, and although this scheduling offers certain advantages, it creates a lifestyle that leaves little time for personal self-care activities. A 12-hour shift easily stretches to 14 or more hours when considering report time, paperwork, and commuting. The work is physically and mentally taxing and, at the end of the day, nurses arrive home with little time or energy left to care for their families, let alone themselves.

Nurses in general are a resilient group capable of dealing with work-related stress and thriving in the demanding healthcare environment. Unfortunately, it is easy for our professional lives to overrun our personal lives with the result that we lack a positive balance between work, home, and personal interests. Maintaining this pace for prolonged periods can have untoward effects on one's health, relationships, and overall quality of life. The effects of stress are multiple and varied and can affect the following:

- Feelings, including anxiety, irritability, fear, anger, and moodiness
- Thoughts, including self-criticism, difficulty concentrating and making decisions, forgetfulness or mental disorganization, preoccupation with the future, repetitive thoughts, and fear of failure
- Behaviors, including crying, acting impulsively, nervous laughter, snapping at friends, teeth grinding or jaw clenching, smoking, alcohol or drug abuse
- Physical sensations, including headaches, tight muscles, cold or sweaty hands, back or neck problems, difficulty sleeping, stomach aches, colds and infections, fatigue, rapid breathing or pounding heart, or trembling (Sikorsky & Malaney, 2007)

The means by which we deal with stress become very important. All too often, nurses use coping methods that are detrimental to their overall well-being. Lack of exercise and poor nutrition increase the deleterious effects of stress. Addictive behaviors such as smoking, overeating, self-medication, and substance abuse can develop. Some nurses are attracted to needy people and enter into toxic relationships. The results of these negative behaviors can lead to physical illness, increased risk of injuries, and burnout.

■ Burnout: An Occupational Hazard

Burnout occurs when nurses can no longer cope with the stresses and strains of professional nursing and choose to leave the profession to seek employment elsewhere. Symptoms of burnout include physical, psychological, and emotional exhaustion; lack of enthusiasm and decreased interest in work-related activities; and depression, negativism, and anger. Nurses experiencing burnout withdraw emotionally from both clients and coworkers. They might experience an increase in physical symptoms that results in absenteeism. Nurses who continuously give of themselves physically and emotionally without sufficient effective rest and recreation eventually become depleted and develop burnout. Savvy employers recognize this danger and implement measures and programs designed to identify nurses at risk and intervene to prevent burnout from occurring. All too often,

> Nurses who continuously give of themselves physically and emotionally without sufficient effective rest and recreation eventually become depleted and develop burnout.

however, this workplace crisis is overlooked until nurses resign in frustration. Ultimately, we as nurses are responsible for our own physical and mental health. It is imperative that nurses understand the effects of workplace stress and the symptoms of burnout to prevent this occupational hazard.

■ Stress Management and Self-Care

To survive and thrive in the profession, nurses must be as attentive to their own needs as they are to the needs of their clients. **Self-care** means acknowledging and meeting your own physical, psychological, social, and spiritual needs. It means caring for yourself before you care for others, not after you have tended to everyone else. In an emergency, airline attendants always advise individuals traveling with young children to place the oxygen masks over their own faces before placing them on the children. We cannot help others if we are starved and depleted ourselves.

Individuals are happiest and function at their best when there is balance in their lives. Meeting one's physical needs is a good place to begin. Nurses understand the importance of nutrition on wound healing and illness recovery in their clients; therefore, they must similarly nourish their own bodies with healthy, balanced, nutritious meals for optimal performance. Problems with overweight and obesity should be addressed through programs of sound nutrition and planned exercise. One of the cruel ironies of nursing is that, although the work is physically demanding, it is not particularly good exercise. Nurses must make time in their busy schedules for aerobic activities such as walking, jogging, swimming, tennis, spinning, bicycling, or dancing in addition to basic weight training to strengthen muscles and build stamina. Habits such as smoking, consuming alcohol, and taking nonprescription medications must be avoided.

Rest is as important as diet and exercise in dealing with stress. Most people require a minimum of 8 hours of sleep at night. Nurses who rotate shifts or work nights often have problems sleeping during the day and fail to get adequate rest. Sleep aids can offer temporary relief; however, most sleep-inducing medications cause dependency and have side effects. Melatonin is a naturally occurring hormone that induces sleep and can be purchased over the counter in drugstores or health food stores. To date, melatonin has not been shown to have negative side effects when taken as directed for short-term relief of sleeplessness. The most effective sleep aid, however, is good nutrition, physical exercise, and an environment conducive to rest and relaxation.

Fulfilling psychological, social, and spiritual needs is as important to one's well-being as taking care of physical needs. Unfortunately, these are often sacrificed when time and energy are at a premium. Whether one considers nursing a vocation, an occupation, or a career, it remains only one aspect of an individual's life and must not become all-consuming. Time away from the job is as important as time spent on the job. Socializing with people we

KEY COMPETENCY 7-4

Examples of Applicable
*Nurse of the Future: Nursing
Core Competencies*

Professionalism:

Knowledge (K8b) Recognizes
the relationship between
personal health, self renewal,
and the ability to deliver sustained quality care

Source: Massachusetts Department
of Higher Education (2010), p. 15.

love and who contribute positively to our lives is crucial; however, not all relationships with friends or family members are healthy. When you regularly leave social encounters feeling worse than before, it is time to reevaluate that relationship. By all means, address interpersonal issues and resolve conflict whenever possible; seek counseling if necessary, but if the relationship remains toxic, you must limit your exposure to that person. We are social beings who rely on each other for validation, stress relief, and sheer enjoyment of life. Without positive social relationships, we lose perspective and problems can rapidly become overwhelming.

Human beings naturally strive to find meaning in their existence. All of us have spiritual needs, but for nurses who deal with life and death on a daily basis, spirituality becomes particularly important as we struggle to come to terms with these issues. Belief in a higher being, in a planned universe, and in a rich afterlife helps provide context for the joys and tragedies we witness regularly. Regardless of one's personal spiritual beliefs, participation in prayer, religious services, and fellowship with others sharing your beliefs is important to maintain balance and perspective.

■ Time Management Is Key to Life Management

For most of us, the greatest challenge and key to life balance is time management. Each of us has 24 hours a day, 168 hours per week, or 8,760 hours per year to manage. If a third of your daily allotment is spent sleeping and another third working, that leaves only 8 hours to attend to all of the other activities of daily living—shopping, meal preparation, dining, housekeeping, laundry, errands, childcare, carpooling, commuting, and so on. Precious little time remains at the end of the day for quiet reflection, recreation, reading, relaxing, or relationships; yet, these are the activities that are vital to restoring our physical and mental health. The more activities we cram into our day, the more the stress builds. It is impossible to do it all! Yes, we can have it all—career, friends, family relationships, children, home—we just might not be able to have it all at the same time or manage it all by ourselves.

Many people approach the challenge of time management by attempting to become more organized, employing to-do lists, daily planners, or personal assistive devices to gain control over multiple demands for time and attention. These strategies can help you organize your activities, but they cannot add hours to the day. An alternative approach to time management is life management. **Life management** entails determining what is truly important to you and making positive choices about how, where, and with whom you spend your precious hours. Life management means letting go of the minutiae that clutter our lives and sap our strength. It involves simplifying our environments, our commitments,

> **Life management entails determining what is truly important to you and making positive choices about how, where, and with whom you spend your precious hours.**

and our relationships to eliminate the physical and psychological baggage that weighs us down.

The popular press abounds with books written by life coaches and time management specialists with suggestions on how to identify your values, formulate personal mission statements, and set priorities that allow you to incorporate the relationships and activities that nourish and enrich your life into your schedule. Take advantage of whatever tools are available to you to learn to put into place the people and systems that assist you to accomplish that which is truly important.

> **www CRITICAL THINKING QUESTION** *
>
> Think about what it is that is truly important to you. Do the choices you make about how, where, and with whom you spend your time reflect what is important to you? *

Conclusion

As nurses, our professional lives are both challenging and rewarding. Simply by introducing yourself as a nurse, you are invited into the lives of others in a way that rarely happens in other disciplines. People entrust you with the most intimate details of their lives and literally place their lives and the lives of their loved ones in your hands. On a daily basis, you have the opportunity to make a difference in the life of another human being. Few professions offer this level of interaction. This is, at the same time, a rare privilege and an awesome responsibility. As members of a widely respected profession, we must keep in mind the responsibility that we bear and strive to uphold continuously the standards of excellence that our profession holds.

One crucial aspect of this responsibility lies in caring for ourselves both personally and professionally. We must attend to our own needs first so that we can address the needs of our clients and of our profession. This chapter has discussed the importance of career management, life management, and personal self-care. As individuals make the decision to enter the nursing profession, they also choose whether nursing, for them, will be an occupation or a career. The future of nursing depends on members caring for themselves and choosing to approach nursing as a lifelong profession. We hope that you will choose wisely.

Classroom Activity: Nursing School Survival Game

Before class the instructor will prepare the board game. Spaces on the board will reflect self-care activities and give instructions for moving forward or backward depending on whether the activity reflected in the space promotes self-care or is detrimental. Divide students into small groups to play the Nursing School Survival Game. Students roll the dice to determine how many spaces to move. As they move around the board, they will progress from nursing school admission to second semester, third semester, fourth semester, and then graduation.

As the groups land on different spaces, take time to discuss the self-care activity and why it will help them to be successful in nursing school. Activities might include things such as buying a planner to get organized, reading assignments before class, finding a study group, getting regular exercise, eating nutritious meals,

and employing specific stress management techniques. This game is a good one to use at the beginning of the first semester to help students get to know one another as well as discuss ways in which students can begin using self-care strategies from the very beginning of their nursing school career.

Spaces on the board may alternately reflect categories if verbal questions will be asked during the game. If this approach is used, the group will answer questions about self-care categories to progress around the board. Another approach to this game that is fun is to have different colored pieces of paper labeled as categories of self-care questions on the floor, creating a game board effect and letting the students (either alone or in groups) move around the "game board" as they answer questions related to self-care. www.

References

American Association of Colleges of Nursing. (2002). *White paper on the professional practice setting*. Retrieved from http://www.aacn.nche.edu/Publications/positions/hallmarks.htm

Covey, S. R. (1989). *The 7 habits of highly effective people*. New York, NY: Simon & Schuster.

Joel, L. A. (2003). Career management. In L. A. Joel (Ed.), *Kelly's dimensions of professional nursing* (9th ed.). New York, NY: McGraw-Hill.

Massachusetts Department of Higher Education. (2010). *Nurse of the future: Nursing core competencies*. Retrieved from http://www.mass.edu/currentinit/documents/NursingCoreCompetencies.pdf

Miller, T. W. (2003). Work versus career. In T. W. Miller (Ed.), *Building and managing a career in nursing*. Indianapolis, IN: Sigma Theta Tau International.

Oxford University Press. (1996). *The Oxford English dictionary*. New York, NY: Oxford University Press.

Riley, J. B. (2004). Feedback. In J. B. Riley (Ed.), *Communication in nursing* (5th ed.). St. Louis, MO: Mosby.

Sikorski, E., & Malaney, K. (2007). Personal and financial health. *Vermont Nurse Connection, 10*(3), 9.

Tappan, R. M. (2001). Individual evaluation procedures. In R. Tappen & C. Lynn (Eds.), *Nursing leadership and management concepts and practice* (4th ed.). Philadelphia, PA: F. A. Davis.

Vance, C., & Olson, R. (1998). *The mentor connection in nursing.* New York, NY: Springer.

Professional Nursing Practice and the Management of Patient Care

The Healthcare Delivery System and the Role of the Professional Nurse

8

Sharon Vincent

Perhaps you wonder why hospitals are called healthcare delivery systems and not just hospitals, or why nurses are referred to as professional nurses and not just nurses? This chapter explores what the healthcare delivery system means to us and some of the roles nurses play that define what it means to be a professional nurse. Various models of nursing care delivery are discussed so that the graduate nurse possesses a greater understanding of the healthcare delivery environment. The method used to assign staff nurses and technicians might seem like a distant concept at this moment, but as a baccalaureate entry-level nurse, you could be making assignments soon after graduation.

All nurses today are managers. Registered nurses (RNs) manage the care of specific groups of patients, perform care themselves, direct others to provide care, and collaborate with other healthcare providers. Nurses must know how to delegate, supervise, evaluate, motivate, and communicate with other disciplines, nurses, and unlicensed personnel. Nurses must also lead teams. In the management of care, each nurse directs the nursing care within a delivery setting to protect the clients, significant others, and healthcare personnel.

Learning Objectives

After completing this chapter, the student should be able to:

1. Describe how health care is delivered and how the system is changing.
2. Describe nursing care delivery models.
3. Analyze factors that affect collaboration in the healthcare delivery system.
4. Analyze the role of the professional nurse.
5. Describe the advocacy role of the professional nurse.
6. Explain how effective delegation can benefit both the client and the healthcare delivery system.
7. Identify the need for consultation and collaboration with other healthcare providers.
8. Describe the importance of continuity of care and interdisciplinary collaboration between healthcare providers.
9. Discuss the need for continuous quality improvement in the provision of patient care.

The professional nurse uses critical thinking skills to assess clients and to evaluate the expertise of nursing staff when making assignments. The nurse's role encompasses collaboration in the continuity of care from admission to discharge and rehabilitation. This chapter clearly defines some of the concepts that are needed for the entry-level nurse to maintain safe and competent entry-level nursing practice.

Healthcare Delivery System

The **healthcare delivery system** has changed profoundly over the past several decades for many reasons. Population shifts (demographic changes), cultural diversity, the patterns of diseases, advances in technology, and economic changes have all affected the practice of nursing. Population changes affect delivery of health care. Health care is needed now more than in the past because the population is growing, the composition of the population is changing, birth rates are decreasing, and the life span is lengthening. People older than 85 years of age, who often require health care for chronic conditions, make up one of the fastest-growing segments of the population: The number was 34 times larger in 1999 than in 1900 (Smeltzer, Bare, Hinkl, & Cheever, 2010). More senior citizens, many of whom are women, are a factor in health care because of the healthcare resources they consume.

Also, a significant portion of the population now resides in urban areas, with a steady influx of ethnic minorities. Homeless persons, including homeless families, are on the rise. Cultural diversity increases as people from different nationalities enter the country. The professional nurse must know how to provide for the diverse needs of people from varied cultural backgrounds. It is projected that by 2030, racial and ethnic minority groups could approach 50% of the population of the United States (Smeltzer et al., 2010). Nursing care must be sensitive to cultural differences. Being culturally aware within the healthcare delivery system helps the nurse avoid imposing personal value systems when the patient has a different point of view.

In the last 50 years, evolving patterns of diseases have brought significant changes to the healthcare delivery system. Diseases such as tuberculosis, acquired immunodeficiency syndrome (AIDS), and sexually transmitted infections are increasing. Because of the widespread inappropriate use of antibiotics, an increasing number of infectious agents are becoming resistant to antibiotic therapy. Obesity is now a major health challenge as are its comorbidities—hypertension, coronary heart disease, diabetes mellitus, and cancer.

Also, the improvement in techniques for trauma and acute care means that more people are living decades longer with chronic conditions. Technology has boosted surgical and diagnostic service areas so that patients can receive sophisticated treatment on an outpatient basis. Communication techniques provide a means to train providers and deliver health care to remote countries or islands by satellite. The Veterans Administration has a program of post-traumatic stress disorder and telemental health for veterans in tribal reservations and on remote islands. Telehealth uses electronic communications and information technology to provide and support health care when distance separates participants.

In the past, the healthcare delivery system was mainly hospital based with an acute care focus. Currently, many clients stay in the hospital for a short time, just 23 hours. Other facets of current healthcare delivery include hospital testing and precertification, telecommunications, home health, mobile vans, and mall clinics. Historically, as healthcare costs became alarmingly high, cost containment mandated by Congress initiated the beginning of diagnosis-related groups (DRGs), a plan to cut costs related to Medicare reimbursement. Treatment became focused on cost and profit, and the quality of nursing care declined. Nurses experienced work-related stress and burnout, and many left nursing as hospitals operated with fewer resources. Because of cost constraints and a shortage of available nurses, cross training became a common practice. For example, one nurse could be cross trained to work in the operating room and the postanesthesia care unit and thus possess the specialized skills to work in either unit when the need arises (Blais, Hayes, Kozier, & Erb, 2006). Nurses are trained to fill two departments or more because fewer nurses are being hired as a result of cost constraints.

Nurses are challenged more than ever to provide quality care with fewer resources. Two major issues are at the forefront of healthcare delivery: cost containment and access to care. Reductions in healthcare personnel have been a major challenge to providing quality care in an era of restructured resources. Many people have limited or no access to health care. Fewer patients are covered by insurance, and many have lower percentages of coverage, copayment problems, or no insurance coverage at all. The uninsured segment of the population is increasing: About 40 million Americans are estimated to be uninsured at a time, and 60 million Americans are without health insurance for a portion of the year (Blais et al., 2006). Many more are underinsured, thus limiting them from receiving health care.

The *chain of command* refers to the hierarchy of authority and responsibility in an organization. Line authority is a type of authority in traditional healthcare delivery systems in which the supervisor directs activities of employees he or she supervises. A chain of command allows employees to understand their tasks and to manage supervisory relationships within the organization. This structure provides an avenue for reporting issues that need management's attention. Nursing students should follow chain of command, first with nursing instructors and then school program directors. Organizational charts with chain of command illustrate flow of responsibility from staff nurse to nurse managers and on up to the chief nursing officer. This is the centralized/decentralized approach (Smeltzer et al., 2010).

Other models of healthcare delivery are emerging as organizations face increasing unpredictability and the need for change. Healthcare organizations (HCOs) are examples of complex systems. The term **complex adaptive systems (CASs)** refers to a collection of individual agents who are free to act in ways not totally predictable and whose actions are interconnected so that one action changes the context for other agents or units (Wilson & Holt, 2001). A CAS is highly adaptive and is characterized by self-organization, emergence of new patterns or behaviors, and distributed rather than centralized control. Patterns and behaviors enable understanding of CASs. Plsek and Wilson (2001) advocate applying CAS concepts to organizational structure. Such application to healthcare organizations would describe a zone of complexity in which CASs range from adaptability of high order to an area of emergence, with the ability to adapt to different conditions (Butts & Rich, 2011). One unit or agent can change the order of behavior, and this change does not necessarily follow a linear hierarchy structure.

In HCOs, the CAS implications are that hospitals are examples of high-order complex systems, and they typically contain systems embedded within systems. New models of organizational development are needed to understand the dynamic and fast-paced unpredictability of healthcare delivery. These new models must replace outdated ones, including models of organizational development and change based on linearity, vertical organization, hierarchical decision making, and controlled change strategies, which are outmoded and no longer work for contemporary HCOs.

Complexity science offers new mental models. Complexity science is a vehicle for change and also creates a lens through which we can understand organizations and change. Mental models are generalizations we make about reality that form patterns that organize how we understand the world. Healthcare professionals must begin to abandon linear models, accept unpredictability and creativity, and respond to emerging opportunities (Plsek & Wilson, 2001). For example, nurses can adopt a new paradigm of complexity of human physiology and can then provide more individualized care that augments adaptive components of the human body.

As organizations struggle to be more responsive to issues, the ability to be flexible, adaptive, and innovative becomes essential for survival. Nurses must understand the framework of CASs if they are to sustain a dynamic organization ready for innovation and change in the complex health environment (Butts & Rich, 2011).

Newer healthcare delivery systems use interdisciplinary teams, collaboration techniques, and case management, whereas in previous eras the physician directed all patient care, and everyone else followed the physician's lead. Currently, professional nurses are career focused, with an interest in continuing their education for specialty training and joining professional organizations, whereas nurses of the past were simply job-focused employees. The care of clients has shifted from care of the sick to health promotion and prevention programs, continuity of care, and complementary health alternatives. The focus on billing with cost containment has shifted to a focus on accountability of caregivers, continuous quality improvement (CQI), and care maps or critical pathways (Blais et al., 2006).

Representing a step in the shift from a centralized biomedical model of caring, community nursing centers are a creative healthcare delivery model with a more holistic nursing model of caring. Over the past century, the focus of the traditional biomedical model of illness has been on discovering the pathology or the cure to one problem, rather than on understanding the illness and its various components (Wade & Halligan, 2004). Community nursing centers located in churches, mobile units, shelters, and schools are set up to meet the underserved populations by providing a range of services to the public that are not normally available. The needs of the patient become the focus, instead of a medical diagnosis and a single cure. These centers offer education and preventive measures for topics of interest to the local community. A nurse or group of caregivers might go to community centers to assess and teach health promotion and prevention strategies for cancer or hypertension. This represents a shift from seeking a single cure to the promotion of health, wellness, and well-being (Blais et al., 2006).

The healthcare delivery system is continuously changing and evolving. Within the healthcare delivery system there are several models of patient care delivery, discussed next.

> **www | CRITICAL THINKING QUESTION** ✳
>
> Positive health promotion is a process of enabling people to improve and increase control of their maximum health potential. Think of positive health promotion behaviors that you have demonstrated (or not) since beginning nursing school. What have you noticed since using these behaviors in your daily routine? ✳

Nursing Models of Patient Care

Nurses are leaders and managers within various **models of patient care delivery**. The methods of care delivery might differ significantly from one organization to another. The purpose of a nursing care delivery system is to provide a framework for nurses to deliver care to a specific group of patients. The delivery of care implements the nursing process and includes assessing and triaging clients so that the order of care can be prioritized, a care plan formulated, and client responses to nursing interventions evaluated in collaboration with other health team members (Wendt, Kenny, & Anderson, 2007).

The methods and models of nursing care have evolved over the years and have included functional nursing (task nursing), team nursing, total patient care, primary nursing, and case management. Team nursing, total patient care, and

> **The purpose of a nursing care delivery system is to provide a framework for nurses to deliver care to a specific group of patients.**

KEY COMPETENCY 8-1

Examples of Applicable
*Nurse of the Future: Nursing
Core Competencies*

Systems-Based Practice:

Knowledge (K3a) Under-
stands the concept of
patient care delivery models

Skills (S3a) Considers
resources available on the
work unit when contributing
to the plan of care for a
patient or group of patients

Attitudes/Behaviors (A3a)
Acknowledges the tension
that may exist between a
goal-driven and a resource-
driven patient care delivery
model

Source: Massachusetts Department
of Higher Education (2010), p. 20.

case management models of nursing care delivery are discussed in this chapter. The continual evaluation of nursing models of care has been prompted by changes in nursing staff availability, reduction in hospital revenue and reimbursement, changes in acuity levels (critical illness levels), shorter stays in the hospital, consumer demands for quality care and lesser charges, and demands by healthcare workers for improvements.

▪ Team Nursing

The **team nursing** model of care is used in the United States most frequently in hospitals and in long-term and extended care facilities. This arrangement evolved after the functional nursing of the 1940s. With this approach, the nursing staff is divided into teams and total patient care is provided to a group of patients who might be grouped according to their diagnoses. A team might consist of an RN, LPN, and two unlicensed assistive personnel (UAPs). The RN is the team leader responsible for making assignments and who has overall responsibility for patient care by team members. The team works collaboratively, with each member performing activities he or she is best trained to do. The team communicates client care needs and possible changes in the care plan to the team leader. The team acts as a whole with a holistic perspective of the personal needs of each client. The team leader takes the lead to resolve problems that the team encounters by updating care plans and communicating with physicians and other healthcare personnel. Often the team leader makes rounds with physicians. The nursing reports communicated at the beginning of each shift are a key feature to high-quality team nursing.

Team nursing has several advantages. One is that UAPs can carry out some of the functions that do not require a registered nurse's expertise. Team nursing also allows for tasks to be carried out that require several persons because an assigned team is readily available. Several disadvantages can surface with a team. If communication skills are not adequate, the holistic view of the patient might be fragmented. Also, UAPs and LPNs might feel resentment if they perceive the RN to be focused totally on paperwork and documentation and less on the physical needs of the client. For a team leader to be effective, delegation, communication, and problem-solving skills are essential.

▪ Total Patient Care

Appearing as early as the 1920s, the first model of patient care delivery was **total patient care** (Sullivan & Decker, 2005). In this model, the RN has responsibility for all aspects of care of the patient or patients. The RN works directly with the client, other nursing staff, and physicians in implementing a plan of care. The objective of total patient care is to have one nurse provide all care to the same patient or patients for the entire shift. Currently, this model is practiced in areas such as critical care units or postanesthesia recovery units where a high level of expertise is required. This system's advantages are that nurses provide holistic continuous care, there is continuity of communication from clients to other healthcare team members, and the nurse has total accountability for that shift. The disadvantage is that some of the tasks could be performed by lesser-skilled persons, which might be more cost effective.

■ Case Management

A current nursing model of nursing care delivery is **case management**, which relies on clinical pathways to evaluate care. The clinical pathway refers to expected outcomes and interventions that the collaborative practice team establishes (Sullivan & Decker, 2005). The professional nurse is responsible for initiating and updating the plan of care, care map, or clinical pathway that is used to guide and evaluate client care. The clinical pathway provides a time frame for expected outcomes of care and involves an interdisciplinary team of caregivers who use the pathway to provide consistent care.

Nursing case management focuses on managing a group (caseload) of clients and the members of the healthcare team caring for those clients. The case manager organizes patient care by major diagnoses or DRGs and focuses on specific time frames to achieve predetermined patient outcomes and contain costs. The case manager makes referrals to other healthcare providers and manages the quality of care. Important characteristics to the role of nursing case managers are collaboration, identification of patient outcomes with time frames, and the use of continuous quality improvement (CQI) analysis. The case manager does not usually provide direct patient care but supervises the provision of care by UAPs and licensed personnel.

A case manager's role in an acute care setting involves the management of a caseload of 10 to 15 patients. Case managers follow patient progression from admission through discharge and solve problems of variances from the expected outcomes. A variance would be, for example, that a total hip surgery patient did not get discharged on day 6 (expected outcome by time frame) as planned. Instead, that person was hospitalized for 10 days. The case manager intervenes and communicates with the team to analyze specific patient progression and outcomes and determine why the patient was not discharged. Usually, case managers have considerable nursing experience and an advanced degree.

To manage the cases of a group of clients, a team is selected that includes clinical experts from the disciplines needed such as nursing, medicine, or physical therapy. The key features of a case management team are support by administration and physicians, a qualified case manager, collaboration of the teams, a CQI system in place, and critical pathways. All members of the team must agree on the critical pathways and accept responsibility and accountability for interventions and patient outcomes. Case management contributes to the reduction of complications that arise during hospitalization. Specific measurable patient outcomes with time frames for the group of clients are determined.

The caseload selected for case management includes high-volume, high-cost, and high-risk cases. One such example is the total hip replacement client population in orthopedics. The number of hip replacement surgeries performed is higher than the number of many other procedures; they cost more and include higher risks such as pulmonary emboli and surgical site infections. The total cost to the client and related departments is higher, so careful monitoring is necessary. Other high-risk clients are those in critical condition, in ICU more than 2 days, or on a ventilator. Baseline data such as length of stay, cost of care, and complications are collected on these groups and analyzed.

The critical path quickly orients the staff to the expected outcomes that should be achieved for that day. Nursing diagnoses identify the outcomes needed. If these are not achieved, the case manager is notified and the situation analyzed. An example of a **collaborative critical pathway** for a patient having a total hip replacement is described here. A critical path for a total hip client on days 1 and 3 postoperatively might include the following:

- Day 1 Operating Room and Postoperative Care
  Activity: Bed rest, turn/cough/deep breath q 2 hrs
  NSG: VS q h × 4, then q 4 hrs, circulation/neuro checks q h × 4, then q 4 hrs, Hemovac: Check q hr × 4, then q 4 hrs, I & O
  Medications: Antibiotics, pain control
  Nutrition: NPO to clear liquids as tolerated
  Teaching: Pain control, assist devices, incentive spirometry, mobility plan, D/C plan, home health evaluation

- Day 3 Postoperatively
  Activity: Continue mobility plan, turn/cough/deep breath q 2 hrs, skin protocols
  NSG: VS q 8 hrs, D/C assessment, D/C hemovac, ck drainage, I & O q 8 hrs, D/C Foley, continue elastic hose
  Medications: Antibiotics, p.o. pain control, continue stool softeners, IV to heplock, continue Coumadin
  Nutrition: Diet as tolerated, repeat teaching as needed
  D/C plans: Review transfer orders, D/C needs

Normally, a total hip client would be expected to be discharged on the sixth day after surgery. The critical path continues all 6 days, with potential nursing diagnoses attached, such as pain control deficit or impaired mobility. The critical path is also given to the patient's family so that they know what to expect during an uncomplicated total hip surgery hospitalization. Case management is one role of professional nursing. The following sections further define some of the many roles that nurses assume.

Role of the Professional Nurse

The role of the professional nurse is one of the most exciting areas to discuss for entry-level nurses. Think about it. You go from high school student to professional in zero to 4 years or so! The role of the professional nurse has expanded in response to changing populations and the philosophical shift toward health promotion rather than illness cure. Several roles of nurses include **practitioner, caregiver, advocate, educator, leader, manager, collaborator, and researcher**. Placing *RN* after your name means that you are committed to the legal, ethical, and moral responsibilities that define professional roles. These responsibilities are based on the American Nurses Association's (ANA's) *Nursing Scope and Standards of Professional Practice*, the ANA's *Nursing Code of Ethics*, and the ANA's *Nursing Social Policy Statement*. You are the fulcrum of patient care and patients' safety net as well as their advocate. You have a legal obligation to explain the physician's orders to your patients! Documentation is a legally important role of the registered nurse (Smeltzer et al., 2010).

This section examines the most important aspects of the entry-level nurse role and also defines basic concepts of care management. Nurses practice health promotion (primary prevention or illness prevention) through education of clients and their families.

> The role of the professional nurse has expanded in response to changing populations and the philosophical shift toward health promotion rather than illness cure.

■ Caregiver

The role of the nurse as caregiver has changed tremendously during the past century. The role as a dependent person to the physician who only provided personal care has evolved to that of the educated nurse who is an autonomous and informed professional. As a caregiver, the nurse practices nursing as a science. The nurse provides interventions to meet physical, psychosocial, spiritual, and environmental needs of clients and families using the nursing process and critical thinking skills. Holistic care is a philosophical approach that emphasizes the uniqueness of the individual and in which interacting wholes are more important than the sum of each part. That is, the whole person is greater than merely each component part of the client—biophysical, psychological, social, and spiritual parts. The science (knowledge base) of nursing becomes the art of nursing through caring, where the nurse is concerned for the client. The nurse and client are connected. The nurse as a caregiver is skilled and empathetic, knowledgeable and caring.

KEY COMPETENCY 8-3

Examples of Applicable
*Nurse of the Future: Nursing
Core Competencies*

Patient-Centered Care:

Knowledge (K6) Demonstrates understanding of the diversity of the human condition

Skills (S6b) Provides holistic care that addresses the needs of diverse populations across the life span

Attitudes/Behaviors (A6) Values the inherent worth and uniqueness of individuals and populations

Source: Massachusetts Department of Higher Education (2010), p. 10.

KEY COMPETENCY 8-4

Examples of Applicable
*Nurse of the Future: Nursing
Core Competencies*

Systems-Based Practice:

Knowledge (K4) Understands the role and responsibilities as patient advocate, assisting patient in navigating through the health care system

Skills (S4a) Serves as a patient advocate

Attitudes/Behaviors (A4a) Values role and responsibilities as patient advocate

Source: Massachusetts Department of Higher Education (2010), p. 20.

■ Advocate

As the nurse–client relationship develops, the nurse needs professional knowledge to assist clients in their decision making. The nurse fills the role of client advocate in healthcare delivery, intervening in crises of AIDS, homelessness, drug and alcohol abuse, teenage pregnancy, child and spouse abuse, and increasing healthcare costs. A client advocate is a person who pleads the cause for clients' rights. The purpose of this role is to respect client decisions and boost client autonomy. Client advocacy includes developing a therapeutic nurse–client relationship to secure patient self-determination, protection of patients' rights, and acting as an intermediary among patients and their significant others and healthcare providers (Blais et al., 2006). A client advocate is mainly concerned with empowering the client through the nurse–patient relationship. The nurse represents the interests of the client, who has needs that are unmet and are likely to remain unmet without the nurse's special intervention. The professional nurse speaks for the client as if the client's interests were the nurse's own.

In numerous situations the nurse can speak up for the patient. Examples are pain control, the clients' refusal of treatment, or issues of resuscitation status. Ethical challenges face the nurse as client advocate. To be an effective client advocate, the nurse must do the following:

- Be assertive.
- Recognize the client's values as more important than the healthcare providers'.
- Ensure adequate information so that clients and families can make decisions.
- Be aware that moral or ethical conflicts can arise that require consultation or negotiation among healthcare providers.

Nurses need to assist clients in the clarification of their values as they relate to a particular health problem or end-of-life issue. The nurse and the client are equally responsible for the outcomes of care, but the nurse is responsible for assisting the client to use his or her strengths to obtain the highest level of health possible. Advance directives should be addressed early in the course of patient hospitalizations while the patient is capable of making personal choices.

■ Manager

In exploring the concept of management in practice, all nurses are managers. They direct the work of professionals and nonprofessionals to achieve expected outcomes of care. All nurses need to learn management and leadership skills to be efficient and effective in their respective fields. In the healthcare setting, a *manager* is an individual who is employed by an organization and is responsible and accountable for the goals of that organization (Sullivan & Decker, 2005). In practice, nurses are expected to manage the care of each patient assigned to them for that shift. So, imagine you've just received a report on your patients. Where do you begin? Assessments and medicines are due. Patients need to go to surgery and radiology. Breakfast trays are being distributed. Insulin is past due. Charting is needed. Student nurses want report. So much to do, and so little time! How can you get everything done, provide quality care, and still be standing? Well, *delegation* is a terrific concept!

It is easy to say delegate, but delegation is a difficult leadership role for nurses to adopt and one that is not readily learned during nursing education. Both experienced nurses and entry-level nurses struggle to develop delegation and prioritization skills. Nurse managers must continually expand delegation skills to survive. Nurses must also learn to delegate without the threat of litigation. With cost containment, it is necessary now more than ever to delegate effectively. **Delegation** is defined as the process by which responsibility and authority for performing a certain task are transferred to another individual. This individual accepts that authority and responsibility (Sullivan & Decker, 2005). When accepting responsibility, a nurse has the obligation to intervene and accomplish a task. Nurses become accountable when they accept ownership for the results, or the lack of results, depending on the situation. When delegating, responsibility can be transferred to another individual and both individuals are held accountable. Accountability is a shared concept. It is the quality or state of being accountable, especially the obligation or willingness to accept responsibility or to account for one's actions. To delegate, the person delegating (delegator) must be the one who is responsible for the task.

It is important to understand the acceptance of delegation. The one to whom a task is being delegated (delegatee) must realistically decide whether he or she has the skills and abilities for the task being assigned and the time to do it. If not, the individual must inform the person delegating that he or she does not have the skills. The next step is to see if the delegator has the time and willingness to train and assist in accomplishing the task. If the delegator cannot do this, the delegatee must refuse the assignment. When delegation is accepted, responsibility is accepted for outcome benefits and also for liabilities. The delegator has the option to delegate parts of a task, but the one delegated to also has the option to negotiate for the parts of the task that can be accomplished. New skills can be obtained in the process. After the participants agree on the responsibilities to be assumed, they must clarify the time frame and other expectations. The delegatee must communicate with the delegator effectively throughout the completion of the task. If a nurse declines a task, he or she should thank the delegator and indicate a desire to help him or her in the future.

It is important to examine the liability issues of delegation. The National Council of State Boards of Nursing suggests five "rights of delegation":

- Right task
- Right circumstances
- Right person
- Right direction and communication
- Right supervision (Sullivan & Decker, 2005)

It is important to use these five rights of delegation. According to the ANA (2001) *Code of Ethics for Nurses with Interpretive Statements*, the nurse is responsible for using informed judgment and basing the decision to delegate on the person's competencies and qualifications. If the nurse fails to do this, it is considered negligence. So, the delegating nurse must follow the steps of delegation when defining the task. The procedure should be communicated with clear instructions and guidelines. The nurse must delegate to accomplish the goals of care. After tasks have been delegated, the nurse must evaluate the tasks to ensure correct completion of each activity. Delegation is definitely a skill that can be learned and requires practice. Successful nurses learn the process of delegation. Nurses accomplish more by delegating than if they try to do everything themselves.

To summarize the concept of delegation, it is a contractual agreement in which authority and responsibility for a task are transferred by the delegator, who is accountable for the task, to another person. Delegation necessitates proficiency in determining the task and level of responsibility, determining who has the skills required, communicating expectations clearly to assigned personnel, and monitoring the performance of assigned tasks. When nurses carefully select a qualified person as a delegatee and provide supervision, liability is minimized. All nurses and managers must learn to delegate to be successful.

▪ Collaborative Practice

Health care has become so complex today that it takes several professional providers delivering care in a collaborative environment to improve client health outcomes. All members of the healthcare team must combine their skills, knowledge, and resources to improve outcomes; nurses and physicians must modify their traditional roles and work more collaboratively as colleagues. One of the many roles of the professional nurse is participating in collaborative practice. The purpose of collaboration is to achieve high-quality client care and client satisfaction. A collaborative framework with an interdisciplinary team can also limit costs. Other goals of collaboration are to the following:

- Enhance continuity across the continuum of care from wellness and prevention, through acute episodes of illness, to discharge or transfer and rehabilitation
- Improve client and significant others' satisfaction with care

- Provide research-based, high-quality, cost-effective care that is driven by expected outcomes
- Promote mutual respect and communication among client, nurse, and caregiver to form a coalition
- Provide opportunities to solve issues and problems

> **The purpose of collaboration is to achieve high-quality client care and client satisfaction. A collaborative framework with an interdisciplinary team can also limit costs.**

The level of collaboration achieved and nature of decisions are the primary outcomes. This leads to secondary outcomes of goal attainment and autonomy. Collaborative practice in caregiving can include nurse–physician interaction, nurse–nurse interaction, or the interaction of interdisciplinary teams or committees (Blais et al., 2006). Collaborative teams provide extensive care by providing a full range of expertise through each of the team members, and thus contributing to outcomes. Nurse–physician collaboration is essential to maximize quality patient care and requires knowledge sharing with joint responsibility for patient care. On some occasions, collaboration between nurses and physicians can involve fleeting encounters in patient areas. In this situation, there is no second chance to collaborate effectively on a committee, but the volume of these professional encounters might be increasing. The challenge is to make the most of all interactions to use the best knowledge and abilities of all healthcare team members and produce positive client outcomes (Lindeke & Seickert, 2005). Bottom-line attention is given to compassionate and humanitarian patient care. Interdisciplinary collaboration can keep this central despite economic pressures. Motivated teams must work together to thrive by being optimistic and positive, thus inspiring hope in others.

As discussed previously, critical pathways are implemented by collaboration with input from various departments. Critical pathways are also called interdisciplinary plans, or action plans. The **interdisciplinary healthcare team** can be especially effective in outpatient services. The teams deal with client-related problems and help the patient progress through the clinic and hospital efficiently. The physician or nurse practitioner sees the client and recommends **consultations** as needed. Professional nurses practice consultations on a day-to-day basis. The primary nurse's role is to assess the need for consultations and identify expected outcomes of consultation, along with the need for revising care as client needs change. For example, nurse–nurse consulting might occur between a staff nurse and an enterostomal therapist for the care of a client's excoriated ostomy site secondary to radiation and chemotherapy. This type of consultation is documented in the patient record by obtaining a physician's order for an enterostomal therapist consult; then, the enterostomal nurse intervenes and documents the care rendered. The primary nurse changes the current plan of care with continuous evaluation of outcomes.

The ability to collaborate is particularly important for staff nurses. Collaboration is one of the key skills required in nursing. The advent of group practice, managed care, and practice standards has driven the need for collaboration and consultation. On a continuum, collaboration at the lowest level begins with communication among all involved disciplines and the client, with everyone asking similar questions (Blais et al., 2006). Each professional has separate interventions with a separate plan of care, and decision making is independent. Coordination and consultation represent a middle-range level of collaboration, where the professionals seek to make best use of the resources. Comanagement and referral represent the highest level of collaboration, in which providers are responsible and accountable for their own aspects of care, and then patients are directed to other providers when the problem is beyond a particular provider's expertise. The main levels of the continuum of collaboration are represented in Figure 8-1.

Successful consultation becomes apparent when each person making a contribution is recognized so that a unified plan can be put into practice. Nurses collaborate with clients, peers, and other persons in the healthcare delivery system. Specifically, the nurse's role as a collaborator with the client includes acknowledging and supporting the client in healthcare decisions, encouraging client autonomy, helping clients set goals for care, and providing client consultation in a collaborative fashion. With other healthcare professionals, the nurse's role is to recognize the contribution and expertise of each member of the interdisciplinary team, listen, share responsibilities in exploring options and setting goals, and participate in collaborative interdisciplinary research to increase knowledge of a particular clinical problem. A nurse can also collaborate within professional organizations by serving on committees at the local, state, national, or international level to create solutions for professional and healthcare concerns.

Key elements needed for collaboration of the interdisciplinary healthcare team include effective communication skills, mutual respect and trust, the ability to give and receive feedback, decision-making skills, and conflict resolution skills. Each professional group must focus on common ground: the client's needs. A person-centered approach is essential Brown, 2005). Mutual

Figure 8-1 Levels of the continuum of collaboration

respect develops in the team when individuals show honor or give credit to one another. When one team member is confident in the actions of another, trust occurs. Hospitals have not always fostered mutual caring and respect among professionals, so nurses must strive to promote positive relationships with team members despite lingering negative attitudes from the past. Also, when professionals work closely together on a team, giving and receiving timely and relevant feedback are some of the most difficult challenges but important to the team process. Type of feedback given can be affected by a person's perceptions, roles, confidence, beliefs, and environment. Helpful feedback is characterized by warm, caring, and respectful communication. Opportunities to practice listening and giving and receiving feedback can enhance professional communication skills. Giving and receiving feedback helps the professional collaborative team develop an understanding and effective working relationship.

Another key element of collaboration by the interdisciplinary team involves responsibility for the expected outcome. To achieve a solution, team decision making must begin with a clear definition of the problem and be directed at the objectives of the specific effort. By focusing on the client's priority needs first, organization of interventions can be planned accordingly. The discipline best able to address the client's highest needs at the moment is given priority in planning and is responsible for providing its interventions in a timely manner. Often, nurses can help the team identify priorities and focus on areas that require further referral or attention. Take, for example, a terminal oncology patient who requires care post abdominal surgery to correct a bowel obstruction caused by an invasive tumor. Cancer has affected the patient's spine, causing neurologic deficits of the extremities. The patient has an implanted port for chemotherapy, parenteral nutrition, and requires multiple antibiotic infusions. Several decubiti have developed. The primary nurse ensures total patient care by communicating with the client and significant others. The nurse then collaborates with the physician for pain control and postoperative care. The nurse ensures expert intravenous lines for chemotherapy and multiple antibiotic infusions, collaborating with peers if necessary. The nurse consults per physician orders with the enterostomal therapist for wound care of the decubiti and consults with the dietician for hyperalimentation (total parenteral nutrition) needs. The nurse collaborates with physical therapy for resumption of activity for neurologic deficits. Each member of the interdisciplinary team contributes his or her own expertise to common goals of care.

Interpersonal conflict might occur when individuals are working together and their expectations are incompatible. Conflicts between people can affect interdisciplinary collaboration. To reduce conflict, team members can conduct

---

www | CRITICAL THINKING QUESTION ✳

One of the most difficult challenges in promoting collaboration among professionals is giving and receiving feedback. What is your experience in giving and receiving timely and helpful feedback with a team? Think of an example of receiving both negative and positive feedback. Compare the effect of the negative and positive feedback. Compare the experiences. ✳

KEY COMPETENCY 8-6

Examples of Applicable *Nurse of the Future: Nursing Core Competencies*

Teamwork and Collaboration:

Knowledge (K2) Describes scope of practice and roles of interdisciplinary and nursing health care team members

Skills (S2) Functions competently within own scope of practice as a member of the health care team

Attitudes/Behaviors (A2) Values the perspectives and expertise of all health care team members

Source: Massachusetts Department of Higher Education (2010), p. 31.

interdisciplinary conferences, take part in interdisciplinary educational programs, and recognize and accept personal responsibility for teamwork. Sometimes the failure of professionals to collaborate is because they lack the skills necessary to contribute to effective teamwork. In the past, nursing has been interested in emphasizing nursing research and nursing practice. Attention is now shifting to focus on interdisciplinary collaboration and the recognition of different points of view. Collaboration among disciplines requires that nurses have the ability to articulate their own theories while considering different perspectives, a mutual give-and-take to determine the best approach to specific problems. Sometimes organizational structure affects role conflict. Delivery systems that maintain a hierarchy of authority do not support interdisciplinary collaboration. In situations where a traditional authority figure is strong, the organization can promote collaboration between physicians and nurses. Whatever the organizational hierarchy or delivery system, the relationship among all members of an effective collaborative team must reflect trust and respect.

Conflict can be overt or covert. Reactive behaviors include whining, complaining, passive-aggressive behavior, and gossiping. Conflict can be an engine of innovation and change if nurses confront it properly. Possible causes of conflict include incorrect facts, lack of trust, unclear position descriptions, unclear goals, inadequate action plans, unstable leadership, lack of leadership, or limited staff participation in decision making. Nurses need to take steps to avoid conflicts. Recognizing causes of conflict can assist organizations to develop strategies to prevent conflict. Nurses should deal with conflicts as they occur. Collaboration is a positive approach to conflict. Strategies for conflict resolution can be to first identify the problem and collect facts, documenting each fact and its sources. An explanation of behaviors should give opportunity for discussion of issues and expectations. Counseling sessions should give opportunity for growth with encouragement of active participation. The counseling session and action plan with a timeline should be reported to the appropriate supervisor with appropriate documentation of all events and facts.

Continuous Quality Improvement

Continuous quality improvement (CQI) is defined as a structured organizational process that involves personnel in planning and implementing the continuous flow of improvements in the provision of quality health care that meets or exceeds expectations. CQI generally includes the following common set of characteristics: a link to key elements of the organization's strategic plan, a quality council composed of the organization's leadership, training programs for personnel, mechanisms for the selection of improvement opportunities, formation of process improvement teams, staff support for process analysis and redesign, policies that motivate and support staff participation in process improvement, and application of current and rigorous techniques of scientific method and statistical process control (Sollecito & Johnson, 2013, pp. 4–5).

The nurse's role in CQI is especially important in hospitals that promote a culture of patient safety and view quality-related activities as priority "safety checks." Ensuring high-quality patient care and safety cannot be overstated. Quality care results from caregivers doing the right thing the right way the first time.

Collaboration and evidence-based practice are key elements of successful quality improvement programs (Caramanica, Cousino, & Petersen, 2003). In the 1980s, hospitals and agencies implemented ongoing quality assurance programs. Quality assurance programs were required for reimbursement of services and for accreditation by the Joint Commission. In 1992, the revised Joint Commission standards identified continuous quality improvement as a mechanism of health care. This differed from previous quality programs by purposely identifying the causes of problems or systems that needed improvement in health care. In 2002, the Joint Commission standard amendments further specified that patients have the right to age-specific and considerate health care that preserves dignity and respects cultural, psychosocial, and spiritual values (Smeltzer et al., 2010).

Evidence-based practice in performance improvement includes the use of standardized care plans and outcome assessments such as clinical pathways or algorithms. A current national initiative is the bundling of care for various problems that have been identified by the National Quality Forum and other organizations. These problems include ventilator-associated pneumonia (VAP), sepsis protocols, and infections related to central venous catheters. Bundling is a listing of care criteria necessary to reduce infections such as a checklist or graph for nurses to use at the bedside. These data are tracked by the performance improvement council.

The monthly exchange (collaboration) among physicians and nurses and other healthcare personnel fosters mutual trust and respect. When the need for quality improvement is identified by the performance improvement council, the registered nurse at the bedside uses quality techniques that were once employed only by quality assurance personnel. The nurse might utilize Excel spreadsheets, flow diagrams, computer programs, or control charts to record data when analyzing a clinical problem or situation. Trended data collected by nurses are provided by the risk management department or performance improvement council and disseminated to the units.

Quality improvement is tied into each nurse's performance. Individual nurse and team goals for quality and safety are important components of each staff member's annual review. As nursing leadership and staff foster a culture of safety and quality, they emphasize reporting near misses and unintended outcomes as a means to identify and fix the weak link in processes of care. For example, the anonymous reporting of medication adverse events in some institutions has led to an increased number of incident reports being

KEY COMPETENCY 8-8

Examples of Applicable *Nurse of the Future: Nursing Core Competencies*

Quality Improvement:

Knowledge (K1) Describes the nursing context for improving care

Skills (S1a) Actively seeks information about quality in their own settings and organization; (S1b) Actively seeks information about quality improvement in the care setting from relevant institutional, regulatory and local/national sources

Attitudes/Behaviors (A1) Recognizes that quality improvement is an essential part of nursing

Source: Massachusetts Department of Higher Education (2010), p. 36.

made by bedside caregivers. This has resulted in the identification of areas of the medication use system that need improvement, and this ultimately leads to prevention of other possible near misses and more serious unintended or negative outcomes in medication administration (Caramanica et al., 2003).

Continuous quality improvement has proved to be beneficial in promoting client safety, but conflicts involving groups or individuals might occur. Intergroup conflicts can occur when the group disagrees about policies governing practice, such as when a nurse is asked to float to another unit. Whatever the conflict, resolution strategies are essential to success. Problem solving can be achieved with open discussion and an investigation of all dimensions of the conflict. When each professional's goal has a positive outcome, success is more likely. Negotiating or bargaining occurs when the top priority need and optimal outcome are identified followed by reaching a final agreement that is close to each person's position. All parties must be sincere in the effort to negotiate, and the goals of negotiation should be seen as fair and reasonable to each side. For example, the nurses working in an outpatient surgery unit plan the on-call schedule at a monthly staff meeting with their nurse manager. When a change in schedule is needed, the nurses must plan a meeting to discuss strategies and negotiate the change. Successful negotiation occurs when the nurses reach a favorable schedule and view the outcome as fair, reasonable, and aligned with their personal goals.

Professional nurses have expertise in a wide variety of roles to practice client-driven care. The concepts of consultation, continuity of care, collaboration, and referral are interrelated. To provide continuity of care from admission to discharge and rehabilitation, the nurse collaborates with other services and agencies to provide care. The old cliché that discharge plans begin with admission makes more sense now than ever before, even for the acute care patient. With shortened lengths of hospital stay, nurses must evaluate all clients for their ability to manage at home. The referral source prior to discharge might be a physician, nurse, social worker, or discharge planner. This person supplies the agency with details about the client's needs. The nurse's role is to assess the need to refer clients for assistance with actual or potential problems and identify community resources, such as respite care, social services, or shelters, for the client, family, and significant others (Wendt et al., 2007).

If the nurse refers the patient to a home health agency and the agency believes that the client qualifies for services, the agency usually contacts the client's physician and requests a referral on the client's behalf (LeMone & Burke, 2007). The nurse can refer a client to hospice, a community resource, or support group. The kinds of agencies that provide care in the community and home have increased because of the more complex needs of patients. Technologies that were once limited to the acute care setting such as ventilatory support, dialysis, and intravenous or parenteral nutrition therapy have been adapted to the home care setting. Home care nurses function as acute care nurses in the home, providing "high-tech, high-touch" services to patients with acute healthcare needs. They are responsible for family teaching and collaborating with community resources in the continuity of care to promote and maintain patient self-care management. The nurse can consider the following questions when assessing the client being discharged from acute care to home care (LeMone & Burke, 2007):

- Does the client need follow-up treatments or additional education?
- What equipment or supplies are necessary?
- What teaching materials do the clients need, and are they at an acceptable reading level for the client?
- Are there any sensory deprivations that might impede learning?
- Who is going to be the principal caregiver in the home? If he or she is not comfortable, what support does the caregiver need?
- Was the caregiver present during instructions in the hospital setting? Did he or she comprehend the instructions?
- Has a devastating prognosis just been determined?
- Is high-technology intervention necessary?
- Are community resources available where this patient lives?

In every instance, the nurse should not make assumptions. Well-educated or financially secure clients can be just as overwhelmed by illness as clients who appear less educated or poor. Every client is a referral candidate. If the family believes that no help is necessary but the nurse believes otherwise, the nurse can suggest an evaluation visit by an agency once the client is at home. If a referral is made to a home care agency, it must proceed with a physician-approved treatment plan, which is a legal requirement. If physical therapy or other services are needed, the nurse or social worker arranges for these visits.

The nursing process used in home care settings is the same as that practiced in any other healthcare setting. The nurse is responsible for maintaining continuity of care between and among healthcare agencies. This includes providing and receiving reports on assigned clients and using appropriate documents such as medical records or transfer forms to record and communicate client information. Accurate transcription of primary healthcare provider orders is also necessary.

Home care nursing is a specialty area that requires advanced knowledge and high-level assessment skills, critical thinking, and decision-making skills where other healthcare professionals are not available to validate conclusions and decisions about care. Because of this, the scope of home care nursing encompasses not only the acute care setting in the hospital but also the acute care setting as it expands into the community.

Collaborative practice should be a primary goal for nursing. This goal promotes shared participation, responsibility, and accountability in a healthcare environment that is striving to meet the complex healthcare needs of the public. Nurses with a significant practice that empowers others are those who value collaboration and develop the ability to associate effectively and positively with other healthcare personnel (Ponte et al., 2007). An influential professional nurse works well with others, is fair, and has perspectives that are sought out by other healthcare personnel. Leading and participating in interdisciplinary teams and partnering with others are essential to sound nursing practice.

Conclusion

This chapter has introduced healthcare delivery systems and the role of the professional nurse. It explored various models of nursing care delivery. All nurses are managers of the care of a specific group of patients and collaborate with other healthcare providers in the delivery of client-centered and safety-focused care. Nurses must possess the skills of critical thinking, delegation, supervision, collaboration, evaluation, motivation, and communication to work with other disciplines of care. This chapter has defined some of the concepts that are necessary for the entry-level nurse to maintain safe and competent entry-level nursing practice.

Classroom Activity

You are planning the discharge of an 82-year-old man who has heart failure and chronic obstructive pulmonary disease (COPD). Divide the class into small groups of students to discuss how the case manager would intervene for the client and family and provide continuity of care from ICU to home. Have a spokesperson for each group briefly present each group's plan. www

References

American Nurses Association. (2001). *Code of ethics for nurses with interpretive statements*. Washington, DC: Author.

Blais, K. K., Hayes, J. S., Kozier, B., & Erb, G. (2006). *Professional nursing practice concepts and perspectives* (5th ed.). Upper Saddle River, NJ: Pearson Prentice Hall.

Brown, F. (2005). Nurse consultations: A person-centered approach. Retrieved from http://tcmdiscovery.com/2007/6-24/200762416820.html

Butts, J., & Rich, K. (2011). *Philosophies and theories for advanced nursing practice*. Sudbury, MA: Jones & Bartlett Learning.

Caramanica, L., Cousino, J. A., & Petersen, S. (2003). Four elements of a successful quality program, alignment, collaboration, evidence-based practice, and excellence. *Nursing Administration Quarterly, 27*(4), 336–343.

LeMone, P., & Burke, K. (2007). *Medical-surgical nursing critical thinking in client care* (4th ed.). Upper Saddle River, NJ: Pearson Prentice Hall.

Lindeke, L. L., & Seickert, A. M. (2005). Nurse–physician workplace collaboration. Retrieved from http://www.nursingworld.org/ojin

Massachusetts Department of Higher Education. (2010). *Nurse of the future: Nursing core competencies*. Retrieved from http://www.mass.edu/currentinit/documents/NursingCoreCompetencies.pdf

North Carolina Concept-Based Learning Editorial Board. (2011). *Nursing: A concept-based approach to learning* (Vols. 1 and 2). Upper Saddle River, NJ: Pearson.

Plsek, P. E., & Wilson, T. (2001). Complexity, leadership and management in healthcare organisations. *British Medical Journal, 323,* 746–749.

Ponte, P. R., Glazer, G., Dann, E., McCollum, K., Gross, A., Tyrrell, R., . . . Washington, D. (2007). The power of professional nursing practice: An essential element of patient and family centered care. *Online Journal of Issues in Nursing, 12.* Retrieved from http://nursingworld.org/ojin

Smeltzer, S. C., Bare, B. G., Hinkl, J. L., & Cheever, K. H. (2010). *Brunner & Suddarth's textbook of medical-surgical nursing* (12th ed.). Philadelphia, PA: Lippincott Williams & Wilkins.

Sollecito, W. A., & Johnson, J. K. (2013). *McLaughlin and Kaluzny's continuous quality improvement in health care* (4th ed.). Burlington, MA: Jones & Bartlett Learning.

Sullivan, E. J., & Decker, P. J. (2005). *Effective leadership and management in nursing* (6th ed.). Upper Saddle River, NJ: Pearson Prentice Hall.

Wade, D. T., & Halligan, P. W. (2004). Do biomedical models of illness make for good healthcare systems [Electronic version]? *British Medical Journal, 329,* 1398–1401. Retrieved from http://www.bmj.com/content/329/7479/1398.full

Wendt, A., Kenny, L., & Anderson, J. (2007). National Council of State Boards of Nursing 2007 NCLEX-RN detailed test plan. Retrieved from https://www.ncsbn.org/2007_NCLEX_RN_Detailed_Test_Plan_Candidate.pdf

Wilson, T., & Holt, T. (2001, September). Complexity and clinical care. *British Medical Journal, 323,* 685–688.

Critical Thinking and Clinical Judgment in Professional Nursing

9

Jill Rushing

The responsibilities of a professional registered nurse have increased significantly over the years. Nurses and nursing students must be able to function within the complicated environment of the healthcare system. The impact of advanced technology, the increased acuity level and complexity of patients, combined with the accountability and responsibility nurses have in the delivery of safe and effective care, make it essential, more now than ever, for nurses to possess the ability to think critically. In nursing, critical thinking is the ability to think in a systematic and logical manner, solve problems, make decisions, and establish priorities in the clinical setting. Critical thinking is the competent use of thinking skills and abilities to make sound clinical judgments and safe decision making.

Critical thinking in nursing is an essential component of professional accountability and quality nursing care. Concern for patient safety has grown as high rates of error and injury continue to be reported. To improve patient safety, nurses must be able to recognize changes in patient condition, perform independent nursing interventions, anticipate orders, and prioritize.

New nurses need to be prepared to practice safely, accurately, and compassionately, in varied settings, where knowledge and innovation increase at astonishing rates (Benner, Sutphen, Leonard, & Day, 2010). Nursing students must use a complex array of nursing skills and knowledge at the same time and practice thinking in changing situations, always for the good of the patient (Benner et al., 2010).

Key Terms and Concepts

» **Critical thinking**
» Clinical judgment
» Reflective thinking
» Nursing process
» Concept mapping
» Journaling

Learning Objectives

After completing this chapter, the student should be able to:

1. Define critical thinking.
2. Describe important critical thinking skills.
3. Explore characteristics of critical thinking.
4. Describe the characteristics of a critical thinker.
5. Explain why critical thinking is important in nursing practice.
6. Explore the process involved in critical thinking.

Recent studies indicate new nursing graduates have deficiencies in critical thinking ability including recognition of problems, reporting of essential clinical data, initiating independent nursing interventions, anticipating relevant medical orders, providing relevant rationale to support decisions, and differentiating urgency (Fero, Witsberger, Wesmiller, Zullo, & Hoffman, 2009). New graduate nurses practice at the novice or advanced beginner level (Benner, 1984). New graduate nurses are at the early stage of developing a skill set and applying critical thinking. For the novice, the beginning nursing student, the difficulty encountered in setting priorities is that all tasks, requests, and concerns seem to be of equal weight or importance and they must all be done (Benner et al., 2010). Determining which tasks are most important or urgent requires deliberate thought because the student has not yet learned to see the big picture or gained the skill to recognize quickly what is most urgent, most important in each clinical situation; this level of thinking is often difficult for the novice, the beginning nursing student (Benner et al., 2010). For example, you are about to administer medications to a patient. What is the bigger picture? Why is the patient being given these medications? Or you have a patient who has just returned from surgery. What should be carried out in the first hours post operation?

To ensure quality care for patients, we must implement strategies to help nursing students develop the essential skill of critical thinking. There should be a progression through their education tenure in nursing students' ability to think critically.

What Is Critical Thinking?

Critical thinking is an integral part of nursing practice and promotes quality nursing care and positive patient outcomes. Although critical thinking is widely regarded as a component of clinical reasoning and decision making, it is difficult to define, and there is no single, simple definition that explains critical thinking. In nursing, **critical thinking** for clinical decision making is the ability to think in a systematic and logical manner, with openness to question and reflect on the reasoning process used to ensure safe nursing practice and quality care. It is providing effective care based on sound reasoning (Scriven & Paul, 2011). Critical thinking in nursing is an essential component of professional accountability and quality nursing care. Critical thinkers exhibit the following habits of mind: confidence, contextual perspective, creativity, flexibility, inquisitiveness, intellectual integrity, intuition, open-mindedness, perseverance, and reflection. In nursing, critical thinkers practice the cognitive skills of analyzing, applying standards, discriminating, information seeking, logical reasoning, predicting, and transforming knowledge (Scheffer & Rubenfeld, 2000).

There is a strong link between critical thinking and **clinical judgment**. The following definition offers a comprehensive description of elements incorporating critical thinking from a nursing prospective. Critical thinking and clinical judgment in nursing: (1) are purposeful, informed, outcome-focused thinking; (2) carefully identify key problems, issues, and risks; (3) are based on principles of nursing process, problem solving, and the scientific method; (4) apply logic, intuition, and creativity; (5) are driven by patient, family, and community needs; (6) call for strategies that make the most of the human potential; and (7) require constant reevaluating (Alfaro-Lefevre, 2009). Thus, critical thinking, problem solving, and decision making are processes that are interrelated. Decision making and critical thinking need to occur concurrently to produce reasoning, clarification, and potential solutions.

Competence in critical thinking is one of the expectations of nursing education. Critical thinkers are described as well informed, inquisitive, open minded, and orderly in complex matters. Critical thinking competence is an outcome for quality nursing care and for the development of clinical judgment. The ability to think critically is also described as reducing the research–practice gap and fostering evidence-based nursing (Wangensteen, Johansson, Bjorkstrom, & Nordstrom, 2010).

Learning to be a nurse requires more than memorizing facts. It requires that you learn to think like a nurse, to think through and reason on a greater depth, and to draw a more sophisticated or deeper understanding of what you are doing in clinical practice so that you provide safe, quality patient care. Nursing is not a careless, mindless activity. All acts in nursing are deeply significant and require the nurse's mind to be fully engaged. The following illustration shows nursing is both thinking and doing: The physician has ordered an IV to be placed in a patient. How do you choose between a butterfly or an IV intracath? First, you have to consider why the line is being placed. You take into consideration whether it is a short-term, keep-open IV with limited medications; if so, then the butterfly IV is more comfortable and presents less of a threat of phlebitis. Doctors vary in their preferences as well, and this has to be considered. Also, the condition of the patient and his or her veins makes a great deal of difference. For example, with older patients special skill is required. The

> **Decision making and critical thinking need to occur concurrently to produce reasoning, clarification, and potential solutions.**

www] CRITICAL THINKING QUESTION ✳

You are assigned to care for Ms. C., an 81-year-old patient who was admitted today with symptoms of increasing shortness of breath over the last week. She is currently receiving oxygen through a nasal cannula at 3 L/minute. You go into the room to assess her. You find that she is sitting up in bed at a 60-degree angle. She is restless and her respirations appear labored and rapid. Her skin is pale with circumoral cyanosis. You ask if she feels more short of breath. Because she is unable to catch her breath enough to speak, she nods her head "yes." What action should you take first?

- Listen to her breath sounds.
- Ask when the shortness of breath started.
- Increase her oxygen flow rate to 6 L/min.
- Raise the head of the bed to 75 to 85 degrees

Based on knowledge you have learned, you realize the patient's symptoms indicate acute hypoxemia, so improving oxygen delivery is the priority. The other actions also are appropriate, but they are not as critical as the initial action. ✳

> **All acts in nursing are deeply significant and require the nurse's mind to be fully engaged.**

www. CRITICAL THINKING QUESTION *

What do all of the following scenarios have in common?

- An elderly male becomes acutely confused and refuses to follow directions for his safety.
- A teen comes into an urgent care setting requesting information about STDs.
- A mother visits a school nurse and requests information about how the school handles sex education.
- A team leader needs to rearrange assignments when one team member goes home sick.
- Nursing staff in an ICU need to develop an evacuation plan.

Answer: They all require critical thinking skills. *

veins look as they are going to be easy to get because they look large, but they are very fragile. If you do not use a very slight tourniquet, the vein will pop open (Benner, 1984).

Characteristics of Critical Thinking

How do you know when critical thinking is taking place? Critical thinking has some of the following characteristics (Wilkinson, 2007):

- Critical thinking is rational and reasonable.
- Critical thinking involves conceptualization.
- Critical thinking requires reflection.
- Critical thinking involves cognitive (thinking) skills and attitudes (feelings).
- Critical thinking involves creative thinking.
- Critical thinking requires knowledge.

Critical thinking is rational and reasonable. It is based on reasons rather than preferences, prejudice, or self-interest. It uses facts and observations to draw conclusions. For example, suppose during an election you decide to vote for the Democratic candidate because your family has always voted for Democrats. This decision is based on preference, prejudice, and, possibly, self-interest. By contrast, suppose you took time to reflect on what the candidate in the election said about the issues and based your choice on that. Even though you still might vote for the Democrat, you would be thinking rationally, using facts and observations to draw your conclusions (Wilkinson, 2007).

Critical thinking involves conceptualization. Conceptual thinking is the ability to understand a situation by identifying patterns or connections, and focusing on key underlying issues and integrating them into a conceptual framework. It involves using professional training and experience, creativity, and inductive reasoning that lead to solutions or alternatives that may not be easily identified. Conceptual thinking involves a willingness to explore and having an openness to a new way of seeing things or "looking outside of the box." Consider, for example, a case in which a patient with heart failure is coughing up yellow sputum. If the nurse suspects that the patient is short of breath from infection, he or she will evaluate other indicators of infection. The nurse will check the patient for an elevated temperature and will assess the last white

www. CRITICAL THINKING QUESTION *

You will be taking care of a patient in a nursing home for the first time. Your assignment is to care for an older man who has heart disease. In addition, he has five other medical problems and takes 20 medications. While developing a plan of care for this patient, you can identify 8 to 10 nursing problems. You have no previous experience with nursing homes, and most of what you have heard and read about them is negative. Will you find yourself dreading the clinical day and expecting a negative experience before you even begin? *

blood cell count in the patient's chart to see if it is elevated. The nurse will also consider factors that may place the patient at risk for infection, such as immobility, poor nutrition, or immune suppression (Craven & Hirnle, 2007).

Critical thinking uses reflection. **Reflective thinking** is deliberate thinking and careful consideration. It is the process of analyzing, making judgments, and drawing conclusions. Reflective thinking involves creating an understanding through one's experiences and knowledge and exploring potential alternatives—assessing what you know, what you need to know, and how to bridge that gap. Processes of reflective thinking involve the following:

- Determine what information is needed (what you need to know) for understanding the issue.
- Examine what you have already experienced about an issue.
- Gather the available information.
- Synthesize the information and opinions.
- Consider the synthesis from different perspectives and frames of reference.
- Create some meaning from the relevant information and opinions.

Reflective thinking is important during complex problem-solving situations because it provides an opportunity to step back and think about how to actually solve problems and how problem-solving strategies are used for achieving set goals. Reflection allows students to observe and reflect, pulling together what they learn in the clinical and classroom settings in taking care of patients. Students can build and integrate knowledge and skills. Reflecting on a nursing experience or situation can assist nurses in critically reflecting on their practice. Choose a clinical situation and ask yourself some of the following questions:

- What was my role in this situation? Did I feel comfortable or uncomfortable? Why?
- What actions did I take? How did I and others respond? Was it appropriate?
- How could I have improved the situation for myself, the patient, and others involved? What can I change in the future?
- What have I learned through this situation?
- Did I expect anything different to happen? What and why?
- Has this situation changed my way of thinking in any way?
- What knowledge from theory and research can I apply in this situation?
- What broader issues, for example, ethical, social, or political, arise from this situation?

Through reflection, students manage to be more organized and effective because they have a better understanding of who the patient is and what his or her care needs are. Reflection on practice helps the student develop a self-improving practice (Benner et al., 2010).

Critical thinking involves cognitive (thinking) skills and attitudes (feelings). Critical thinking involves having thinking skills as well as the motivation to use them. It involves the willingness to utilize complex thought processes compared to easily understood ones. Critical thinkers do not oversimplify. Critical thinking is about being willing and able to think.

Critical thinking involves creative thinking. Creativity is part of the thinking process. When you brainstorm potential problem solutions or possible decisions, you are using creativity. Creative and critical thinkers combine ideas and information in ways that form new solutions or innovative ideas. A creative thinker is an open-minded thinker. Nurses can utilize creative thinking when encountering a patient situation in which traditional methods are not effective. For example, a pediatric nurse is caring for 9-year-old Pauline, who has ineffective respirations following abdominal surgery. The physician has ordered incentive spirometry breathing treatments, but Pauline is frightened by the equipment and she quickly tires during the treatments. The nurse offers Pauline a bottle of soap bubbles and a blowing wand. The nurse knows that the respiratory effort in blowing bubbles will promote alveolar expansion and suggests that Pauline blow bubbles between incentive spirometry treatments (Wilkinson, 2007).

Critical thinking requires knowledge. In most academic disciplines, the educational system uses an expert to deliver a body of knowledge to the unpracticed novice, who will later be expected to go out and apply the knowledge and rules learned in school to various work situations. In nursing, a specific educational knowledge base is required before applying that knowledge in patient care. It is important to know that the process is being applied correctly. In essence, to become a nurse you must learn the knowledge to think like a nurse. On the "flip side" of this, as the level of experience of the nurse increases, so will the scientific knowledge base that the nurse applies. For example, you are caring for a patient with heart failure. After obtaining the vital signs, what heart rate would prevent you from performing ambulation on this patient? If you did not have knowledge regarding heart failure or did not know that the normal heart rate was 60–100 beats per minute, you could not make the good decision that ambulation should be postponed if the heart rate is above 100 beats per minute for this patient.

KEY COMPETENCY 9-1
Examples of Applicable *Nurse of the Future: Nursing Core Competencies*
Leadership:
Knowledge (K2) Understands critical thinking and problem-solving processes
Skills (S2a) Uses systematic approaches in problem solving
Attitudes/Behaviors (A2) Values critical thinking processes in the management of client care situations
Source: Massachusetts Department of Higher Education (2010), p. 17.

What Are the Characteristics of a Critical Thinker?

Nurses are required to think critically in all settings. Nurses' ability to think critically is one of their most important skills, and a commitment to think critically benefits the nurse's ability to care for patients most effectively. A critical thinker has many characteristics, including the following:

- Critical thinkers are flexible—they can tolerate ambiguity and uncertainty.
- Critical thinkers base judgments on facts and reasoning, not personal feelings. They identify inherent biases and assumptions. Critical thinkers separate facts from opinions.

- Critical thinkers don't oversimplify.
- Critical thinkers examine available evidence before drawing conclusions.
- Critical thinkers think for themselves and do not simply go along with the crowd.
- Critical thinkers remain open to the need for adjustment and adaptation throughout the inquiry stages.
- Critical thinkers accept change.
- Critical thinkers empathize; they appreciate and try to understand others' thoughts, feelings, and behaviors.
- Critical thinkers welcome different views and value examining issues from every angle.
- Critical thinkers know that it is important to explore and understand positions with which they disagree.
- Critical thinkers discover and apply meaning to what they see, hear, and read.

Approaches to Developing Critical Thinking Skills

As students develop in their nursing role, they learn and build critical thinking skills and apply them to real healthcare situations. Critical thinking requires conscious, deliberate effort. Critical thinking does not just come naturally, and people tend to believe what is easy to believe or what those around them believe (Wilkinson, 2007). With effort and practice, everyone can achieve some level of critical thinking to become an effective problem solver and decision maker. As the elements of critical thought develop into a habit, nurses improve their ability to assess complex situations and engage in the practice of nursing. The objectives for critical thinking in nursing include the ability to ask pertinent questions, analyze multiple forms of evidence, and evaluate options before coming to a conclusion. Following are examples that can be used as approaches to developing critical thinking skills.

> **KEY COMPETENCY 9-2**
>
> Examples of Applicable *Nurse of the Future: Nursing Core Competencies*
>
> Professionalism:
>
> Knowledge (K1b) Justifies clinical decisions
>
> Skills (S1b) Exercises critical thinking within standards of practice
>
> Attitudes/Behaviors (A1b) Shows commitment to provision of high quality, safe, and effective patient care
>
> *Source:* Massachusetts Department of Higher Education (2010), p. 13.

■ The Nursing Process

The American Nurses Association standards have set forth the framework necessary for critical thinking in the application of the nursing process. The **nursing process** is the tool by which all nurses can become equally proficient at critical thinking. The nursing process contains the following criteria: (1) assessment, (2) identifying the problem (nursing diagnosis), (3) planning, (4) implementation, and (5) evaluation. Through the application of each of these components the nurse can become proficient at critical

> The nursing process is a systematic problem-solving approach toward giving nursing care that allows the nurse to be accountable by using critical thinking before taking actions.

thinking. Nurses use critical thinking in each stage of the nursing process. This approach to critical thinking entails purposeful, informed, outcome-focused thinking, which requires identification of nursing and healthcare needs of clients (Knapp, 2007).

The nursing process is a systematic problem-solving approach toward giving nursing care that allows the nurse to be accountable by using critical thinking before taking actions. Nurses provide effective care based on sound reasoning, which is the reasonable reflection about nursing problems before selecting one of a variety of solutions. This is accomplished by regularly employing the elements of critical thought, such as defining the problem, identifying the goal, and analyzing the evidence (Caputi, 2010).

Each of the thinking skills listed in this category is commonly used when a nurse gathers data (Caputi, 2010). These skills include the following:

- Assessing systematically and comprehensively
- Checking accuracy and reliability
- Clustering related information
- Collaborating with coworkers
- Determining the importance of information
- Distinguishing relevant from irrelevant information
- Gathering complete and accurate data and then acting on that data
- Judging how much ambiguity is acceptable
- Recognizing inconsistencies
- Using diagnostic reasoning

Each one of the following thinking skills is commonly used when nurses provide care to patients (Caputi, 2010):

- Applying the nursing process to develop a treatment plan
- Communicating effectively
- Predicting and managing potential complications
- Resolving conflicts
- Resolving ethical dilemmas
- Setting priorities
- Teaching others

■ Assessment

The nursing assessment answers the questions: "What is happening?" or "What could happen?" It involves systematically collecting, organizing, and analyzing information about the client. Once data or information has been collected and it is determined that the data are accurate and complete,

KEY COMPETENCY 9-3

Examples of Applicable *Nurse of the Future: Nursing Core Competencies*

Patient-Centered Care:

Knowledge (K1) Identifies components of nursing process appropriate to individual, family, group, community, and population health care needs across the life span

Skills (S1a) Provides priority-based nursing care to individuals, families, and groups through independent and collaborative application of the nursing process

Attitudes/Behaviors (A1a) Values use of scientific inquiry, as demonstrated in the nursing process, as an essential tool for provision of nursing care

Source: Massachusetts Department of Higher Education (2010), p. 9.

the nurse performs data analysis or data interpretation. What are the client's actual and/or potential problems? A problem list is then developed based on the data, and the nurse prioritizes the client's problems. The nurse performs an ongoing assessment throughout the implementation of the nursing process.

■ Diagnosis

The nurse analyzes and derives meaning from the assessment information and selects a diagnosis. Diagnosis is the identification of a problem. It is a statement that describes a specific response to an actual or potential health problem. For example, a nursing diagnosis for a selected patient might be "decreased cardiac output related to inability of the heart to pump effectively, and occlusion and constriction of vessels impairing blood flow."

■ Planning

During planning, the nurse develops a plan to provide consistent, continuous care that meets the client's unique needs. Planning includes developing expected outcomes and working with the client to identify goals and to determine appropriate nursing actions and interventions that will reduce the identified problem. The nurse uses critical thinking to develop goals and nursing interventions for problems that require an individualized approach. Nurses use judgment to determine which interventions have a probability of achieving desired outcomes. To continue with the previous example, expected outcomes might include the following:

1. Patient will be free of chest pain during my shift.
2. Patient will maintain O_2 sat of 90% during my shift.
3. Vital signs will remain stable: T < 99.0°F, HR > 60 < 110 beats/min, R > 12 < 24 breaths/min, and SBP > 90 mm Hg while under my care.
4. Patient will have no further weight gain and will have a decrease in edema during my shift.

■ Implementation

Implementation is carrying out the plan of care and depends on the first three steps of the nursing process. These steps provide the basis for nursing actions performed during the implementation phase of the nursing process. The nurse carries out nursing interventions individualized to the patient, reassesses the client, and validates that the plan of care is accurate and successful. In this stage, to each patient care situation the nurse applies knowledge and principles from nursing and from related courses. The ability to apply, not just memorize, principles is a component of critical thinking (Wilkinson, 2007).

For the patient with decreased cardiac output, the nurse could implement some of the following individualized interventions:

- Assess LOC—confusion, anxiety.
- Provide reassurance to the patient.
- Monitor vital signs every 4 hours.
- Assess heart rate and rhythm; monitor telemetry or electrocardiography.
- Monitor for jugular vein distension.
- Monitor for chest pain.
- Monitor peripheral pulses; assess capillary refill.
- Auscultate lung sounds; monitor respiratory rate and rhythm; monitor oxygen saturation; assess for cough and sputum.
- Look at skin color and temperature.
- Monitor for fatigue and activity tolerance.
- Assess intake and output, daily weight, and edema in dependent areas.
- Assess abdomen for distension or bloating, ascites, and bowel function.
- Monitor lab and X-rays: CBC, PT/PTT, electrolytes, cardiac enzymes, arterial blood gases, and chest X-ray.
- Elevate head of bed to improve gas exchange.
- Administer oxygen as ordered to improve gas exchange.
- Administer morphine sulfate as prescribed to relieve chest pain, provide sedation and vasodilation, and monitor for respiratory depression and hypotension after administration.
- Administer diuretics as prescribed to reduce preload, enhance renal excretion of sodium and water, reduce circulating blood volume, and reduce pulmonary congestion; closely monitor potassium level, which might decrease as a result of diuretic therapy.
- Provide teaching: Identify precipitating risk factors of heart failure and prescribed medication regimen; notify physician if unable to take medications because of illness; avoid large amounts of caffeine; cardiac diet instruction; signs of exacerbation; monitor fluids; balance periods of activity and rest; avoid isometric activities that increase pressure in the heart.

▪ Evaluation

During evaluation, the nurse compares the patient's current status to the patient goals. Were the goals achieved? The nurse analyzes outcomes to determine if the interventions worked, and if not, why? The information provided during evaluation can be used to begin another plan of care sufficient to meet patient needs. Continuing with the previous example, the evaluation might include the following:

- Patient denies chest pain on my shift. Patient rates pain 0 on pain scale.
- Patient's O_2 saturation dropped to 85% when oxygen at 3 L nasal cannula was removed. With oxygen on, patient's O_2 saturation remained 92%.

- Vital signs were: T, 101.0°F; HR, 100–110 beats/min; R, 32 breaths/min and labored; BP, 90/50 mm Hg.
- Patient's weight was 241 lbs with 2+ edema in lower extremities.

▪ Concept Mapping

Concept mapping is a visual representation of the relationships among concepts and ideas. The concepts are represented by boxes and linked with lines. In nursing, concept maps are used to organize and link information about a patient's health problems. This allows the nurse to see relationships among the patient's problems and helps plan interventions that can address more than one problem.

To begin a concept map, start in the center of the page with the main idea or central theme, and work outward in all directions, producing a growing organized structure composed of key words or pictures. Place words or pictures around the main idea to illustrate how they relate to each other and the central theme. Pictures, words, or a combination of both can be used to create a map.

Concept maps are useful for summarizing information, consolidating information from different sources, thinking through complex problems, and presenting information in a format that shows the overall structure of your subject.

Figure 9-1 illustrates mind mapping techniques used by students with a patient case.

> In nursing, concept maps are used to organize and link information about a patient's health problems. This allows the nurse to see relationships among the patient's problems and helps plan interventions that can address more than one problem.

▪ Journaling

Keeping a journal of clinical experiences that were meaningful or troubling to you is a recommended way to help enhance and develop reasoning skills. Think about and record experiences that bother you, and consider what you could and would do differently in the future. This is a form of reflection and allows you to view your own thinking, reasoning, and actions. It helps create and clarify meaning and new understandings of a particular experience. When you encounter a similar situation, you should be able to recall what you did or would do differently as well as the reasoning behind your actions (Raingruber & Haffer, 2001. Some suggestions you should try to address when **journaling** your nursing experience include the following:

- What happened? What are the facts?
- What was my role in the event?
- What feelings and senses surrounded the event?
- What did I do?
- How and what did I feel about what I did? Why?
- What was the setting?

Figure 9-1   Mind mapping techniques

1. Decreased cardiac output related to inability of the heart to pump effectively, occlusion and constriction of vessels

Dx; Exacerbation of CHF	Sacral edema	ALB 3.0	I & O	Digoxin
HX; HTN, CAD, MI, CABG	Yellow secretions	PCO2 32	Foley	Lasix
Family HX: CVA, MI, diabetes	HX; Smoking × 20 years	EKG NSR old infarct	Tele	Potassium
C/O SOB, productive/congested cough,	Wt. 240 lbs.	CXR – Bil. inflt, enlarged heart	D-stick's	Prinivil
Swelling in legs, chest pain	HR 100, BP 88/60	BR w BRP	Egg crate	Humulin R & NPH
Obese pt,	K+ 2.9	HOB 40°	Ted hose	Heparin
3+ edema	RBC 4.0	1800 cal ADA, low, NA,	O_2 3 L/NC	Albuterol
Lungs w rales	H & H 11.0 & 35	low chol, & low fat	O_2 Sat	Morphine
O_2 sat 86%	Glucose 210	Fluid restriction 1200 cc	EKG for CP	Colace
JVD	PT 31.0, PPT 80	Daily wt.	Daily lab;	
		VS Q4h	H & H, PT/PTT	

Chief medical diagnosis:

Exacerbation of
CHF & pneumonia

Secondary diagnosis
Type I diabetes
HTN
CAD
Hypothyroidism
PVD

3. Altered Nutrition related to inability of pancreas to secrete insulin

Dx; Exacerbation of CHF	RBC 4.0	I & O
Hx: Diabetes type I, CAD, PVD, MI	Glucose 210	Foley
Family Hx: Diabetes, MI, CABG, CVA	ALB 2.9	D – Stick's
C/O SOB, CP	Prot. 5.6	Egg crate
Obese – 240 lbs.	BR	Ted hose
Labored resp, chest pain	1800 cal ADA, low, NA	Morphine
T - 99°	low chol, & low fat	Colace
WBC 14,000	FR 1200 cc	Potassium
K+ 2.9	Daily wt.	Humulin R & N
H & H 11.0 & 35	VS Q4	Lasix
	Daily H & H	
	BC for T > 101	

2. Impaired gas exchange related to mucous build-up in alveoli impairing oxygen movement

DX exacerbation of CHF & pneumonia	HGB 11.0	Daily H & H
Hx: CAD, PVD, CABG	PCO2 32	BC for T > 101
C/O SOB, productive cough, chest pain	CXR – Bil Infl & enlarged heart	O_2 3L/NC
Obese	BR w BRP	O_2 Sat
3+ Edema	HOB 40°	EKG prn CP
Lungs w rales	Fluid Rest 1200 cc	Lasix
O_2 Sat 86%	Daily Wt.	Heparin
JVD	I & O	Albuterol via HHN
Yellow secretions	Foley	Morphine
Hx: Smoking × 20 yrs.	Telemetry	
Wt. 240 lbs.	Egg crate	
HR - 100, R – 34	Ted hose	

- What were the important elements of the event?
- What preceded the event, and what followed it?
- What should I be aware of if the event recurs?

It is important that you write in your journal as soon as possible after an event to capture the essence of what happened in the clinical experience. The following is an example of a journal excerpt that illustrates reflection on events and the feelings elicited by those events over the course of many patient care encounters during the career of a nurse.

> I have learned, not so easily, that my job is not just about saving a life, trying to keep people well, or helping them get well when they are ill, but importantly, it also entails providing that same dedicated care to them as they take their last breaths in life. It is my job, my duty, and I have learned, my privilege. As I care for a dying patient, listening to the rise and fall of methodical machines imitating life, I hope I never get calloused to the point that I say, "I do this every day. It is just another patient." I want to appreciate that every individual's life has been remarkable in some way—that they are remarkable in some way. I want to make my patient's journey through this last chapter in their life a little easier, provide comfort, recognize their fears, hold their hand, and always realize this is not another patient, but a person.

■ Group Discussions and Reflection

Another way to enhance critical thinking skills is by using group discussions to explore alternatives and arrive at conclusions. Group discussions among nursing students and teachers can take place in the classroom or following clinical experiences. During discussions, students are encouraged to formulate alternatives to clinical or ethical decisions. Teacher and learner group discussions over clinical and ethical scenarios should encourage questions, analysis, and reflection. Group discussions can assist nursing students in connecting clinical events or decisions with information obtained in the classroom. This form of cooperative learning occurs when groups work together to maximize their own and each other's learning. For example, following a clinical experience, students and teacher use reflection and discussion on a certain clinical experience that a student encountered. Together they discuss different scenarios of "What if?," "What else?," and "What then?" to encourage the formulation of alternatives or clinical decisions. Other examples of this process include the following:

- You are going into a patient's room—what are you going to do? When you go in there, what are you going to do? Walk yourself through it step by step.
- What are you going to do first? What should you get done first? Which one takes importance and then where do you go from there?
- This is the patient, and this happens. What do you do next?
- These are your assessment findings. What else do you need to know?

KEY COMPETENCY 9-4

Examples of Applicable *Nurse of the Future: Nursing Core Competencies*

Professionalism:

Knowledge (K4c) Understands the importance of reflection to advancing practice and improving outcomes of care

Skills (S4b) Demonstrates ability for reflection in actions, reflection for action, and reflection on action

Attitudes/Behaviors (A4c) Values and is committed to being a reflective practitioner

Source: Massachusetts Department of Higher Education (2010), p. 13.

www▸ CRITICAL THINKING QUESTIONS ✳

Think about a clinical experience that was troubling to you. Reflect on what bothered you about the experience. What could you have done differently? What were the reasons behind your actions? Try to create and clarify meaning or a new understanding of the particular situation. ✳

Why Is Critical Thinking Important in Nursing Practice?

Nursing competence plays a large role in ensuring patient safety. In 2008, the Robert Wood Johnson Foundation and the Institute of Medicine (IOM) launched a 2-year initiative to respond to the need to assess and transform the nursing profession. The IOM report points out nurses are going to have a critical role in the future, especially in producing safe, quality care and coverage for all patients in our healthcare system (Institute of Medicine [IOM], 2011). The Agency for Healthcare Research and Quality (2008) (AHRQ) and the Robert Wood Johnson Foundation developed a handbook for nurses on patient safety and quality. This is a wealth of information for nursing that provides background research and tools for improving the quality of care. In 2008, the American Association of Colleges of Nursing (AACN) revised its *The Essentials of Baccalaureate Education for Professional Nursing Practice* based on early discussion of IOM reports and the necessity of building a safer healthcare system (American Association of Colleges of Nursing [AACN], 2008). A majority of sentinel events, unexpected occurrences involving death or serious physical or psychological injury, occur in acute care settings, where new graduate nurses traditionally begin their professional nursing careers. The inability of a nurse to set priorities and work safely, effectively, and efficiently can delay patient treatment in a critical situation and result in serious life-threatening consequences. Critical thinking is essential to providing safe, competent, quality nursing care.

> The inability of a nurse to set priorities and work safely, effectively, and efficiently can delay patient treatment in a critical situation and result in serious life-threatening consequences.

New realities of health care require nurses to master complex information, to coordinate a variety of care experiences, to use advanced technology for healthcare delivery and evaluation of patient outcomes, as well as assist patients with managing and navigating an increasingly complex system of care. Some of the trends that have added to the complexities of the healthcare environment, and nursing specifically, include increases in longevity; markedly shortened hospital stays, which are moving patients out of the hospital "quicker and sicker"; scientific advances; major advances in technology; an increase in population; increased diversity in the U.S. population; and an increased incidence of chronic diseases and infectious diseases (AACN, 2008).

To prepare nursing students for the multifaceted role of professional nurse, the learning process involves components that will provide a solid foundation for developing clinical judgment skills. One of these components or core competencies is critical thinking. Course work or clinical experience should provide the nursing student and graduate with knowledge and skills to do the following:

- Use appropriate nursing theories and models and appropriate ethical frameworks in practice.
- Use research-based knowledge from nursing and the sciences as the basis for practice.
- Use sound clinical judgment and decision-making skills.
- Engage in processes such as self-reflection and shared educational dialogue about professional practice.
- Evaluate nursing care outcomes through acquiring data and the questioning of inconsistencies, allowing for the revision of actions and goals.
- Engage in creative thinking and problem solving.

You are working in an acute care clinical situation. After receiving report, you have started your morning routines. Everything is going as planned, and you are about to start preparing your medications. The wife of one of your patients reports that the oxygen is burning his nose and wants you to get an oxygen humidifier. All of a sudden, the daughter of your other patient, Mr. Peary, rushes toward you and informs you that her father is spitting up blood. He looked fine when you observed him a few minutes ago. You walk rapidly toward the patient's room, thinking, "What am I going to do when I get there? I have to get the oxygen humidifier for room 202. His nose was burning, and his wife was waiting for me. What could be happening with Mr. Peary?"

You enter the room, and the first thing you think is: "He's lying flat," and you think to yourself, "I need to elevate his head. That is what I did on the respiratory unit where I recently worked." The daughter tells you that Mr. Peary coughed up some blood in the emesis basin. There is a small amount of bright red blood in it. You do not know what to do next. An RN stops by the room and tells you that the wife of the patient in room 202 is asking about the burning in her husband's nose again. Your mind doesn't seem to be able to think about anything. Do you feel scattered and things seem out of control at this point? Do you feel a little overwhelmed and can't think what to do next? The RN says she will take over with Mr. Peary while you follow up with the patient in room 202. Later, you recall the situation and can't believe you didn't think to take Mr. Peary's blood pressure, count respirations, ask about pain, or listen to his lungs or anything else. All you did was just raise his head. You wonder why you missed so many things.

- What do you think was going on in the situation that influenced what happening and caused you to lose your ability to think and plan what to do next?

www. **CRITICAL THINKING QUESTIONS** ✳

Beginning nursing students often tend to focus primarily on their routines, such as to get their list of tasks done, such as assessments, ordered treatments, daily care, and charting. What if an unexpected situation occurred during the day? Do you think you would be able to reason, plan, and take appropriate action—think critically? ✳

- What would you do differently in this situation after having a chance to reflect on it? Prioritize the order in which you would have done things.
- If this had happened to you and no one helped you through it, what would you have done to mobilize yourself to think about what to do?

Conclusion

In nursing, critical thinking is the ability to think in a systematic and logical manner, solve problems, make decisions, and establish priorities in the clinical setting. Nurses need to develop critical thinking skills to make sound clinical judgments and to provide safe, competent patient care. Nursing requires constant decision making. What should I do first? What is the most important thing to do at this time? Prioritizing nursing actions involves recalling important nursing information as well as using complex problem-solving skills to make decisions in providing safe and effective patient care. As a nurse, you will constantly have to demonstrate good judgment in analyzing facts and situations and applying nursing knowledge.

Classroom Activity 1

Critical thinking gives you the power to make sense of something by deliberately choosing how to respond to events that you encounter. You take in information, examine and ask questions about it, look at new perspectives, and identify a plan. You use problem-solving and decision-making strategies.

- Choose a decision that you need to make soon, and write it down.
- What goal or desired outcomes do you seek from this decision? Prioritize goals or desired outcomes, and write them down.

- Identify who and what will be affected by your decision, and indicate how your decision will affect them.
- Identify any available options you might have.
- Taking into account and evaluating your information, identify a plan or decide what you are going to do.
- After you have made your decision, evaluate the result. www

Classroom Activity 2

You are receiving morning reports on the following patients from the night-shift nurse. After receiving the following report, which patient would you choose to see first? As you make your decision, think about your thought processes and how you made your decision.

1. A woman who is scheduled to have a biopsy on a breast lump this morning, and who is scared and crying

2. An 85-year-old man who was admitted during the night because of increased confusion who remains disoriented this morning

3. A woman who had lung surgery the previous day, and who has two chest tubes in place with minimal drainage

4. A man who is scheduled to have a colon resection in 2 hours and is complaining of chills

Answer: You should have answered the client who is scheduled for surgery and is exhibiting symptoms of infection. This patient needs to be assessed immediately for infection, and the doctor notified. If an infection is present, the surgery needs to be postponed. The other patients are stable, and their needs do not have to be addressed immediately. www

www CASE STUDY ■ JIM FULLER

Jim Fuller is a 40-year-old male patient. He is currently in the recovery room following an inguinal hernia repair under general anesthesia. His vital signs are: T, 99.0°F; BP, 120/80 mm Hg; HR, 80 beats/min; R, 18 breaths per minute.

Case Study Questions

- Are Mr. Fuller's vital signs within normal limits? List normal adult ranges.
- What factors might affect body temperature?
- List sites where a nurse might take a patient's pulse. What sites are most commonly used?
- What factors might influence respiratory rate?

Two hours postoperative, Mr. Fuller begins to complain of abdominal pain. Vital signs at this time are:

T, 99.5°F; BP, 90/60 mm Hg; HR, 122 beats/min; R, 24 breaths/min.

Case Study Questions

- What could Mr. Fuller's vital signs indicate?
- What nursing interventions are indicated? What should the nurse assess in Mr. Fuller at this time?
- What clinical signs associated with an elevated temperature might the nurse assess?
- If Mr. Fuller's fever persists and increases, what might the nurse suspect is happening, and what might be done? ■

References

Agency for Healthcare Research and Quality. (2008). *Patient safety and quality: An evidence-based handbook for nurses* (Vols. 1, 2, 3). Rockville, MD: U.S. Department of Health and Human Services. Retrieved from www.ahrq.gov/qual/nurseshdbk

Alfaro-Lefevre, R. (2009). *Critical thinking and clinical judgment: A practical approach to outcome-focused thinking* (4th ed.). St. Louis, MO: Saunders Elsevier.

American Association of Colleges of Nursing. (2008). *The essentials of baccalaureate education for professional nursing practice*. Washington, DC: Author.

Benner, P. (1984). *From novice to expert*. Menlo Park, CA: Addison-Wesley.

Benner, P. E., Malloch, K., & Sheets, V. (2010). *Nursing pathways for patient safety, NCSBN*. St. Louis, MO: Mosby Elsevier.

Benner, P. E., Sutphen, M., Leonard, V., & Day, L. (2010). *Educating nurses: A call for radical transformation*. San Francisco, CA: Jossey-Bass.

Caputi, L. (2010). Developing critical thinking in the nursing student. In L. Caputi (Ed.), *Teaching nursing: The art and science* (2nd ed.). Glen Ellyn, IL: College of DuPage Press.

Craven, R. F., & Hirnle, C. J. (2007). *Fundamentals of nursing: Human health and function* (5th ed.). Philadelphia, PA: Lippincott Williams & Wilkins.

Fero, L., Witsberger, C., Wesmiller, S., Zullo, T., & Hoffman, L. (2009). Critical thinking ability of new graduate and experienced nurses. *Journal of Advanced Nursing, 65*(1), 139–148.

Institute of Medicine. (2011). *The future of nursing: Leading change, advancing health*. Washington, DC: National Academies Press.

Knapp, R. (2007). Nursing education—the importance of critical thinking. Retrieved from http://www.articlecity.com/articles/education/article_1327.shtml

Massachusetts Department of Higher Education. (2010). *Nurse of the future: Nursing core competencies*. Retrieved from http://www.mass.edu/currentinit/documents/NursingCoreCompetencies.pdf

Raingruber, B., & Haffer, A. (2001). Using your head to land on your feet: A beginning nurse's guide to critical thinking. Philadelphia, PA: F. A. Davis.

Scheffer, B. K., & Rubenfeld, M. G. (2000). A consensus statement on critical thinking in nursing. *Journal of Nursing Education, 39*(8), 352–359.

Scriven, M., & Paul, R. (2011). Defining critical thinking. Retrieved from http://www.criticalthinking.org/pages/defining-critical-thinking/410

Wangensteen, S., Johansson, I. S., Bjorkstrom, M. E., & Nordstrom, G. (2010). Critical thinking dispositions among newly graduated nurses. *Journal of Advanced Nursing, 66*(10), 2170–2181.

Wilkinson, J. (2007). *Nursing process and critical thinking* (4th ed.). Upper Saddle River, NJ: Pearson.

Evidence-Based Professional Nursing Practice

10

Kathleen Masters

Evidence-Based Practice: What Is It?

Evidence-based practice—it is more than the most recent buzzword in nursing. Evidence-based practice allows nurses to provide high-quality patient care based on research evidence and knowledge rather than tradition, myths, hunches, advice from peers, outdated textbooks, or even what the nurse learned in school 5, 10, or 15 years ago. Evidence-based practice provides a strategy to ensure that nursing care reflects the most up-to-date knowledge available. Nursing practice that is based on evidence is now the accepted standard for practice as well as one of the six core competencies for all registered nurses identified in the Quality and Safety Education for Nurses project (Cronenwett et al., 2007). Nurses are accountable for interventions they provide to patients. Evidence-based practice provides a systematic approach for decision making and provides a framework for the nurse to use to incorporate best nursing practices into the clinical care of patients (Pugh, 2012).

Key Terms and Concepts

» **Research utilization**
» Quality improvement
» Evidence-based practice
» PICO
» Clinical practice guidelines

www

> **Nursing practice that is based on evidence is now the accepted standard for practice.**

Learning Objectives

www

After completing this chapter, the student should be able to:

1. Describe the importance of evidence-based nursing care.
2. Identify barriers to the implementation of evidence-based nursing practice.
3. Identify strategies for the implementation of evidence-based nursing practice.
4. Describe how and where to search for evidence.
5. Identify methods to evaluate the evidence.
6. Discuss approaches to integrating evidence into practice.
7. Identify models of evidence-based nursing practice.

> Evidence-based practice assumes that evidence is used in the context of patient preferences, the clinical situation, and the expertise of the clinician.

Most nurses want to provide care for their patients based on the most current knowledge, but for many nurses trying to integrate evidence-based practice into patient care in the clinical environment it raises many questions:

- What exactly is evidence-based practice, and how is it relevant to my practice?
- Is evidence-based practice different from research utilization?
- Is evidence-based practice different from quality improvement?

Although they may be widely used and related processes, evidence-based practice is not research utilization or quality improvement.

- **Research utilization** involves critical analysis and evaluation of research findings and then determining how these findings fit into clinical practice. In research utilization, the research findings are the only source of evidence. In evidence-based practice, research is only one of the sources of evidence (Levin, 2006a).
- **Quality improvement** focuses on systems, processes, satisfaction, and cost outcomes, usually within a specific organization. These projects can contribute to understanding best practices for the processes of care in which nurses are involved, but typically quality improvement efforts are not designed to develop nursing practice standards or nursing science.

Evidence-based practice is a framework for clinical practice that incorporates "the conscientious, explicit, and judicious use of the current best evidence in making decisions about the care of individual patients" (Beyea & Slattery, 2006). Put another way, evidence-based practice is "the integration of best research evidence with clinical expertise and patient values" (Sackett, Straus, Richardson, Rosenberg, & Haynes, 2000). In other words, evidence-based practice assumes that evidence is used in the context of patient preferences, the clinical situation, and the expertise of the clinician.

Evidence-based practice is relevant to nursing practice because it does the following:

- Helps resolve problems in the clinical setting
- Results in better patient outcomes
- Contributes to the science of nursing through the introduction of innovation to practice
- Keeps practice current and relevant by helping nurses deliver care based on current best research
- Decreases variations in nursing care and increases confidence in decision making

- Supports Joint Commission readiness because policies and procedures are current and include the latest research
- Essential for high-quality patient care and achievement of magnet status (Beyea & Slattery, 2006; Spector, 2007)

Barriers to Evidence-Based Practice

Because evidence-based practice is now the standard for professional nursing practice, one would think that practice based on evidence is commonplace. However, this is not the case. Practicing nurses cite many barriers to evidence-based practice. Common barriers to implementing evidence-based practice include the following:

- Lack of value for research in practice
- Difficulty in changing practice
- Lack of administrative support
- Lack of knowledgeable mentors
- Insufficient time
- Lack of education about the research process
- Lack of awareness about research or evidence-based practice
- Research reports and articles not readily available
- Difficulty accessing research reports and articles
- No time on the job to read research
- Complexity of research reports
- Lack of knowledge about evidence-based practice
- Lack of knowledge about the critique of articles
- Feeling overwhelmed by the process
- Lack of sense of control over practice
- Lack of confidence to implement change
- Lack of leadership, motivation, vision, strategy, or direction among managers (Beyea & Slattery, 2006; Spector, 2007)

Strategies to Promote Evidence-Based Practice

Despite barriers, nurses are making a difference in patient outcomes through the use of evidence-based practice. Strategies that can be useful in the promotion of evidence in practice generally fall into two categories: strategies for individual nurses and organizational strategies.

Strategies for individual nurses include the following:

- Educate yourself about evidence-based practice through avenues such as online sites, books, articles, and conferences.
- Conduct face-to-face or online journal clubs that can be used to educate yourself about critiquing articles, share new research reports and guidelines with peers, and provide support to other nurses.
- Share your results through posters, newsletters, unit meetings, or a published article to support a culture of evidence-based nursing practice within the organization and the profession.
- Adopt a reflective and inquiring approach to practice by continuously asking yourself and others within your organization questions such as, "What is the evidence for this intervention?" or "How do my patients respond to this intervention?" (Beyea & Slattery, 2006)

Strategies for organizations include the following:

- Developing a center for evidence-based practice
- Administrative support for evidence-based practice by providing the time and the funds for necessary resources
- Access to electronic resources in the workplace
- Enhancement of job descriptions to include criteria related to evidence-based practice
- Offering incentives such as a paid registration to a conference for the best clinical question in a unit-wide or facility-wide contest
- Providing opportunities for nurses to collaborate with nurse researchers or faculty with nursing research expertise

www | CRITICAL THINKING QUESTIONS ✳

How is new evidence disseminated to the bedside nurse in the organization in which you practice as a nursing student? How does the organization promote evidence-based practice? Do the nurses in the organization use current evidence in practice? ✳

Whichever strategies are incorporated, it is important to note that passive dissemination of results within an organization is ineffective in changing practice. Multifaceted interventions are much more likely to be effective in facilitating evidence-based practice within an organization.

Searching for Evidence

■ Asking the Question

Nurses must learn to ask questions in a format that facilitates searching for evidence. It has been suggested that all nurses should learn how to use the PICO format to ask clinical questions. **PICO** is simply an acronym that assists in the formatting of clinical questions. Using this format helps the nurse to ask pertinent clinical questions, focus on asking the right questions, and choose relevant guidelines.

P = Patient, Population, or Problem
- How would I describe a group of patients similar to mine?
- What group do I want information on?

I = Intervention or Exposure or Topic of Interest
- Which main intervention am I considering?
- What event do I want to study the effect of?

C = Comparison or Alternate Intervention (if appropriate)
- What is the main alternative to compare with the intervention?
- Compared to what? Better or worse than no intervention at all, or than another intervention?

O = Outcome
- What can I hope to accomplish, measure, improve, or affect?
- What is the effect of the intervention? (Levin & Feldman, 2006)

Some researchers also add the element of time or time frame to the PICO question format and refer to the format as PICOT, although the time frame might not be applicable to all questions.

T = Time or Time Frame
- How much time is required to demonstrate an outcome?
- How long are participants observed?

After determining the patient, intervention, comparison, and outcome of interest, the nurse then combines these four elements into a single question in combinations such as the following examples:

- In (patient or population), what is the effect of (intervention or exposure) on (outcome) compared with (comparison)? (Levin, 2006b)
- For (patient or population), does the introduction of (intervention or exposure) reduce the risk of (outcome) compared with (comparison intervention)? (Levin, 2006b)

■ Electronic Indexes

Electronic indexes provide options for narrowing or broadening a topic to identify relevant literature. Most electronic indexes provide citation information and will indicate if the selected articles are available locally in print form or if the items are available in an electronic format. Three of the most common electronic indexes used in health care are the Cumulative Index to Nursing and Allied Health Literature (CINAHL), available at www.cinahl.com; MEDLINE, available at www.nlm.nih.gov; or PubMed, a web-based format of Medline available at www.pubmed.gov.

■ Electronic Resources

Many other helpful Internet resources are available that can assist the nurse in uncovering the most current evidence for practice. Some of the most commonly used include these:

- National Library of Medicine: www.nlm.nih.gov
- Cochrane Library: www.cochrane.org
- National Guideline Clearinghouse: www.ngc.gov
- Joanna Briggs Institute: www.joannabriggs.edu.au
- Agency for Healthcare Research and Quality: www.effectivehealthcare.ahrq.gov
- Centre for Health Evidence: www.cche.net
- Registered Nurses' Association of Ontario: rnao.ca/bpg
- McGill University Health Centre's Research and Clinical Resources for Evidence Based Nursing: www.muhc-ebn.mcgill.ca

The Cochrane Library is a collection of databases that contain high-quality, independent evidence to inform healthcare decision making. Cochrane reviews represent the highest level of evidence on which to base clinical treatment decisions. In addition to the Cochrane systematic reviews, the Cochrane Library also offers other sources of information, including the Cochrane Database of Systematic Reviews, Database of Abstracts of Reviews of Effects, Cochrane Controlled Trials Register, Cochrane Methodology Register, NHS Economic Evaluation Database, Health Technology Assessment Database, and the Cochrane Database of Methodology Reviews (CDMR).

The National Guideline Clearinghouse includes structured summaries containing information about each guideline, including comparisons of guidelines covering similar topics that show areas of similarity and differences; full text or links to full text; ordering details for full guidelines; annotated bibliographies on guideline development, evaluation, implementation, and structure; weekly email updates; and guideline archives.

> **KEY COMPETENCY 10-2**
>
> Examples of Applicable *Nurse of the Future: Nursing Core Competencies*
>
> Evidence-Based Practice:
>
> Knowledge (K3) Describes reliable sources for locating evidence reports and clinical practice guidelines
>
> Skills (S3) Locates evidence reports related to clinical practice topics and guidelines
>
> Attitudes/Behaviors (A3) Appreciates the importance of accessing relevant clinical evidence
>
> *Source:* Massachusetts Department of Higher Education (2010), p. 37.

Evaluating the Evidence

Regardless of the source, we always need to evaluate the evidence. Begin by asking such questions as follow:

- What is the source of the information?
- When was it developed?
- How was it developed?
- Does it fit the current clinical environment?
- Does it fit the current situation?

Best evidence for practice includes empirical evidence from randomized controlled trials, evidence from descriptive and qualitative research, and information from case reports, scientific principles, and expert opinion. When insufficient research is available, healthcare decision making is derived principally from nonresearch evidence sources such as expert opinion and scientific principles (Titler, 2008).

> **Regardless of the source, we always need to evaluate the evidence.**

Several classification systems exist to evaluate the level or strength of the evidence. The Agency for Healthcare Research and Quality (AHRQ) serves as the recognized authority regarding the assessment of clinical research in the United States. The AHRQ levels of evidence include classifications 1–5 listed here (Melnyk & Fineout-Overholt, 2005). Other sources (Di Cesenso, Guyatt, & Ciliska, 2005) also include additional classifications or levels of evidence (6–7).

- 1A Meta-analysis or systematic reviews of multiple well-designed controlled studies
- 1 Well-designed randomized controlled trials
- 2 Well-designed nonrandomized controlled trials (quasi-experimental)
- 3 Observational studies with controls (retrospective, interrupted time, case-control, cohort studies with controls)
- 4 Observational studies without controls (cohort studies without controls and case series)
- 5 Systematic review of descriptive, qualitative, or physiologic studies
- 6 Single descriptive, qualitative, or physiologic study
- 7 Opinions of authorities, expert committees

Using this classification system, the strongest evidence comes from the first level, representing systematic reviews that integrate findings from multiple well-designed controlled studies. The weakest evidence is represented by the seventh level and is based on opinion (Polit & Beck, 2008).

In addition, grading the strength of a body of evidence should incorporate three domains that include quality, quantity, and consistency. Quality has to do with the extent to which a study minimizes bias in the design, implementation, and analysis. Quantity refers to the number of studies that have evaluated the research question, as well as the sample size across the studies and the strength of the findings. The category of consistency refers to both the similarity and differences of study designs that investigate the same research question and report similar findings (Agency for Healthcare Research and Quality [AHRQ], 2002; LoBiondo-Wood, Haber, & Krainovich-Miller, 2006).

KEY COMPETENCY 10-3

Examples of Applicable *Nurse of the Future: Nursing Core Competencies*

Evidence-Based Practice:

Knowledge (K4) Differentiates clinical opinion from research and evidence summaries

Attitudes/Behaviors (A4) Appreciates that the strength and relevance of evidence should be determinants when choosing clinical interventions

Source: Massachusetts Department of Higher Education (2010), p. 37.

Using the Evidence

■ Clinical Practice Guidelines

Clinical practice guidelines are developed to guide clinical practice and represent an effort to put a large body of evidence into a manageable form. Clinical practice guidelines are usually based on systematic reviews and give specific recommendations for clinicians. Guidelines usually attempt to address all the issues relevant to a clinical decision, including risks and benefits.

There is an ongoing collaboration that focuses on improving the quality and effectiveness of clinical practice guidelines. The group has established a framework for determining the quality of guidelines for diagnoses, health promotion, treatments, or clinical interventions. The instrument can be used with new, existing, or updated guidelines and is known as the Appraisal of Guidelines for Research and Evaluation (AGREE) instrument. The instrument, first published in 2003 by the AGREE Collaboration, has been revised and is now known as AGREE II (AGREE Next Steps Consortium, 2009). The AGREE II replaces the original instrument and is the preferred tool. The full version of the AGREE II instrument and training materials are available at: www.agreetrust.org. The AGREE instrument is composed of six categories comprising the 23 items listed here:

- Scope and purpose
    - Overall objectives of the guideline are specifically described.
    - The health questions covered by the guideline are specifically described.
    - The population (patients, public, etc.) to whom the guideline is meant to apply is specifically described.
- Stakeholder involvement
    - Guideline development group includes individuals from all relevant professions.
    - The views and preferences of the target population (patients, public, etc.) have been sought.
    - Target users of the guideline are clearly defined.
- Rigor of development
    - Systematic methods were used to search for evidence.
    - The criteria for selecting the evidence are clearly described.
    - The strengths and limitations of the body of evidence are clearly described.
    - The methods used for formulating the recommendations are clearly described.
    - The health benefits, side effects, and risks have been considered in formulating recommendations.

- There is an explicit link between the recommendations and the supporting evidence.
  - The guideline has been externally reviewed by experts prior to publication.
  - A procedure for updating the guideline is provided.
- Clarity and presentation
  - Recommendations are specific and unambiguous.
  - Different options for management of the condition or health issue are clearly presented.
  - Key recommendations are easily identifiable.
- Application
  - The guideline describes facilitators and barriers to its application.
  - The guideline provides advice and/or tools on how the recommendations can be put into practice.
  - The potential resource implications of applying the recommendations have been considered.
  - Guideline presents monitoring and/or auditing criteria.
- Editorial independence
  - The views of the funding body have not influenced the content of the guideline.
  - Competing interests of guideline development group members have been recorded and addressed (AGREE Next Steps Consortium, 2009, pp. 2–3).

The usefulness of a guideline depends on whether the actual recommendations in the guideline and meaningful and practical. Recommendations should be practical in relation to implementation, be as unambiguous as possible, address frequency of screening and follow-up, and address clinically relevant actions. Other questions that the clinician must address in relation to guidelines must include such factors as the setting of care, the patient population, and the strength of the recommendations (Beyea & Slattery, 2006).

Models of Evidence-Based Nursing Practice

Differences exist among evidence-based practice models, but most models do have common elements that include selection of a practice topic, critique and synthesis of evidence, implementation, evaluation of the impact on patient care and provider performance, and consideration of the context in which the practice is implemented (Titler, 2008). No one model of evidence-based practice is a perfect fit for every organization. Some models focus on the perspective of the individual clinician, or the researcher, while others focus on institutional efforts. Therefore, before embarking on this journey, the nurse or organization should consider several models and select or adapt one that fits the nurse's or organization's needs.

■ ACE Star Model of Knowledge Transformation

The Academic Center for Evidence-Based Nursing (ACE) Star Model of Knowledge Transformation, developed by Dr. Kathleen Stevens, is available at www.acestar.uthscsa.edu/acestar-model.asp. The model involves five steps that include knowledge discovery, evidence summary, translation into practice recommendations, integration into practice, and evaluation. Discovery refers to the original research. During the second step, the task is to synthesize all the related research into a meaningful whole. It is during this step that information is reduced to a manageable form. During the step of translation, the scientific evidence is considered in the context of clinical expertise and values. This results in clinical practice guidelines, best practices, protocols, standards, or clinical pathways. During the stage of implementation, changes take place in practice. During evaluation, the impact of the change is measured. Variables such as specific health outcomes, length of stay, or patient satisfaction are examples of possible outcomes that might be examined.

■ The Iowa Model of Evidence-Based Practice

The Iowa Model of Evidence-Based Practice resembles a decision-making tree that identifies either problem-focused or knowledge-focused triggers that initiate the process in the organization. Additional information and a diagram of the Iowa Model of Evidence-Based Practice are available at www.conehealth.com/documents/public/Nursing%20Research/Iowa%20 Model%201998.pdf.

Problem-focused triggers within an organization can include risk management data, process improvement data, benchmarking data, financial data, or the identification of clinical problems. Knowledge-focused triggers within an organization can include the publication of new research or literature, a change in organizational standards and guidelines, changes in philosophies of care within the profession or organization, or questions from an institutional standards committee.

Once there is either a problem-focused or knowledge-focused trigger within the organization, a team must identify whether the topic is a priority for the organization. If the topic is indeed a priority, evidence is examined, and the change in practice can be piloted. This process is followed by monitoring and analysis of both the process and the outcome data and finally by dissemination of the results.

■ Agency for Healthcare Research and Quality Model

A model for maximizing and accelerating the transfer of research results from the Agency for Healthcare Research and Quality (AHRQ) patient safety research portfolio to healthcare delivery has recently been developed. The three major stages of knowledge transfer in the AHRQ model include: (1) knowledge creation and distillation, (2) diffusion and dissemination, and (3) organizational adoption and implementation. More specifically, knowledge creation and distillation refers to the conducting of research and then packaging relevant research findings into usable form such as practice recommendations. The diffusion and dissemination stage involves partnering with professional leaders, professional organizations, and healthcare organizations to disseminate knowledge to potential users such as nurses, physical therapists, or physicians. During the final stage of the process, the focus is on organizational adoption and implementation of evidence-based research findings and innovations in practice. In this model, the stages of knowledge transfer are viewed from the perspective of the researcher or the creator of new knowledge and begin with decisions about what research findings ought to be disseminated (Titler, 2008).

■ Johns Hopkins Nursing Evidence-Based Practice Model

The process used in the Johns Hopkins Nursing Evidence-Based Practice Model is known as PET, which refers to asking a practice question, finding the evidence, and translating the evidence to practice (Newhouse, Dearholt, Poe, Pugh, & White, 2007). In the model, questions are stated in the PICO format. Next, the research and nonresearch evidence undergoes appraisal. Nonresearch evidence includes not only expert opinion, patient experience data, and guidelines, but also evidence gathered from organizational experience such as quality improvement reports, program evaluations, and financial data analysis. The final step of the PET process is translation, assessing the evidence-based

Mr. P. is a 52-year-old married, Hispanic male who is approximately 100 pounds overweight. Mr. P. has developed hypertension and adult-onset diabetes. He is currently being followed in a clinic setting. As a nurse working in the clinic setting, you have noticed that many of the patients you see in the clinic who are demographically similar to Mr. P. have poorer health outcomes as compared with some other patient populations.

Case Study Questions

1. What PICO(T) questions can you ask to generate evidence for the patient population represented in the case study?

2. Based on a search of the literature, your expertise, and what you know about the preferences of this patient population, what are some evidence-based nursing interventions that you might want to translate into clinical practice in this setting? ■

recommendations for transferability to the practice setting. During this process, practices are implemented, evaluated, and communicated, leading to a change in nursing processes and outcomes (p. 129).

Conclusion

Currently, the greatest challenge we face in fully implementing evidence-based practice in nursing as a profession is how to get the evidence to the practicing nurse. Nurses are very busy taking care of patients. From the perspective of the individual it can indeed be daunting, especially when many practicing nurses are not knowledgeable about evidence-based nursing practice. But daunting or not, the impetus for evidence-based practice will continue to grow. As healthcare costs continue to climb, consistent, data-based answers to patient care problems will be an expectation. Patients will eventually demand evidence-based nursing care. Patients now have access to many computerized databases and reports, and they have the incentive and the time to read the reports. If patients are able to discern best practices, they will expect that nurses can as well (Simpson, 2004).

Classroom Activity 1

Create clinical questions in PICO(T) format for a patient in a case study provided by the instructor or a patient recently cared for in the clinical setting. www

Classroom Activity 2

Go to the computer lab and access evidence from resources such as CINAHL, the National Guideline Clearinghouse, or Cochrane Library to plan evidence-based care based on the questions created in Classroom Activity 1. www

Classroom Activity 3

Partner with a local clinical facility to work jointly on a PET project. Collaborate to identify PICO(T) questions, find evidence, and plan the process of translation of evidence into practice within the facility or on a nursing unit within the facility. www

References

Agency for Healthcare Research and Quality. (2002). *Systems to rate the strength of scientific evidence.* File inventory, Evidence Report/Technology Assessment No. 47, AHRQ Publication No. 02-E016. Rockville, MD: Author.

AGREE Collaboration. (2003). Development and validation of an international appraisal instrument for assessing the quality of clinical practice guidelines: The AGREE project. *Quality and Safety in Health Care, 12,* 18–23.

AGREE Next Steps Consortium. (2009). *Appraisal of guidelines for research and evaluation.* Ottawa, Ontario: AGREE Research Trust.

Beyea, S. C., & Slattery, M. J. (2006). *Evidence-based practice in nursing: A guide to successful implementation.* Marblehead, MA: Healthcare Compliance Company.

Cronenwett, L., Sherwood, G., Barnsteiner, J., Disch, J., Johnson, J., Mitchell, P., ... Warren, J. (2007). Quality and safety education for nurses. *Nursing Outlook, 55*(3), 122–131.

Di Cesenso, A., Guyatt, G., & Ciliska, D. (2005). *Evidence-based nursing: A guide to clinical practice.* St. Louis, MO: Mosby.

Levin, R. F. (2006a). Evidence-based practice in nursing: What is it? In R. F. Levin & H. R. Feldman (Eds.), *Teaching evidence-based practice in nursing: A guide for academic and clinical settings.* New York, NY: Springer.

Levin, R. F. (2006b). Teaching students to formulate clinical questions: Tell me your problems and then read my lips. In R. F. Levin & H. R. Feldman (Eds.), *Teaching evidence-based practice in nursing: A guide for academic and clinical settings.* New York, NY: Springer.

Levin, R. F., & Feldman, H. R. (Eds.). (2006). *Teaching evidence-based practice in nursing: A guide for academic and clinical settings.* New York, NY: Springer.

LoBiondo-Wood, G., Haber, J., & Krainovich-Miller, B. (2006). The research process: Integrating evidence-based practice. In G. LoBiondo-Wood & B. Haber (Eds.), *Nursing research: Methods and critical appraisal for evidence-based practice* (6th ed.). St. Louis, MO: Mosby.

Massachusetts Department of Higher Education. (2010). *Nurse of the future: Nursing core competencies.* Retrieved from http://www.mass.edu/currentinit/documents/NursingCoreCompetencies.pdf

Melnyk, B. M., & Fineout-Overholt, E. (2005). *Evidence-based practice in nursing and healthcare: A guide to best practice.* Philadelphia, PA: Lippincott Williams & Wilkins.

Newhouse, R. P., Dearholt, S. L., Poe, S. S., Pugh, L. C., & White, K. M. (2007). *Johns Hopkins nursing evidence-based practice: Model and guidelines.* Indianapolis, IN: Sigma Theta Tau International.

Polit, D. F., & Beck, C. T. (2008). *Nursing research: Generating and assessing evidence for nursing practice* (8th ed.). Philadelphia, PA: Lippincott Williams & Wilkins.

Pugh, L. C. (2012). Evidence-based practice: Context, concerns, and challenges. In S. L. Dearholt and D. Dang (Eds.), *Johns Hopkins nursing evidence-based practice: Model and guidelines* (2nd ed.). Indianapolis, IN: Sigma Theta Tau International.

Sackett, D. L., Straus, S., Richardson, S., Rosenberg, W., & Haynes, R. B. (2000). *Evidence-based medicine: How to practice and teach EBM* (2nd ed.). London, England: Churchill Livingstone.

Simpson, R. L. (2004). Evidence-based nursing offers certainty in the uncertain world of healthcare. *Nursing Management, 35*(10), 10, 12.

Spector, N. (2007). *Evidence-based health care in nursing regulation.* Chicago, IL: NCSBN.

Titler, M. G. (2008). The evidence for evidence-based practice implementation. In R. G. Hughes (Ed.), *Patient safety and quality: An evidence-based handbook for nurses.* Rockville, MD: Agency for Healthcare Research and Quality.

Ethical Issues in Professional Nursing Practice

Karen Rich and Janie B. Butts

11

In the previous 100 years great technological and medical advances have helped shape the world of bioethics, health care, and nursing practice. However, there has been a human price for the progress that has been made. New and intriguing moral dilemmas have surfaced related to professional healthcare practice, patient care, and the meaning of moral standing for individuals.

Learning Objectives

After completing this chapter, the student should be able to:

1. Explain important ethical issues related to nurses' relationships with others, such as patients, families, and colleagues.

2. Identify and discuss key ethical concepts involved in nurses' work, such as boundaries, dignity, and advocacy.

3. Discuss the concept of patient rights in health care.

4. Compare and contrast the meaning and details of end-of-life documents—living will, medical directive, and durable power of attorney.

5. Identify complex problems in determining healthcare allocation and explore standards of distributive justice.

6. Discuss three major ethical issues that are involved with organ transplantation.

7. Compare and contrast active, passive, voluntary, and nonvoluntary euthanasia.

8. Define key concepts related to end-of-life care.

9. Identify appropriate decision-making standards when patients have lost decision-making capacity.

10. Identify moral dilemmas that occur during end-of-life care and decision making.

Relationships in Professional Practice

Although professional healthcare practices are made credible because of formal expert knowledge, relationships arising from natural human conditions, such as illness, are at the foundation of these practices (Sokolowski, 1991). If nurses take seriously the guidance of the American Nurses Association's (ANA) 2001 *Code of Ethics for Nurses with Interpretive Statements*, patients

Key Terms and Concepts

- » **Unavoidable trust**
- » Boundaries
- » Dignity
- » Advocacy
- » Moral right
- » Informed consent

are to be the central focus of nursing and nursing relationships. However, the quality of patient care that nurses render often depends on the existence of harmonious relationships between nurses and physicians, other nurses, and other healthcare workers. Nurses who are concerned about providing compassionate care to patients must be concerned about their relationships with colleagues as well as with their direct relationships with patients. If nurses view life as a network of interrelationships, all of a nurse's relationships can potentially affect patients' well-being. Therefore, these relationships have a moral nature.

■ Nurse–Physician Relationships

In 1967, Stein, a physician, wrote an article characterizing a type of relationship between physicians and nurses that he called "the doctor–nurse game" (Stein, Watts, & Howell, 1990). The game is based on a hierarchical relationship, with doctors being in the position of the superior. The hallmark of the game is that open disagreement between the disciplines is to be avoided. Avoidance of conflict is achieved when an experienced nurse, who is able to provide helpful suggestions to a doctor regarding patient care, cautiously offers the suggestions so that the physician does not directly perceive consultative advice as coming from a nurse. In the past, student nurses were educated about the rules of "the game" while attending nursing school. Over the years, other people have given credence to the historical accuracy of Stein's characterization of doctor–nurse relationships (Fry & Johnstone, 2002; Jameton, 1984; Kelly, 2000).

Stein, along with two other physicians, wrote an article revisiting the doctor–nurse game in 1990, 23 years after the phrase was first coined (Stein et al., 1990). They proposed that nurses unilaterally had decided to stop playing the game. Some of the reasons for this change and some of the ways the change was accomplished involved nurses' increased use of dialogue rather than gamesmanship, the profession's goal of equal partnership status with other healthcare professionals, the alignment of nurses with the civil rights and women's movements, the increased percentage of nurses who are receiving higher education, and the joint demonstration projects on collaboration between nurses and physicians. In conjunction with the dismantling of the doctor–nurse game, some nurses have taken an adversarial stance with physicians. These nurses believe that they need to continue fighting for freedom from physician domination to establish nursing as an autonomous profession.

However, rather than taking an adversarial stance that generates conflict, the nursing profession might be better served if nurses take a communitarian approach with physicians. It is within communities that morality in general

> **Although professional healthcare practices are made credible because of formal expert knowledge, relationships arising from natural human conditions, such as illness, are at the foundation of these practices.**

and bioethics in particular receive their meaning (Engelhardt, 1996). A community works toward a common good and is held together by moral traditions. Nurses and physicians, as members of the healthcare community, must work together for the health and well-being of patients whether those patients are individuals, groups, or communities. When overt or covert battles are waged between nurses and physicians, moral problems arise, and patients can be the losers. Some ethicists have contended that the best approach for healing actually involves bringing patients into the community of healthcare providers (Hester, 2001). If nurses and physicians do not see themselves as members of a common community, the best interests of patients might not be served.

■ Nurse–Patient–Family Relationships

Unavoidable Trust

When patients enter the healthcare system, they are usually entering a foreign and forbidding environment (Chambliss, 1996; Zaner, 1991). Intimate conversations and activities, such as touching and probing, that normally do not occur between strangers, are commonplace between patients and healthcare professionals. Patients are frequently stripped of their clothes, subjected to sit alone in cold and barren rooms, and made to wait anxiously on frightening news regarding the continuation of their very being. When patients are in need of help from nurses, they frequently feel a sense of vulnerability and uncertainty. The tension that patients feel when accessing health care is heightened by the need for what Zaner (1991) calls **unavoidable trust**. This concept represents Zaner's contention that patients, in most cases, have no option but to trust nurses and other healthcare professionals when the patient is at the point of needing care.

This unavoidable trust creates an asymmetrical, or uneven, power structure in nurse–patient and family relationships (Zaner, 1991). Professional nurses' responsiveness to this trust must include promising to be the most excellent nurses that they can be. According to Zaner, healthcare professionals must promise "not only to take care of, but to care for, the patient and family—to be candid, sensitive, attentive, and never to abandon them" (p. 54). It is paradoxical that trust is necessary before health care is rendered, but it can be evaluated only in terms of whether the trust was warranted after care is rendered. Nurses must never take for granted the fragility of patients' trust.

> **Nurses must never take for granted the fragility of patients' trust.**

Boundaries

A discussion of professional boundaries is specifically covered in provision 2.4 of the *Code of Ethics for Nurses with Interpretive Statements* (ANA, 2001). In addition to the issues of trust discussed in the previous section, **boundaries** in nursing can be thought of in terms of appropriate professional behavior that serves to maintain trust between patients and nurses and to maintain nurses' good standing within their profession. Again, by keeping in mind that the primary concern of nurses' care is "preventing illness, alleviating suffering, and protecting, promoting, and restoring the health of patients," nurses can find guidance in maintaining professional boundaries (p. 11). The nature of nurses' work with both patients and colleagues has a very personal element but must not be confused with the common definition of friendship. Nurses are not discouraged from caring for patients, families, or colleagues. However, caring for patients and jeopardizing professional boundaries are two distinct issues.

Concepts that underlie nurse–patient boundaries include power, choice, and trust (Maes, 2003). The asymmetry of power in favor of the nurse must prompt nurses to ask if they are inappropriately influencing the decisions of patients. Patients must be provided with complete information to make choices, and nurses must facilitate in the process of patients receiving the information that they need. Patients trust nurses to have the knowledge and skill necessary to provide them with competent care; nurses must be faithful to that trust.

Potential violations of nurse–patient boundaries can involve gifts, intimacy, limits, neglect, abuse, and restraints (Maes, 2003). The gifts that patients give to nurses must be considered in terms of the implication of why the gift was given, its value, and whether the gift might provide therapeutic value for the patient but not influence the level of care provided by the nurse. Gifts generally lead to boundary violations and need to be discouraged most of the time. In addition to an obvious violation of intimacy through inappropriate sexual relationships, a violation of intimacy might occur if a nurse inappropriately shares information with other people in ways that violate patients' privacy. Nurses and patients must observe limits that prevent either person from becoming uncomfortable in their relationship. Nurses must take care to provide reasonable care to all patients according to appropriate ethical codes and state nurse practice acts so as not to be neglectful in the provision of nursing care, and they must do everything possible to prevent or intervene to stop patient abuse in whatever form it occurs. Finally, physically, chemically, and environmentally restraining patients can provide a major pitfall for nurses in terms of boundary violations. Nurses must know the policies of their employer as well as the standards set by accrediting agencies to safeguard patients.

Dignity

In the first provision of the *Code of Ethics for Nurses with Interpretive Statements*, the ANA (2001) included the standard that a nurse must have "respect for human dignity" (p. 7). However, Shotton and Seedhouse (1998) propose that the term *dignity* has been used in vague ways. They characterize dignity as being related to persons being in a position to use their capabilities. In general terms, a person has **dignity** "if he or she is in a situation where his or her capabilities can be effectively applied" (p. 249). For example, nurses can enhance dignity when caring for elders by assessing their priorities and determining what the elder has been capable of in the past and what the person is capable of in the present.

A lack of or loss of capability is frequently an issue when caring for patients such as children, elders, and people who are physically and mentally disabled. Having absent or diminished capabilities is consistent with what MacIntyre (1999) refers to in his discussion of human vulnerability. According to MacIntyre, people generally progress from a point of vulnerability in infancy to achieving varying levels of independent practical reasoning as they mature. However, all people, including nurses, would do well to realize that all persons have been or will be vulnerable at some point in their lives. Taking a "there but for the grace of God go I" stance can prompt nurses to develop what MacIntyre calls the virtues of acknowledged dependence. These virtues include just generosity, *misericordia*, and truthfulness and are exercised in communities of giving and receiving. Just generosity is a form of giving generously without "keeping score" of who gives or receives the most; *misericordia* is a Latin word that signifies giving based on urgent need without prejudice; and truthfulness involves not withholding information from others that is needed for their own good. Nurses who cultivate these three virtues can move toward preserving patient dignity and toward the common good of the community.

Patient Advocacy

Nurses acting as patient advocates try to identify unmet patient needs and then follow up to address the needs appropriately (Jameton, 1984). **Advocacy**, as opposed to advice, involves the nurse's moving from the patient to the healthcare system rather than moving from the nurse's values to the patient. The concept of advocacy has been a part of the International Council of Nursing's *Code of Ethics* and the ANA's code since the 1970s (Winslow, 1988). In the *Code of Ethics for Nurses with Interpretive Statements*, the ANA (2001) continues to support patient advocacy in elaborating on the "primacy of the patient's interest" (p. 9) and requiring nurses to work collaboratively with others to attain the goal of addressing the healthcare needs of patients and the public. Nurses are called on to ensure that all appropriate parties are involved in patient care decisions, that patients are provided with the information needed to make informed decisions, and that collaboration is used to increase the accessibility and availability of health care to all patients who need it. The International Council of Burses (2006), in the *Code of Ethics for Nurses*, affirms that the nurse must share "with society the responsibility for initiating and supporting action to meet the health and social needs of the public, in particular those of vulnerable populations" (p. 2).

> The *Code of Ethics for Nurses with Interpretive Statements* continues to support patient advocacy in elaborating on the "primacy of the patient's interest."

KEY COMPETENCY 11-1

Examples of Applicable
*Nurse of the Future: Nursing
Core Competencies*

Professionalism:

Knowledge (K6) Understands
role and responsibilities as
patient advocate

Skills (S6) Serves as a
patient advocate

Attitudes/Behaviors (A6)
Values role and responsibilities as patient advocate

Source: Massachusetts Department
of Higher Education (2010), p. 14.

■ Nurse–Nurse Relationships

As in the case of nurse–physician relationships, nurse–nurse relationships can be thought of as relationships within a community. Nurses in a nursing community might be what Engelhardt (1996) calls moral friends. According to Wildes (2000), moral friends exist together within communities and use similar moral language. They "share a moral narrative and commitments [and] common understandings of the foundations of morality, moral reason, and justification" (p. 137). Communities are strongest when moral friends share "common moral traditions, practices, and [a] vision of the good life" (p. 137). In putting patients first in nurses' priorities, nurses in a community work together for a common good, using professional traditions to guide the communal narrative of nursing.

Unfortunately, nurses often treat other nurses in hurtful ways through what some people have called lateral or horizontal violence (Kelly, 2000; McKenna, Smith, Poole, & Coverdale, 2003). Lateral or horizontal violence involves interpersonal conflict, harassment, intimidation, harsh criticism, sabotage, and abuse among nurses. Some people believe that this oppression among nurses occurs because nurses feel oppressed by other dominant groups such as physicians or institutional administrators. Kelly (2000) reports that some nurses have characterized the violence perpetrated against nurses who excel and succeed as the "tall poppy syndrome." Nurses who succeed are ostracized, thereby creating a culture among nurses that discourages success.

Lateral violence in nursing is very counterproductive for the profession. A more productive path for nurses might be to cultivate the virtue of sympathetic joy. *Sympathetic joy* refers to experiencing happiness in regard to the good things experienced by others. The nursing community does not benefit from lateral violence, but nurses who cultivate the virtue of sympathetic joy can strengthen the sense of community among nurses. Nurses must support other nurses' success rather than treat colleagues as "tall poppies" that must be cut down.

However, there are occasions when unpleasant action must be taken in regard to nursing colleagues. In addition to advocating directly for patients' unmet needs, nurses are advocates when they take appropriate action to protect patients from the unethical, incompetent, or impaired practice of other nurses (ANA, 2001). When nurses are aware of these situations, they must deal compassionately with the offending coworkers while ensuring that patients receive safe, quality care. Concerns must be expressed to the offending nurse when personal safety or patient safety is not jeopardized in doing so and appropriate guidance must be obtained from supervisory personnel and institutional policies. Although action must be taken to safeguard patients' care, the manner in which a nurse handles situations involving unethical, incompetent, or impaired colleagues must not be a matter of gossip, condescension, or unproductive derogatory talk.

Moral Rights and Autonomy

In a society that is perfectly just, moral rights and legal rights would overlap; however, the two types of rights are not the same in our society (Brannigan & Boss, 2001). A **moral right** can be defined as "the right to perform certain activities (a) because they conform to the accepted standards or ideas of a community (or of a law, or of God, or of conscience), or (b) because they will not harm, coerce, restrain, or infringe on the interests of others, or (c) because there are good rational arguments in support of the value of such activities" (Angeles, 1992, p. 264).

Generally, moral rights are separated into welfare rights and liberty rights (Brannigan & Boss, 2001). Welfare rights allow persons to pursue their legitimate interests or those personal interests that do not interfere with the interests of other persons' that are similar and equal to one's own. "Welfare (positive) rights entail the right to receive basic goods such as education, medical care, and police protection, as well as a duty on the part of others such as the government to provide these social goods" (p. 33).

As opposed to welfare rights, liberty (negative) rights involve the right to noninterference from any person or governmental entity when pursuing one's legitimate interests (Brannigan & Boss, 2001). "Liberty or negative rights include autonomy, privacy, freedom of speech, and freedom from harassment, confinement, unwanted medical treatment, or participation in experiments without our informed consent" (p. 33). Although the World Health Organization has proposed that every person has a fundamental right to health without prejudice, in the United States, liberty rights are emphasized over welfare rights, except in cases of elders and the poor.

■ Informed Consent

Considerations of informed consent fall within the overview of respect for autonomy, or self-direction (Beauchamp & Childress, 2009; Veatch, 2003). Although nurses often facilitate informed consent and have a role in terms of patient advocacy, the actual responsibility for ensuring informed consent historically has belonged to the physician. However, with the increased numbers of advanced practice nurses and the increased complexity of nurses' roles, informed consent has become more of a direct ethical issue for nurses. A liberally applied concept of **informed consent** includes the rule that "meaningful information must be disclosed even if the clinician does not believe that it [the information] will be beneficial" (Veatch, 2003, p. 75). This definition is in contrast to the rule applied under the Hippocratic Oath that allowed for healthcare professionals to withhold information if they believed that it would harm or upset a patient.

It must be noted that a patient's signature on a consent form proves neither that a patient read the form nor that the patient understands what is written on it (Veatch, 2003). It would be impossible to inform each patient of everything about a procedure. In an attempt to deal with this reality, two standards are often applied. The first is the reasonable person standard that states the health-care professional will disclose information that a reasonable person would want to know. The second is the subjective standard that states that disclosure must be based on the subjective interests of a particular patient rather than a hypothetical reasonable person. The ideal standard, therefore, adjusts what a reasonable person would want to know with what the healthcare professional knows that a particular patient is or might be interested in knowing.

■ Patient Self-Determination Act

The **Patient Self-Determination Act** of 1990, enacted in 1991, was designed to facilitate the knowledge and use of advance directives (Guido, 2001). Under the act, healthcare providers must ask patients if they have advance directives and must provide patients with advance directive information according to patients' wishes. This act provides nurses with a good opportunity to take an active role in facilitating the moral rights of patients in regard to end-of-life decisions. In addition to responding to the direct questions that patients ask about advance directives and end-of-life options, nurses would do well to "listen" for the subtle cues that patients give that signal their anxieties and uncertainty about end-of-life care. It would be a practice of compassion for nurses to listen deeply to patients and to actively try to alleviate patients' suffering and fears in regard to end-of-life decision making.

Advance Directives

An **advance directive** is "a written expression of a person's wishes about medical care, especially care during a terminal or critical illness" (Veatch, 2003, p. 119). Said another way, individuals lose control over their lives when they lose their decision-making capacity, and advance directives become instructions about health care for the future (Devettere, 2000). Advance directives may be self-written instructions or may be prepared by someone else as instructed by the patient.

There are three types of advance directives: living will, medical care directive, and durable power of attorney (Devettere, 2000). A **living will** is a formal legal document that provides written directions concerning medical care that is to be provided in specific circumstances (Beauchamp & Childress, 2009; Devettere, 2000). The living will gained recognition in the 1960s, but the Karen Ann Quinlan case in the 1970s brought public attention to the living will and subsequently prompted legalization of the document (Devettere, 2000). Although at the time, they were a good beginning, today living wills are inadequate. Living wills often consist of vague language, only instructions for unwanted treatments, and a lack of legal penalties for people who choose to ignore to follow the living wills. Also, living wills might be legally questionable in regard to their authenticity.

A **medical directive** is not a formal legal document but provides specific written instructions concerning the type of care and treatments that individuals want to receive if they become incapacitated (Devettere, 2000). One advantage to medical directives is that physicians can use them as a guide to know what the incapacitated patient wants in terms of specific healthcare treatments. Some attorneys believe that medical directives are only a minimal improvement over living wills. Their rationale is that they think that medical directives are only an elaborate informed consent. Also, other weaknesses of medical directives are that people cannot possibly anticipate every medical problem that might occur in their future, and people change over time and can change in regard to their future wishes. A **durable power of attorney**, the legal document with the most strength, is a written directive in which a designated person is allowed to make either general or healthcare decisions for a patient (Devettere, 2000).

Families and healthcare professionals can experience fear about making the wrong decisions regarding a patient who is incapacitated. Advance directives help to reduce emotional stress but at the same time can produce ethical dilemmas.

Social Justice

■ Definition and Theories of Social Justice

A Sicilian priest first used the term *social justice* in 1840, and then in 1848, the term was more popularized by Antonio Rosmini-Serbati (Novak, 2000). Since then, **social justice** has been defined as (Center for Economic & Social Justice, n.d.):

> A virtue that guides us in creating those organized human interactions we call institutions. In turn, social institutions, when justly organized, provide us with access to what is good for the person, both individually and in our associations with others. Social justice also imposes on each of us a personal responsibility to work with others to design and continually perfect our institutions as tools for personal and social development. (p. 2)

A large portion of the use of the term has been related more to competing powers of social systems and regulative principles on an impersonal basis, such as "high unemployment," "inequality of incomes," "lack of a living wage," and "social injustice" (Novak, 2000, p. 1). The term also has been related to the question of what makes the common good for everyone (Brannigan & Boss, 2001). People who take a communitarian approach put common goods of the community over individual freedoms.

In his social contract book, *A Theory of Justice*, John Rawls (1971) views fairness and equality under a "veil of ignorance." This concept

KEY COMPETENCY 11-2

Examples of Applicable *Nurse of the Future: Nursing Core Competencies*

Patient-Centered Care:

Knowledge (K3) Integrates understanding of multiple dimensions of patient-centered care: patient/family/community preferences, values

Skills (S3a) Communicates patient values, preferences, and expressed needs to other members of the health care team; (S3b) Seeks information from appropriate sources on behalf of patient when necessary

Attitudes/Behaviors (A3c) Respects and encourages the patient's input into decisions about health care and services

Source: Massachusetts Department of Higher Education (2010), p. 9.

means that if people had a veil to shield their own or others' economic, social, and class standing, each person would be more likely to make justice-based decisions from a position that is free from all biases and would view the distribution of resources in impartial ways. Under the veil, people would view social conditions neutrally because they would not know what their own position might be at the time the veil is lifted. This "not knowing" or ignorance of persons about their own position means that they cannot gain any type of advantage for themselves by their choices. Based on this "ignorance" principle, Rawls stated that this view is just (cited in Brannigan & Boss, 2001). Rawls (1971) advocates two principles of equality and justice: Everyone should be given equal liberty no matter what adversities exist for people, and differences should be recognized among people by making sure that the least advantaged people are given their desert for improvements.

Nozick (1974, cited in Brannigan & Boss, 2001) presents the idea of an entitlement system in his book *Anarchy, State, and Utopia*, meaning that if individuals could pay for insurance, only then are they entitled to health care. Nozick emphasizes that in order for a system to be just and fair, it must reward people who contribute to the system (Brannigan & Boss, 2001). Then later, Daniels explores Rawls's concept of justice further by basing his book *Just Health Care* (1985; cited in Brannigan & Boss, 2001) on the liberty principle, as he espouses that every person should have equal opportunity. Daniels emphasizes equal health care and reasonable access to healthcare services and recommends national healthcare reform.

■ Allocation and Rationing of Healthcare Resources

The cost of health care is spiraling out of control worldwide, and therefore, healthcare resources and deciding how to allocate them remain at the forefront of peoples' concerns. The unfortunate and troublesome experiences with healthcare reimbursements are played out through narratives on the front page of almost every newspaper. A central question that healthcare professionals, economists, and politicians have asked themselves for years is what makes up a just and equitable healthcare system? The question continues to be unanswered.

The health care of people in the United States is not the best in the world, yet in 2005, U.S. healthcare expenditures were $2 trillion (Kaiser Family Foundation, 2007). The federal government's second major goal in *Healthy People 2010* was to eliminate health disparities. This remains a major goal in the Healthy People 2020 document, yet the disparities continue to occur without much, if any, improvement in the health of people in the United States. It is believed that inequalities in health care exist because of complex differences in socioeconomic status, racial and ethnic backgrounds, education levels, and healthcare access. These differences underlie many of the health disparities in the United States. As a result, health-promoting behaviors are not as likely to be practiced.

As healthcare costs increase, resources become more limited for people. Distributive justice has become a critical issue in the healthcare system. Guidelines in how scarce resources are distributed must be clearly delineated. Some guiding questions that members of society need to explore in terms of distributive justice include the following:

- Does every person have a right to health care?
- Is health care a right or a privilege that must be earned?
- How should resources be distributed so that everyone receives a fair and equitable share for health care?
- Should healthcare rationing ever be considered as an option in the face of scarce healthcare resources? If so, how?

There might never be clear and concise answers to these complex questions. Brannigan and Boss (2001) outline criteria that could be used when rationing is considered. The criteria include standards of distribution by market or according to people who could afford to pay, social worth, medical needs, age, a first-come, first-served basis, and randomization. From the 1990s to the present, systems of managed care have been operating in the United States as one strategy to improve the use of services based on needs and to maximize health and well-being while reducing overall healthcare costs to individuals (Sugarman, 2000). However, the public has responded very poorly to managed care. Some people have labeled managed care as an ethical disaster. Before such complaints are made, however, healthcare professionals and nurses need to address the sources of the problems.

Sugarman (2000) discusses the enormous travesty that occurred with the Medicaid and Medicare systems from 1965 to 1990. Big money was made available by the U.S. federal government based on the autonomous practice of physicians—meaning that physicians could redirect large amounts of money from taxpayers to the care of sick people through Medicaid and Medicare. Sugarman terms this period as "the good old days," when physicians were not required to justify or show evidence for their medical care for sick people. Since 1990, however, times have changed, and criticism is plentiful. Sugarman contends that no matter what healthcare system is in place, physicians and the public would be critical. Engelhardt (1996), a bioethicist, states this about the current healthcare system:

> Concepts of adequate care are not discoverable outside of particular views of the good life and of proper medical practice. In nations encompassing diverse moral communities, an understanding of what one will mean by an adequate level or a decent minimum of health care will need to be fashioned, if it can indeed be agreed to, through open discussion and by fair negotiation. (p. 400)

KEY COMPETENCY 11-4

Examples of Applicable *Nurse of the Future: Nursing Core Competencies*

Systems-Based Practice:

Knowledge (K5a) Understands that legal, political, regulatory, and economic factors influence the delivery of patient care; (K5b) Is aware that different models of health care financing and regulation can influence patient access to care

Skills (S5a) Provides care based upon current legal, political, regulatory, and economic requirements

Attitudes/Behaviors (A5a) Appreciates that legal, political, regulatory, and economic factors influence the delivery of patient care; (A5b) Values the need to remain informed of how legal, political, regulatory, and economic factors impact professional nursing practice

Source: Massachusetts Department of Higher Education (2010), p. 20.

Promoting open dialogue for expressing moral views in the community and in institutions, negotiating policy change for better allocation and an improved healthcare system, and maintaining a firm commitment for better patient health outcomes are just a few ways that nurses can assist with supporting good health for the common good of the community.

Ethics and Organ Transplantation

A dramatic social allocation issue that involves scarce resources is organ transplantation. In the United States, patients can "opt in" by signing a donor card as potential donors of one or more organs in the event of their death (Perrin & McGhee, 2001). If patients choose not to sign donor cards, they are free from any obligation to donate organs. Three ethical issues are involved with organ transplantation: the moral acceptability of transplanting an organ from one person to another, procurement, and allocation of the organs (Veatch, 2003).

For the first ethical issue, Veatch (2003) poses this question: "Is performing transplants 'playing God'?" (p. 136). This phrase has become quite common in the last few decades with transplants, genetics, and human reproduction technologies being so popular. Many people view transplantations as unacceptable based on religious or cultural beliefs, or just basic beliefs, such as the association that the human heart has with romance and as the "seat of the soul" (Veatch, 2003, p. 137).

The second ethical issue is procurement of organs. In some countries other than the United States, organs can be routinely salvaged without the consent of the patient or anyone in the family with the basic belief that organs, once the person is dead, become the property of the state or country (Veatch, 2003). In the United States, it is believed that donation and informed consent are based on the rights and autonomy of each person.

The third ethical issue is organ allocation, which is one of the most debated issues in health care today because of the scarcity of donor organs. There is a national waiting list established by the United Network for Organ Sharing (UNOS) Committee (U.S. Department of Health and Human Services, 2003). At least 98,151 people in the United States are awaiting organs for transplant (Organ Procurement and Transplantation Network, 2007). Because of the demand for organs and the prospect of money that can be made, the organ black market is thriving. The U.S. organ donor system is organized so that allocation decisions are coordinated by UNOS, and the system is designed to be driven by the principle of justice. UNOS or the organ transplant team should never deny organs based on perceived social worth; rather, allocation of resources should be distributed fairly and equally based on need.

Five major focus areas of health disparities are known to affect racial and ethnic groups in all ages: cardiovascular disease, diabetes, cancer screening and disease management, and immunizations (U.S. Department of Health and Human Services, 2003). People who suffer the most from health disparities between populations often have diseases that eventually result in a need for organ transplants. For instance, a health conditions report from the Office of Minority Health (2007) reveals that in 2004 high blood pressure occurred 1.5 times more in African Americans than in non-Hispanic whites and in 2002, African American men were 2.1 times as likely to start treatment for end-stage renal disease related to diabetes as were non-Hispanic white men. One primary role for nurses is to assist with attempting to eliminate health disparities. Education programs with substantive content that target particular populations provide a beginning role for nurses, who function on a broad community level.

Other roles for nurses include encouraging patients and families to express their feelings and attitudes about donations and transplantations, especially in regard to ethical issues involving death and dying; supporting, listening, and maintaining confidentiality with patients and families; assisting in monitoring patients for organ needs; continually being aware of inequalities and injustices in the healthcare system, which can affect the care of patients; and assisting in the care of surgical organ transplant and donation patients and their families.

Death and End-of-Life Care

▪ Defining Death

The last words of the great composer Frédéric Chopin were, "The earth is suffocating.... Swear to make them cut me open, so that I won't be buried alive" (Death: The Last Taboo, 2003). In the 1700s and 1800s, especially in Europe, there was widespread fear of premature burial or being buried alive because of the inadequate methods for detecting when a person was dead and because of actual accounts of people being buried alive (Bondeson, 2001). In those days, when a body was exhumed, claw marks sometimes were found on the inside of coffin lids (Mappes & DeGrazia, 2001). Because of the widespread fear, a variety of special safety coffins were invented with detailed devices to help the dead, once they were buried, to communicate with others above the ground (Death: The Last Taboo, 2003). The devices included such things as a rope extending to the surface of the ground with a bell on the other end, a speaking tube to the outer coffin, a shovel, and food and water. In addition to a new law that prevented premature burial, funeral home attendants even went to the extent to have their employees monitor dead bodies for any signs of life during the "wait" time.

For several centuries, when a person became unconscious, physicians or other people would palpate for a pulse, listen for breath sounds with their ears, look for condensation on an object when it was held close to the body's nose, and check for fixed and dilated pupils (Mappes & DeGrazia, 2001). In 1819, fear was reduced when the stethoscope was invented because physicians could listen with greater certainty for a heartbeat through a magnified listening device on the chest of the body. In 1903, Willem Einthoven, a Dutch physician, discovered the existence of the electrical properties of the heart with his invention of the electrocardiograph, which provided sensitive information about whether the electrical activity of the heart was functioning. The artificial respirator of the 1950s brought about more uncertainty of death as physicians kept patients alive in the absence of a natural heartbeat (Death: The Last Taboo, 2003). By the 1960s, when transplants were being performed, it was becoming apparent that a diagnosis of death would not depend necessarily on the absence of a heartbeat. Rather, the definition of death would need to include brain death criteria in the future.

The first attempt to redefine death was made in the United States by the Harvard Medical School ad hoc committee in 1968. The definition was based on the committee members' attempt to identify reliable clinical criteria for respirator-dependent patients who had no brain function (Youngner & Arnold, 2001). Then, in 1981, the President's Commission members sanctioned a definition of death, which included brain death, and recommended its adoption by all states (Mappes & DeGrazia, 2001). The 1981 definition led to the Uniform Determination of Death Act (UDDA), in which death is defined as follows:

> An individual who has sustained either (1) irreversible cessation of circulatory and respiratory functions or (2) irreversible cessation of all functions of the entire brain, including the brain stem, is dead. A determination of death must be made in accordance with accepted medical standards. (President's Commission, 1981; cited in Mappes & DeGrazia, 2001, p. 318)

Since this definition was adopted, criteria for brain death have been integrated in almost every state but have been continually debated. A provocative thought that Veatch (2003) has contributed to the debate on the definition of death concerns the loss of full moral standing of human beings. This statement triggers the question as to when humans should be treated as full members of the human community. Although almost every person has reconciled the thought that some persons have full moral standing and others do not, there is continued controversy about when full moral standing ceases to exist and what characteristics qualify the cessation of full moral standing.

Losing full moral standing is equivalent to ceasing to exist. Presently, various groups have proposed and debated the following four conceptions of death since the enactment of the UDDA in 1981 (Munson, 2004, pp. 692, 693):

- Traditional: A person is dead when he is no longer breathing and his heart is not beating (cardiopulmonary).
- Whole-brain: Death is regarded as the irreversible cessation of all brain functions ... no electrical activity in the brain, and even the brain stem is not functioning (brain death).

- Higher brain: Death is considered to involve the permanent loss of consciousness. Someone in an irreversible coma would be considered dead, even though the brain stem continued to regulate breathing and heartbeat (persistent vegetative state).
- Personhood: Death occurs when an individual ceases to be a person. This can mean loss of features that are essential to personal identity or for being a person.

With whole-brain death, a patient physically can survive for an indeterminate period of time with a mechanical ventilator. With higher brain death, a patient lives in a persistent vegetative state indefinitely but without the need for mechanical ventilation. It is because of these situations that the question exists regarding when a person should be treated as one who has full moral standing within the human community. Society, physicians, and nurses have had difficulty in defining death by the UDDA definition, which includes the traditional and the whole-brain concepts. However, the greatest difficulty has been when they have tried to incorporate the concepts of higher brain death and personhood death (Munson, 2004). No definite criteria for either of these concepts—higher brain or personhood—have been established for defining death. The debate continues, and questions continue about when life begins, when life ends, and what it is that ceases to exist when someone is dead (Benjamin, 2003; Veatch, 2003).

■ Euthanasia

Most people do not want prolonged agony and suffering before their death and would like to keep their emotional, financial, and social burdens to a minimum and their dignity intact. However, dying the "good death" is not always possible (Munson, 2004). *Euthanasia*, meaning "good death" in Greek, has come to mean "easy death" and has developed a strong appeal in recent years. A patient might ponder options of euthanasia if suffering and pain become too much for the person to bear. There are two major types of euthanasia: active and passive. **Active euthanasia** occurs when a person takes an action to end a life (including one's own life). Active euthanasia can include a lethal dose of medication, such as in physician-assisted suicide. **Passive euthanasia** means that a person allows another person to die by not acting to stop death or prolong life. An example of this type of euthanasia includes withholding treatment that is necessary to prevent death at a point in time.

> **Dying the "good death" is not always possible.**

Euthanasia also is recognized by the categories of voluntary and non-voluntary (Brannigan & Boss, 2001). **Voluntary euthanasia** occurs when persons with a sound mind authorize another person to take their life or to assist them in achieving death. Also, this type includes the taking of one's own life. **Nonvoluntary euthanasia** occurs when persons are not able to express their decision about death. A blending of these types of euthanasia can occur, such as voluntary active, nonvoluntary active, voluntary passive, and nonvoluntary passive.

A vigorous debate in the United States continues about whether there is a real moral difference between active euthanasia, such as the intentional taking of someone's life, and passive euthanasia, such as withholding or withdrawing life-sustaining treatments (Brannigan & Boss, 2001; Jonsen, Veatch, & Walters, 1998). The action versus omission distinction many times causes nurses and physicians to ponder this troublesome question: "Is there a moral difference between actively killing and letting die?"

■ Rational Suicide

The thought of morally accepting the act of a person's committing rational suicide weighs heavily on the hearts of most people even today. The very connection of the terms *rational* and *suicide* seems a contradiction (Engelhardt, 1996; Finnerty, 1987). However, suicide is an enormous public health crisis. Worldwide, there are an estimated 877,000 suicides each year (World Health Organization, 2007). In 2004, the occurrence of suicide in the United States was more than 32,000 (Centers for Disease Control and Prevention, 2007). **Rational suicide** is a self-slaying and is categorized as voluntary active euthanasia. In this category, the person has made a reasoned choice of rational suicide, which seems to make sense to others at the time. Siegel (1986) states that the person contemplating rational suicide has a realistic assessment of life circumstances, is free from severe emotional distress, and has a motivation that would seem understandable to most uninvolved people within the person's community.

Endorsing any suicide seems so contradictory to good healthcare practice because nurses and mental health professionals have been intervening for years to prevent suicide. Many times, nurses' responses are guided by their cultural, religious, and personal beliefs. Autonomy and beneficence need to be considered when nurses are deciding about interventions to provide for persons who are planning rational suicide. Also, if the nurse knows of the plan for rational suicide, would care be obligatory toward the patient? What actions could the nurse take at this point? Interventions become unique to each situation and can include everything from being asked to provide information regarding the Hemlock Society to being asked about lethal injections. Because nurses are more closely involved with end-of-life decision making, the issue of nurses' responsibility with voluntary active euthanasia is becoming an increasingly common dilemma.

www | CRITICAL THINKING QUESTIONS *

Does a nurse have the right to try to stop a person from committing rational suicide (to act in the best interest of the patient)? Is a nurse supposed to support the person's autonomous decision to commit rational suicide, even when that decision is morally and religiously incompatible with the nurse's perspective? *

■ Palliative Care

Palliative care is providing comfort rather than curative measures for terminally ill patients. Nurses are actively involved in meeting the palliative needs of dying patients. In the last decade, the palliative care movement has become quite organized through official associations and organizations. The World Health Organization (2003) defines palliative care as follows:

> An approach that improves the quality of life of patients and their families facing the problem associated with life-threatening illness, through the prevention and relief of suffering by means of early identification and impeccable assessment and treatment of pain and other problems, physical, psychosocial, and spiritual. (p. 1)

When a patient chooses to receive this type of care, nurses need to understand that they do not hasten or prolong death for these patients; they provide relief of pain and suffering and attempt to allow the patient to die with dignity. Patients or patients' families may choose to forgo, withhold, or withdraw treatment. Some patients have a do-not-resuscitate order, which is a written physician's order that is placed in the patient's chart in an attempt to ensure that no resuscitative measures are initiated when a patient's cardiopulmonary functions cease. Usually there is one of three reasons for the decision to initiate a do-not-resuscitate order: (1) There is no medical benefit that can come from cardiopulmonary resuscitation (CPR), (2) the person had a very poor quality of life before CPR, or (3) the person's life after CPR is anticipated to be very poor (Mappes & DeGrazia, 2001).

Rule of Double Effect

The **rule of double effect** usually is defined narrowly in health care as the use of high doses of pain medication to lessen the chronic and intractable pain of terminally ill patients even if doing so hastens death (Quill, 2001). The first group to define the rule of double effect was the Catholic Church in medieval times. When the rule is applied, nurses need to be aware that the harmful effect, or the hastening of death, can be foreseen but is not the intended outcome of their actions. According to Quill (2001), critical aspects of the rule are as follows:

1. The act must be good or at least morally neutral.
2. The agent must intend the good effect and not the evil effect (which can be "foreseen" but not intended).
3. The evil effect must not be the means to the good effect.
4. There must be a "proportionally grave reason" to risk the evil effect (p. 167).

Nurses might have conflicting moral values concerning the use of high doses of pain medications, such as morphine sulfate. In times when nurses feel uncomfortable, they need to explore their attitudes and opinions with their supervisor and, when appropriate, in clinical team meetings. In Provision 1.3 of the *Code of Ethics for Nurses with Interpretive Statements*, the ANA (2001) supports nurses in their attempts to relieve patients' pain "even when those interventions entail risks of hastening death" (p. 8).

■ Refusing or Forgoing Treatment

Well-informed patients with decision-making capacity have the autonomous right to refuse or forgo recommended treatments (Jonsen, Siegler, & Winslade, 2002). When a person elects to forgo treatment, most of the time there is no ethical or legal backlash. The courts uphold the right of competent patients to refuse treatment (Jonsen et al., 2002; Mappes & DeGrazia, 2001). Even so, it is of the utmost importance that healthcare professionals make certain that the patient's decision is noncoercive and autonomous and that the decision has been made based on the patient's mentally competent decision-making capacity (Mappes & DeGrazia, 2001). Although nurses and other healthcare professionals might have the assurance of the patient's autonomous and competent decision making, sometimes the patient's decision is difficult to accept. Refusal of medical treatments can occur at any time in life, whether at the end of life or not, such as times when patients might refuse treatment based on religious or cultural beliefs.

> **Well-informed patients with decision-making capacity have the autonomous right to refuse or forgo recommended treatments.**

■ Deciding for Others

When patients are no longer able to make competent decisions, families can experience problems in trying to determine a progressive right course of action. The ideal situation is for patients to be autonomous decision makers, but when autonomy is no longer possible, decision making falls to a surrogate (Beauchamp & Childress, 2009). The surrogate, or proxy, is either chosen by the patient, is court appointed, or has other authority to make decisions.

There are three types of surrogate decision makers (Beauchamp & Childress, 2009; Veatch, 2003). The **standard of substituted judgment** is used to guide medical decisions that involve formerly competent patients who no longer have any decision-making capacity. This standard is based on the assumption that incompetent patients have the exact rights as competent patients to make judgments about their health care (Buchanan & Brock, 1990). Surrogates make medical treatment decisions based on how the surrogates believe that the patients would have decided were the patients still competent and able to express their wishes. In making decisions, the surrogates use their understanding of the patients' previous overt or implied expressions of their beliefs and values (Veatch, 2003). Before losing competency, the patient could have either explicitly informed the proxy of treatment wishes by oral or written instruction or implicitly made clear treatment wishes through informal conversations with the proxy.

Decisions based on the **pure autonomy standard** are made on behalf of an incompetent person and are based on decisions that the formerly competent person made. This type of decision also is called the principle of autonomy extended, meaning that a person's autonomy continues to be honored even when the person cannot exercise autonomy through normal channels.

The **best interest standard** is based on the goal of the surrogate's doing what is best for the patient or what is in the best interest of the patient (Veatch, 2003). This standard is applied when the patient who the proxy represents has never been competent, such as a child.

■ Withholding and Withdrawing Treatment

People in society and healthcare professionals have accepted and ethically justified withholding and withdrawing treatments that have been deemed as futile or extraordinary. When a treatment has no physiologic benefit for a terminally ill person, the treatment is considered to be **futile care** (Beauchamp & Childress, 2009). Medical treatments include cardiopulmonary resuscitation, medications, mechanical ventilation, artificial feeding and fluids, hemodialysis, chemotherapy, and other life-sustaining technologies. Futility issues need to be discussed among nurses, physicians, family members, and patients when possible. A court-appointed or family surrogate decision maker can be the spokesperson for the patient. Nurses need to ensure that a decision-making process between the healthcare team and the decision makers for the patient takes place so that everyone has a chance to express feelings and concerns (Ladd, Pasquerella, & Smith, 2002).

Three legal cases generated landmark decisions about withholding and withdrawing treatments. In 1975, Karen Ann Quinlan's case established the right to discontinue mechanical ventilation (Jonsen et al., 1998; *In re Quinlan*, New Jersey). In 1990, the U.S. Supreme Court established through Nancy Cruzan's case three conditions: the patient has a right to refuse medical treatment; artificial feeding constitutes medical treatment; and if the patient is mentally incompetent, then each state has to document clear and convincing evidence that the patient's desires were for discontinuance of medical treatment (Jonsen et al., 1998; *In re Cruzan*, Missouri).

The third case is a more recent one. It is the case of Terri Schiavo, a young woman in a persistent vegetative state, who died on March 31, 2005. There were a total of 21 legal suits, but the last few cases involved Terri's husband Michael's request to have her feeding tube discontinued, which also would end her artificial nutrition and hydration. Terri's parents fought this request. According to Florida law, Michael Schiavo as a spouse and guardian had a legal right to serve as a surrogate decision maker for Terri Schiavo. In conjunction with this legal standard, substituted judgment was used as the appropriate ethical standard. Because Terri Schiavo had no written advance directive, her surrogate was charged with making an unbiased substituted judgment about her care. The judgment should be based on an understanding of what she would decide for herself and not the values of the surrogate. Michael Schiavo and other people testified that Terri had stated that she did not want to live in a condition in which she would be a burden to anyone else. This evidence served as the basis for many of the court's denials of the Schindlers' requests to continue Terri's artificial nutrition and hydration.

In the *Code of Ethics for Nurses with Interpretive Statements*, Provision 1.3, the ANA (2001) takes the position that nurses ethically support the provision of compassionate and dignified end-of-life care as long as nurses do not have the sole intention of ending a person's life. A special statement concerning the Terri Schiavo case was released to the press by the ANA on March 23, 2005, that upheld the decision for the right of a patient or surrogate to choose forgoing artificial nutrition and hydration. No matter what the outcome of difficult end-of-life decisions, family members and patients need to feel a sense of confidence that nurses will maintain moral sensitivity and good judgment.

▪ Terminal Sedation

Legally permissible yet ethically controversial, **terminal sedation (TS)** seems to be moving toward a social and an ethical acceptance (Quill, 2001). Quill (2001) defines terminal sedation as follows:

> When a suffering patient is sedated to unconsciousness, usually through the ongoing administration of barbiturates or benzodiazepines. The patient then dies of dehydration, starvation, or some other intervening complication, as all other life-sustaining interventions are withheld. (p. 181)

When the word *terminal* is used, there is an understanding among the healthcare team members and family that the outcome, and possibly a desired outcome, is death (Sugarman, 2000). TS has been used in situations when patients need pain relief that requires being sedated to the point of unconsciousness. The ANA (2001) does not address TS directly in the *Code of Ethics for Nurses with Interpretive Statements* but does state that nurses are to give compassionate care at the end of life. There is an emphasis in the code that nurses are not to have the sole intent of ending a person's life.

▪ Physician-Assisted Suicide

Moral outrage toward social acceptance regarding physician-assisted suicide has occurred in society. **Physician-assisted suicide** is defined as "the act of providing a lethal dose of medication for the patient to self-administer" (Sugarman, 2000, p. 213). Oregon and Washington are the only states in the United States that currently allow physician-assisted suicide. The legal basis in Oregon is the Death with Dignity Act, which was passed in 1994. With certain restrictions, patients who are near death can obtain prescriptions to end their lives in a dignified way.

Although the ANA (2001), in the *Code of Ethics for Nurses with Interpretive Statements*, plainly states that nurses are not to act with the sole intent of ending a person's life, the Oregon Nurses Association issued special guidelines for nurses that relate to the Death with Dignity Act (Ladd et al., 2002). The guidelines include maintaining support, comfort, and confidentiality; discussing end-of-life options with the patient and family; and being present for the patient's self-administration of medications and during the death. Nurses may not administer the medications themselves; breach confidentiality; subject others to any type of judgmental comments or statements about the patient; or refuse care to the patient.

■ End-of-Life Decisions and Moral Conflicts

Nurses first must sort out their own feelings about the various types of euthanasia before appropriate guidance and direction can be offered to patients and families. In one Japanese study of 160 nurses, Konishi, Davis, and Toshiaki (2002) studied withdrawal of artificial food and fluid from terminally ill patients. The majority of the nurses supported this act only under two conditions: if the patient requested the withdrawal of artificial food and fluids, and if the act relieved the patient's suffering. Nurses agreed that comfort for the patient was a great concern. One nurse in the study stated this: "[Artificial food and fluid] AFF only prolongs the patient's suffering. When withdrawn, the patient showed peace on the face. I have seen such patients so many times" (Konishi et al., 2002). In the same study, another nurse who was experiencing moral conflict with the decision to withdraw the artificial food and fluid stated this: "Withdrawal is killing and cruel. I feel guilty" (Konishi et al., 2002).

Other end-of-life issues can generate moral conflicts, as well. Georges and Grypdonck (2002) conducted a literature review on the topic of ethical issues in terms of how nurses perceive their care to dying patients. They outlined some of the moral dilemmas that are particularly related to nurses and end-of-life care. Some of the moral problems of nurses found in the literature were the following:

- Communicating truthfully with patients about death because they were fearful of destroying all hope among the patient and family
- Managing pain symptoms because of fear of hastening death
- Feeling forced to collaborate with other health team members about medical treatments that in nurses' opinions are futile or too burdensome

- Feeling insecure and not adequately informed about reasons for treatment
- Trying to maintain their own moral integrity throughout relationships with patients, families, and coworkers because of feeling that they are forced to betray their own moral values

Although the conscientious nurse has an obligation to provide compassionate and palliative care, the nurse also has a right to withdraw from treating and caring for a patient as long as another nurse has assumed care for the dying patient. When care is such that the nurse perceives it as violating personal morality and values, the professional nurse must seek alternative approaches to achieve patients' goals.

Conclusion

Nurses' involvement with bioethical issues becomes more complicated as time passes. Nurses must learn to cultivate good professional relationships while also ensuring that the stresses of their job do not distract them from delivering direct or indirect patient care that is ethical and patient centered. Practicing nursing ethically cannot be based merely on intuitive functioning. To be advocates for patients during difficult and sensitive times, nurses must understand key ethical concepts and seek active involvement in being valuable members of healthcare teams.

www CASE STUDY ■ END-OF-LIFE CARE

Gertrude, an 85-year-old woman, was diagnosed with end-stage renal disease, long-standing adult-onset diabetes, and aortic stenosis. Her renal disease now has led to a terminal condition. Still conscious, she told her youngest daughter that she wanted no life-sustaining measures done. On the next day, she lost consciousness. Then, her other two daughters arrived at the hospital from out of town. The three daughters argued about the treatment for their mother; the youngest wanted to honor the wishes of her mother and the other two wanted full medical treatment to be initiated. The physician and nurse discussed the treatment options and the futility issue with the family. To avoid further disagreement, the youngest daughter decided to go along with the decision of the other two sisters.

Case Study Questions

1. Explain the reason that the physician and nurse discussed futile treatment with the daughters.
2. Do you believe that the mother had a right to choose her course of treatment? Explain.
3. Discuss the end-of-life options that the daughters could have chosen for their mother's care had they chosen the "no treatment" option.
4. Discuss the different types of surrogate decision making. Was there a surrogate decision maker in this family? Explain.
5. What specific nursing support and care could you offer to this family and patient? ■

References

American Nurses Association. (2001). *Code of ethics for nurses with interpretive statements*. Washington, DC: Author.

Angeles, P. A. (1992). *The HarperCollins dictionary of philosophy* (2nd ed.). New York, NY: HarperCollins.

Beauchamp, T. L., & Childress, J. F. (2009). *Principles of biomedical ethics* (6th ed.). New York, NY: Oxford University Press.

Benjamin, M. (2003). Pragmatism and the determination of death. In G. McGee (Ed.), *Pragmatic bioethics* (2nd ed.). London, England: Bradford Book—MIT Press.

Bondeson, J. (2001). *Buried alive: The terrifying history of our most primal fear*. New York, NY: W. W. Norton.

Brannigan, M. C., & Boss, J. A. (2001). *Healthcare ethics in a diverse society*. Mountain View, CA: Mayfield.

Buchanan, A. E., & Brock, D. W. (1990). *Deciding for others: The ethics of surrogate decision making*. New York, NY: Cambridge University Press.

Center for Economic Justice and Social Justice. (n.d.). *Defining economic justice and social justice*. Washington, DC: Author. Retrieved from http://cesj.org/thirdway/economicjustice-defined.htm

Centers for Disease Control and Prevention. (2007). Suicide: Facts at a glance. Retrieved from http://www.cdc.gov/ncipc/dvp/suicide/SuicideDataSheet.pdf

Chambliss, D. E. (1996). *Beyond caring: Hospitals, nurses, and the social organization of ethics*. Chicago: The University of Chicago Press.

Daniels, N. (1985). *Just health care*. Cambridge, England: Cambridge University Press.

Death: The last taboo. (2003). What is death? Australian Museum. Retrieved from http://australianmuseum.net.au/What-is-death.

Devettere, R. J. (2000). *Practical decision making in health care ethics: Cases and concepts* (2nd ed.). Washington, DC: Georgetown University Press.

Engelhardt, H. T. (1996). *Rights to health care, social justice, and fairness in health care allocations: Frustrations in the face of finitude: The foundations of bioethics* (2nd ed.). New York, NY: Oxford University Press.

Finnerty, J. L. (1987). Ethics in rational suicide. *Critical Care Nursing Quarterly, 10*(2), 86–90.

Fry, S., & Johnstone, M. J. (2002). *Ethics in nursing practice: A guide to ethical decision making* (2nd ed.). Oxford, England: Blackwell Science.

Georges, J. J., & Grypdonck. M. (2002). Moral problems experienced by nurses when caring for terminally ill people: A literature review. *Nursing Ethics, 9*(2), 155–178.

Guido, G. W. (2001). *Legal and ethical issues in nursing* (3rd ed.). Upper Saddle River, NJ: Prentice Hall.

Hester, D. M. (2001). *Community as healing: Pragmatist ethics in medical encounters*. Lanham, MD: Rowman & Littlefield.

International Council of Nurses. (2006). *The International Council of Nurses code of ethics for nurses*. Geneva: Author.

Jameton, A. (1984). *Nursing practice: The ethical issues*. Englewood Cliffs, NJ: Prentice Hall.

Jonsen, A. R., Siegler, M., & Winslade, W. J. (2002). *Clinical ethics* (5th ed.). New York, NY: McGraw-Hill.

Jonsen, A. R., Veatch, R. M., & Walters, L. (1998). *Source book in bioethics.* Washington, DC: Georgetown University Press.

Kaiser Family Foundation. (2007). U.S. health care costs. Retrieved from http://www. kff.org/

Kelly, C. (2000). *Nurses' moral practice: Investing and discounting self.* Indianapolis, IN: Sigma Theta Tau International.

Konishi, E., Davis, A. J., & Toshiaki, A. (2002). The ethics of withdrawing artificial food and fluid from terminally ill patients: An end-of-life dilemma for Japanese nurses and families. *Nursing Ethics, 9*(1), 7–19.

Ladd, R. E., Pasquerella, L., & Smith, S. (2002). *Ethical issues in home health care.* Springfield, IL: Charles C Thomas.

MacIntyre, A. (1999). *Dependent rational animals.* Chicago, IL: Open Court Publishing.

Maes, S. (2003). How do you know when professional boundaries have been crossed? *Oncology Nursing Society News, 18*(8), 3–5.

Mappes, T. A., & DeGrazia, D. (2001). *Biomedical ethics* (5th ed.). Boston, MA: McGraw-Hill.

Massachusetts Department of Higher Education. (2010). *Nurse of the future: Nursing core competencies.* Retrieved from http://www.mass.edu/currentinit/documents/ NursingCoreCompetencies.pdf

McKenna, B. G., Smith, N. A., Poole, S. J., & Coverdale, J. H. (2003). Horizontal violence: Experiences of registered nurses in their first year of practice. *Journal of Advanced Nursing, 42*(1), 90–96.

Munson, R. (2004). *Intervention and reflection: Basic issues in medical ethics* (7th ed.). Victoria, Australia: Wadsworth-Thomson.

Novak, M. (2000). Defining social justice. *First Things First, 108,* 11–13.

Nozick, R. (1974). *Anarchy, state and utopia.* New York, NY: Basic Books.

Office of Minority Health. (2007). Data statistics African American profiles: Health conditions. Retrieved from http://www.minorityhealth.hhs.gov/templates/browse. aspx?lvl=3&lvlid=23

Organ Procurement and Transplantation Network. (2007). Waiting list candidates. Retrieved from http://optn.transplant.hrsa.gov/

Perrin, K. O., & McGhee, J. (2001). *Ethics and conflict.* Thorofare, NJ: Slack.

President's Commission for the Study of Ethical Problems in Medicine and Biomedical and Behavioral Research. (1981). *Defining death.* Washington, DC: U.S. Government Printing Office.

Quill, T. E. (2001). *Caring for patients at the end of life: Facing an uncertain future together.* New York, NY: Oxford University Press.

Rawls, J. (1971). *A theory of justice.* Cambridge, MA: Harvard University Press.

Shotton, L., & Seedhouse, D. (1998). Practical dignity in caring. *Nursing Ethics, 5*(3), 246–255.

Siegel, K. (1986). Psychosocial aspects of rational suicide. *American Journal of Psychotherapy, 40*(3), 405–418.

Sokolowski, R. (1991). The fiduciary relationship and the nature of professions. In E. D. Pellegrino, R. M. Veatch, & J. P. Langan (Eds.), *Ethics, trust, and the professions: Philosophical and cultural aspects* (pp. 23–43). Washington, DC: Georgetown University Press.

Stein, L. I., Watts, D. T., & Howell, T. (1990). The doctor–nurse game revisited. *Nursing Outlook, 38*(6), 264–268.

Sugarman, J. (2000). *20 common problems: Ethics in primary care.* New York, NY: McGraw-Hill.

U.S. Department of Health and Human Services. (2003). Organ donation and transplantation. Retrieved from http://www.hhs.gov/

Veatch, R. M. (2003). *The basics of bioethics* (2nd ed.). Upper Saddle River, NJ: Prentice Hall.

Wildes, K. W. (2000). *Moral acquaintances: Methodology in bioethics.* Notre Dame, IN: University of Notre Dame Press.

Winslow, G. R. (1988). *Ethical issues in professional life.* New York, NY: Oxford University Press.

World Health Organization. (2003). WHO definition of palliative care. Retrieved from http://www.who.int/cancer/palliative/definition/en/print.html

World Health Organization. (2007). Mental health: The bare facts. Retrieved from http://www.who.int/mental_health/en

Youngner, S. J., & Arnold, R. M. (2001). Philosophical debates about the definition of death: Who cares? *Journal of Medicine & Philosophy, 26*(5), 527–537.

Zaner, R. M. (1991). The phenomenon of trust and the patient–physician relationship. In E. D. Pellegrino, R. M. Veatch, & J. P. Langan (Eds.), *Ethics, trust, and the professions: Philosophical and cultural aspects* (pp. 45–67). Washington, DC: Georgetown University Press.

Law and the Professional Nurse

Evadna Lyons and Kathleen Driscoll

12

The professions of law and nursing are both devoted to helping patients, clients, and society. A harmonious interaction between the areas of law and nursing is necessary for achieving effective outcomes for both the nurse and the patient. Nurses must understand how the legal system works to be safe and effective practitioners. The advanced state of medical technology creates new legal, ethical, moral, and financial problems for the consumer and the healthcare practitioner. Patients are more aware of their legal rights; hence, nurses must make a concerted effort to practice by the legal and professional standards set forth by federal and state entities.

Law and nursing are both professions devoted to helping patient/clients and society by advocating for healthcare improvements and justice. Law serves as a guiding force for relationships between persons, persons and groups, and groups and other groups. Note the words *guiding* and *force*. For guidance to occur, law must be developed. For implementation to occur, the law must be enforced.

Learning Objectives

After completing this chapter, the student should be able to:

1. Discuss why an understanding of the legal profession is necessary for the nurse.
2. Discuss the functions and sources of law as they relate to health care and professional nursing practice.
3. Discuss what the term *standard of care* means for the nurse.
4. Discuss the elements of malpractice and negligence and how they relate to nursing practice.
5. Describe the trial process in regard to civil procedures including the nurse's role as an expert witness.
6. Examine the functions of the state boards of nursing in relationship to education, practice, and discipline.
7. Discuss the importance of the Nurse Practice Act in regard to safe and effective nursing practice.
8. Apply the concept of professional accountability to professional and legal standards in relationship to informed consent, confidentiality, and privacy.
9. Critique the legal aspects of delegation.
10. Examine strategies for avoiding legal problems.
11. Discuss healthcare reform related to the Patient Protection and Affordable Care Act.
12. Describe the nurse's moral role in confronting bullying in the workplace.

Law evolves by accommodating to changes in society while adhering to the basic principles set forth in a nation's guiding document, which in the United States is the Constitution. Principles set forth in the Constitution include freedom of religion and assembly, freedom from undue interference by government, and the right to trial by jury in criminal cases. Three sources of law are built on the fundamental law of the federal Constitution. They are statutory law, administrative law or regulatory law, and case law. It is important to note that federal law is administered the same in all states. However, each state might vary on how it interprets and implements laws. Hence, interpretation of legal issues for nurses varies from state to state.

Nursing and healthcare law set forth nursing and health policy goals. A nurse practice act has the goal of protecting the safety of the public who receive nursing care. Each state has statutes that govern the practice of nursing, and although some differences exist from state to state, in general the nurse practice acts define who must be licensed, requirements for licensure, duties of the licensed nurse, and grounds on which the license may be revoked or taken away. This chapter discusses the three sources of law, nurse practice acts, delegation standards of care, civil procedures, and professional and legal accountability in nursing practice.

The Sources of Law

▪ Statutory Law

Key Terms and Concepts

» Statutory law
» Lobbyist
» Administrative or regulatory law
» Case law
» Civil law
» Tort
» Expert witness
» Negligence
» Malpractice
» *Respondeat superior*
» Licensure
» Alternative program
» Informed consent
» Privacy
» Confidentiality
» Delegation

In a democratic society such as the United States, the people elect representatives to governing bodies that consider proposed legislation. The states and the federal government have a legislative body that is composed of two houses. The federal government has the House of Representatives and the Senate. Most state legislatures have similar names for their legislative bodies. Together the federal legislative body is termed Congress. Most state legislatures also have inclusive names for their legislative bodies; for example, the combination of two state bodies might carry a designation such as General Assembly.

Statutory law consists of ever-changing rules and regulations created by the U.S. Congress, state legislators, local governments, and constitutional law. The statutes are the rights, privileges, or immunities secured and protected for each citizen by the U.S. Constitution (Fremgen, 2002).

The process of creating legislation is complex. The process can begin with a legislator responding to the interests of a group of persons. A legislator might also initiate action on a problem by convening a group of interested persons or other legislators to consider legislative options for resolving the problem. Interested persons or groups can represent specific concerns. Since the turn of the 21st century, nursing organizations such as the American

Nurses Association (ANA) and the American Association of Colleges of Nursing (AACN) have focused on legislation addressing patient safety, such as specific staffing levels and controlling mandatory overtime. Such organized groups often hire lobbyists rather than relying on group members to promote their interests to legislators.

Lobbyists develop expertise on proposed legislation and learn to present that information to legislators clearly and concisely. Conscientious legislators and their staffs listen to both sides before voting on an issue. On a very important issue, however, organizations also encourage their members to write letters supporting the organization's position or to make an appointment to speak with the legislator or talk with the legislator's staff.

Generally, no action is taken on bills introduced to legislative bodies unless there is a confluence of problems, solutions, and political circumstances that create a climate for passing legislation (Longest, 2002). Many more bills are introduced into Congress and the state legislatures than are passed. Legislative action alone is insufficient for a bill to become law. Congressional bills require the president's signature, and state bills require the signature of the state's governor to be enacted into law. The president and state governors can also choose to veto legislation. This check on legislative power by the executive branch of government is part of the system of balances among the branches of government ensured by the nation's founders.

■ Administrative Law (Regulations)

Once a bill becomes law, that law is subject to further refinement by federal or state agencies, which are part of the executive branch of government. Enacted statutory law states what Congress or a state legislature wants to accomplish and what activities should occur to accomplish the legislative goal. Federal or state agencies carry out that activity by developing regulations that further define the law and establish the procedures for administering the law. For example, a state nurse practice act might provide that advanced practice nurses develop a formulary of medications they may prescribe. The process for developing the formulary will be done through the rule-making or regulatory process.

The regulatory process is itself governed by statutory law called administrative procedure acts at both federal and state levels. These acts provide that before regulations can be adopted a published notice of the proposed rules and where they are available must occur. The published notice and availability of the proposed rules provide concerned persons with the opportunity to comment on and suggest changes to the rules before final adoption. When rules are adopted, they become **administrative (or regulatory) law** within a set period of time. Thus, the process has three steps: (1) proposal of regulations, (2) consideration of proposed regulations, and (3) adoption of regulations with or without changes.

Staffs of executive branch agencies develop proposed regulations. In the case of federal regulations, notice of the proposed regulations is provided through a publication called the *Federal Register*. An example is Medicare regulations that describe conditions for healthcare facilities to receive reimbursement. This is a serious concern for hospitals because a high percentage of hospital revenue comes from Medicare reimbursement. Information on federal statutory and administrative law is available at http://thomas.loc.gov. Information on state law can be found at state websites. These can be accessed by entering terms such as *State of Ohio* or *State of California* in a search.

■ Case Law

Case law is established from court decisions, which can explain or interpret the other sources of law. For example, a court case might explain what the constitution, a statute, or a regulation means. Case law or common law also defines legal rights and obligations. For example, a nurse's obligation to practice as a reasonably prudent nurse is a legal obligation stemming from actual court decisions. Case law is based on precedent, meaning a ruling in one case that is then subsequently applied to later similar cases. When case law is applied, it must be reviewed by the court to determine if it is still relevant; hence, many case laws are changed and updated over the years. The prevailing ruler over case law is ultimately the state supreme court for state laws and the U.S. Supreme Court for federal statutes. When the judicial branch of government becomes involved, it creates case law. The judicial branch of government is the third component of the balance of power in government at both federal and state levels.

Classification and Enforcement of the Law

When people choose not to follow the law, courts have the obligation to enforce the law. Enforcers of the law also include police and prosecutors. The justice department at the federal level and the attorney general's offices at the state level represent federal and state government interests. Judges are also enforcers of the law. In jury trials, they instruct jurors to apply the facts of a case to the law; in cases in which there is no jury, trial judges both examine the facts and apply the law.

Case law is both civil and criminal. **Civil law** involves relationships between individuals or between individuals and the government. Civil laws are divided into six categories: tort, contract, property, inheritance, family, and corporate law. Criminal law protects the public from the harmful acts of others.

■ Civil Law

Civil laws that commonly affect nurses include tort and contract laws. Tort law refers to acts that result in harm to another. Contract law includes enforceable agreements between two or more persons. A **tort** is a wrongful act that is committed against another person or property that results in harm.

To sue for a tort, a patient must have suffered a mental or physical injury that was caused by the nurse. Torts can be intentional or accidental and the patient might recover monetary damages. According to Fremgen (2002), intentional torts can include assault, battery, false imprisonment, defamation, fraud, and invasion of privacy:

- Assault: The threat of bodily harm to another. There does not have to be actual touching (battery) for an assault to take place. For example, threatening to harm a patient or to perform a procedure without the informed consent (permission) of the patient.
- Battery: Actual bodily harm to another person without permission. This is also referred to as unlawful touching or touching without consent. For example, performing surgery or a procedure without the informed consent (permission) of the patient.
- False imprisonment: A violation of the personal liberty of another person through unlawful restraint. For example, refusing to allow a patient to leave an office, hospital, or medical facility when the person requests to leave.
- Defamation of character: Damage caused to a person's reputation through spoken or written word. For example, making a negative statement about another nurse's ability.
- Fraud: Deceitful practice, such as promising a miracle cure.
- Invasion of privacy: The unauthorized publicity of information about a patient. For example, allowing personal information, such as test results for HIV, to become public without the patient's permission.

An unintentional tort usually occurs when the nurse does not act within the reasonable standards of nursing care. A *reasonable standard of care* means that the nurse must implement the type of care that a "reasonably prudent nurse would use in a similar circumstance." Often, unintentional torts result from negligence. Negligence is the failure to perform professional duties to an accepted standard of care. Nurses should focus on preventing negligence rather than trying to defend it during a civil case.

The Trial Process for Civil Procedures

Nurses are most often involved in civil cases related to malpractice or negligence. The patient brings the case against the healthcare facility or nurse, who becomes the defendant. If the defendant loses, the plaintiff receives monetary damages as compensation for the injury. For a civil case to be won, the judge or jury must find a preponderance of evidence for the winning side.

Figure 12-1   Procedure for a civil trial

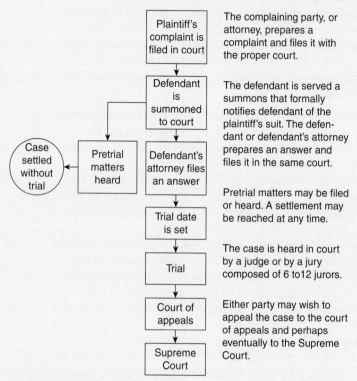

| Plaintiff's complaint is filed in court | The complaining party, or attorney, prepares a complaint and files it with the proper court. |

| Defendant is summoned to court | The defendant is served a summons that formally notifies defendant of the plaintiff's suit. The defendant or defendant's attorney prepares an answer and files it in the same court. |

Case settled without trial ← Pretrial matters heard ← Defendant's attorney files an answer

Pretrial matters may be filed or heard. A settlement may be reached at any time.

Trial date is set

Trial — The case is heard in court by a judge or by a jury composed of 6 to 12 jurors.

Court of appeals

Supreme Court

Either party may wish to appeal the case to the court of appeals and perhaps eventually to the Supreme Court.

Source: Adapted from *A Citizen's Guide to Washington Courts.* State Office of Administrator for the Courts, 1997.

Nurses should have a basic understanding of the proceedings involved in a civil trial because this is the type of trial that involves the nursing profession. In a civil case, if the judge or jury finds in favor of the plaintiff, the defendant will be ordered to pay the plaintiff a monetary award. A plaintiff or defendant may appeal the decision to a higher court (Havinghurst, 1998). See **Figure 12-1** for an illustration of a civil trial procedure.

Nurses as Expert Witnesses

Nurses with advanced degrees and clinical knowledge are often called as expert witnesses during civil trials. An **expert witness** has complex knowledge beyond the general knowledge of most people in the court or on the jury. Most nurses who testify as experts are called to testify as to what the "standard of care" for a patient is in a similar circumstance. Expert witnesses generally do not testify about the exact facts of the case. Instead, they clarify points of knowledge using charts, models, and diagrams.

■ Criminal Law

Criminal laws protect society from the harmful acts of others. Criminal acts are classified as felonies or misdemeanors. A felony carries a punishment of death or imprisonment in a state or federal facility. Felonies often involve murder, rape, robbery, or practicing without a license. Misdemeanors are less serious and include theft, traffic violations, and disturbing the peace. A nurse's license may be revoked by the state board if he or she is convicted of a crime.

A nurse selling or stealing drugs results in a criminal case. In a criminal case, society is the plaintiff, and the nurse becomes the defendant. If the nurse defendant loses, the nurse will have restrictions placed on his or her liberty. Restrictions can include a prison term, probation, or treatment in lieu of conviction. In the last situation, the restriction is compliance with a drug treatment program that includes random drug testing. Failure to comply with the treatment program can result in a criminal punishment such as probation or even incarceration. Criminal cases have a higher standard of evidence. Juries must find the defendant guilty beyond a reasonable doubt. The U.S. justice system is based on the premise that people are innocent until proven guilty. Because the plaintiff is claiming that the nurse violated the law, the burden of proof is placed upon the plaintiff to prove that the defendant is liable.

Boards of nursing also act as enforcers of the law when they discipline a nurse for violation of a provision of the law or rules of the state's nurse practice act. Boards use the preponderance-of-evidence standard.

> **www** | **CRITICAL THINKING QUESTIONS** ∗
>
> What measures are taken when a nurse is summoned to court for a legal action? Is a nurse more responsible than a doctor in that situation if both were involved with the patient's care? ∗

Malpractice and Negligence

The public generally has a very positive view of nurses. Nurses are expected to be of good moral and ethical character because the public has a great deal of trust for nurses. Furthermore, the privilege of obtaining a nursing license is often overlooked as an opportunity, and the right to practice nursing is frequently perceived as an "incidental entitlement" after completing a nursing education (Clevette, Erbin-Rosenmann, & Kelly, 2007). The nurturing aspect of nursing supports a "good will" profile with little, if any, intention of wrongdoing. However, when nurses fail to follow the standards of practice, this can result in claims of malpractice or negligence.

Nurses are citizens who are bound by professional accountability and responsibility. A negligence claim is successful only when the plaintiff proves the required elements of negligence. The first element is duty, which can be defined as "legal obligation that is owed or due to another and that needs to be satisfied; an obligation for which somebody else has a corresponding right" (Garner, 2009).

What are standards? The ANA defines standards as "authoritative statements by which the nursing profession describes the responsibilities for which its practitioners are accountable" (American Nurses Association [ANA], 2004, p. 1). ANA standards of practice are broad and are formatted according to the steps of the nursing process, which is the critical thinking tool of nursing. The steps include assessment, diagnosis, outcomes identification, planning, implementation, and evaluation. The ANA elected to incorporate measurement criteria for each step of the process, thus making the measurement criteria part of the standard. The consistent themes of the measurement criteria permit determining whether the standards are met. They include culturally and ethnically sensitive care, maintaining a safe environment, education of patients, continuity of care, coordination of care, management of information, effective communication, and using technology. Carry out the steps of the nursing process, incorporating the application of the measurement criteria, and the standard of care will be met.

A legal nurse consultant or nurse expert scrutinizing a healthcare record at issue in a lawsuit can use these standards to determine whether there is reason to go forward with a malpractice suit. The nurse will also apply the more specialized and specific standards developed by specialty groups in nursing. For example, the Neonatal Nursing Association, the American Association of Women's Health and Obstetrical and Neonatal Nursing, and the American Association of Critical Care Nurses have their own standards. Standards come from other sources as well. A good example is the Blood-Borne Pathogen Standard promulgated by the Occupational Safety and Health Administration. This standard is an example of a standard for all healthcare providers, not just nurses. Standards evolve over time as research findings are incorporated into practice.

Standards of practice are critical, but there are also standards that are expectations of a professional. Recognizing these expectations, the ANA elected to add professional performance standards to its 1991 standards document. These standards address quality of practice, education, professional practice evaluation, collegiality, collaboration, ethics, research, resource use, and leadership. Because standards of care evolve, one of the ANA's professional performance standards speaks directly to the nurse attaining knowledge and competency that reflects current nursing practice (ANA, 2004). Practice and professional standards can also appear in state practice acts and rules. The legal nurse consultant will expect that the nurses documenting in the medical record demonstrate current knowledge and competency based on general and specialized standards in their area of practice.

KEY COMPETENCY 12-1

Examples of Applicable *Nurse of the Future: Nursing Core Competencies*

Professionalism:

Knowledge (K2) Describes legal and regulatory factors that apply to nursing practice

Skills (S2a) Uses recognized professional standards of practice

Attitudes/Behaviors (A2a) Values professional standards of practice

Source: Massachusetts Department of Higher Education (2010), p. 13.

■ Evidence of Standards of Care Used in Court

The judge decides the issue regarding the element of duty in a negligence claim. The following list included evidence of standards of care that are often used in court:

- Statutes: Common law rules that mandate certain conduct. An example of a statute as evidence of the standard of care is child abuse reporting requirements. These statutes clearly state what a healthcare provider must do when child abuse is suspected.
- Agency regulations: Federal and state administrative agencies promulgate rules and regulations that also can affect the standard of care.
- Accreditation standards: The Joint Commission standards have been recognized in some court cases as evidence for standard of care.
- Facility documents: These might include policies, procedures, job descriptions, and professional nursing guidelines.
- Manufacturer's instructions: In regard to medical equipment or a medication involved in an injury, manufacturer instructions can be examined as standards of care.
- Nursing literature: This includes textbooks and journal articles.
- Expert testimony: Expert witnesses provide testimonial evidence relevant to duty and standard of care.
- It is important to remember that nurses cannot be held as negligent if, when an incident happens, they were performing based on standards of practice. It would be up to their employer to accept liability on their behalf. However, nurses always need to carry liability insurance in case they are charged with negligence or malpractice.

Most nurses are very familiar with the terms *negligence* and *malpractice*. What is the difference between malpractice and negligence? **Negligence** is defined as the failure to act as a reasonably prudent person would have acted in a specific situation (Finkelman, 2006).

Malpractice is the failure of a professional to use such care as a reasonably prudent member of the profession would use under similar circumstances, which leads to harm. For example, a nurse administers the patient's daily dose of Lanoxin without checking the apical pulse and without checking the digoxin level. The patient's pulse drops to 20 beats per minute followed by a full cardiac arrest. Upon inspection of the patient's digoxin level, the nurse discovers that the patient was experiencing digitalis toxicity. A lay person might not know to check the apical pulse and digoxin level prior to Lanoxin administration; but a professional nurse knows that failure to do so prior to Lanoxin administration is a breach of the professional standard of care.

> **Negligence is defined as the failure to act as a reasonably prudent person would have acted in a specific situation.**

> **Malpractice is the failure of a professional to use such care as a reasonably prudent member of the profession would use under similar circumstances, which leads to harm.**

Nurses can be both negligent and guilty of malpractice. According to Finkelman (2006), to prove negligence or malpractice the following four elements must be met:

- There was a duty owed to the patient.
- There was a breach of duty or standard by the healthcare professional.
- There was harm caused by the breach of duty or standard.
- The person (plaintiff) experienced damages or injuries.

Some examples of potential risks for nurses are failure to adequately assess, monitor, and communicate; failure to act as a patient's advocate (for example, not providing proper education for a client with congestive heart failure); or failure to protect the patient when suicidal or at risk for falls. All nurses need to consider these risks when caring for patients.

A question that often comes up with nurses is who is ultimately responsible for the malpractice or negligence: the nurse or the employing institution? *Respondeat superior* is the doctrine that indicates the employer might also be responsible if the nurse was functioning in the employee role at the time of the incident (Grossman, 2005). This implies that both the healthcare organization and the nurse can be sued.

The U.S. Department of Health and Human Services (2003) conducted a study to determine the types of malpractice acts commonly reported to the National Practitioners Data Bank. The results of the study indicated about 1 out of 50 malpractice reports are made for nurses. The report is publicly available at www.npdbhipdb.com. The nursing specializations included in this study were RN, nurse anesthetist, nurse midwife, nurse practitioner, advanced practice nurse, and LVN/LPN (Bolin, 2005). The types of malpractice codes reported are listed in **Table 12-1**.

Can a nurse be brought to court for negligence? Yes. A finding of negligence occurs when the nurse owes a duty to a patient and breaches an ordinary standard of care known by laypersons, and the patient is harmed. An example would be the nurse leaving the side rail down on the bed of a 2-month-old infant. An ordinary person would know that leaving the side rail down is unsafe. Findings of either malpractice or negligence result in the nurse being liable to compensate the harmed person. A malpractice lawsuit requires an expert witness, and a negligence lawsuit does not.

Nurses are rarely individually sued. Malpractice insurance of the facility for which the nurse works will most often cover damages. Nurses, however, can and should purchase malpractice insurance to avoid the risk of losing their personal assets. The nurse might be in a situation in which he or she is viewed as practicing as a nurse and harm occurs. An example might be poor advice given to a friend in failing to recommend further assessment by a healthcare provider when a child is injured in a fall.

Malpractice and negligence are not intentional actions or inactions. They are careless actions or inactions that are more likely to occur in stressful

TABLE 12-1   Malpractice Act or Omission Codes

Diagnosis   Failure, wrong, improper performance, unnecessary, delay, lack of informed consent

Anesthesia   Failure to properly assess, monitor, test, and use equipment, improper choice, intubation, positioning, and failure to obtain informed consent

Surgery   Failure to perform, improper positioning, foreign body, wrong body part, improper performance, unnecessary surgery, delay, improper management, and lack of informed consent

Medication   Wrong med, dosage, improper administration, improper technique, and lack of informed consent

IV and Blood   Failure to monitor, wrong solution, wrong type, improper administration and management

Obstetrics   Improper delivery, delay in delivery, failure to properly manage, delay, abandonment

Treatment   Wrong treatment, improper instruction, improper performance, failure to supervise, failure to refer or seek consult

Monitoring   Failure to monitor, failure to respond and report

Equipment/Product   Improper maintenance, improper use, failure to instruct patient, malfunction or failure

Miscellaneous   Breach of confidentiality, injury to third parties, improper behavior, breach of institutional policies

Source: U.S. Department of Health and Human Services (2003).

circumstances or because the nurse has not maintained knowledge and competency in an area of practice. Montgomery (2007) examines basic principles of human error and sleep physiology and evaluates the evidence for potential effects of fatigued healthcare workers and workload on medical errors. The researchers conducted the study in a pediatric intensive care unit, which is a highly complex environment in which fatigue and excessive workload might allow errors to occur. The results indicated that nursing fatigue and workload have documented effects on increasing intensive care unit errors, infections, and cost. Specific environmental factors such as distractions and communication barriers were also associated with greater errors. The researchers conclude that fatigue, excessive workload, and the pediatric intensive care environment could adversely affect the performance of physicians and nurses working in this type of setting. Castledine (2006) reviews a nursing negligence case in which a registered nurse with 6 months of experience performed a bladder irrigation using a can of cola. The patient suffered major distress, and the nurse was reported to the board of nursing for breach of the code of professional conduct and negligence. The nurse claimed that she thought the cola would break down the "debris" in the bladder. Obviously, this nurse did not follow professional standards of practice relating to bladder irrigation. Because of her inexperience and lack of knowledge, the nurse was only required to receive additional education and support. Nurses must be accountable for their actions while providing patient care. The nurse has a duty to practice competently and possess knowledge, skills, and abilities required for lawful, safe, and effective practice.

Murphy (2004) examines a case (*Logsdon v. Miller*) in which the plaintiff developed reflex sympathetic dystrophy in her left arm and hand after a 7-hour reconstructive jaw surgery in 1999. The circulating nurse positioned, supported, and padded the plaintiff. Postoperatively, the plaintiff woke with numbness and pain in her left arm. The plaintiff suffered permanent nerve damage and sued the physician and the nurse's employer hospital, alleging negligence for failure to properly position the patient. The court ruled that the nurse was not liable because she had followed the appropriate standard of care in positioning the patient. These cases indicate that all nurses need to comply with the guidelines and standards of nursing practice.

> **www CRITICAL THINKING QUESTION ✳**
>
> What does "reasonable and prudent" mean as it relates to standards of care? ✳

Prevention requires learning how to manage stress and adhering to current standards of care. Nurses should learn to leave their personal life stresses at the door of their workplace. They should resist the temptation to self-medicate their stresses with alcohol or other drugs. When they find themselves doing so, they should seek help before their professional practice is affected.

Nurses should also seek to practice in work environments that encourage examination of incidents that might have caused or do cause harm to patients. Often, systems in which the nurse works can be changed to make the environment safer for nurses and patients. The Institute of Medicine (IOM) recommends changing systems to lower the risk of practice errors in several reports. These include *To Err Is Human: Building a Safer Health System*, *Crossing the Quality Chasm: A New Health System for the 21st Century*, and *Keeping Patients Safe: Transforming the Work Environment of Nurses* (IOM, 2000, 2001, 2004). In addition the IOM has released a report entitled *Informing the Future: Critical Issues in Health* that addresses quality of patient care in the United States (IOM, 2007). Changing systems is not the sole solution. Patterns of substandard practice still require the facility to either help the nurse improve practice or make a complaint to the state board of nursing so that disciplinary action can remove the nurse from being in a position to harm patients either through revocation, suspension, or a monitored practice improvement program.

> **www CRITICAL THINKING QUESTION ✳**
>
> You have been asked by a charge nurse on a medical surgical unit to discuss the importance of the legal system for nurses. What are the important aspects regarding law and nursing that you will include in your presentation? ✳

A frequent question about legal issues from practicing nurses at conferences is "Should I carry my own malpractice insurance even though I am covered under my employer's insurance?" The answer is "Never leave home without it!" Nurses should carry their own malpractice insurance because there is a difference and separation between the nurse's liability for a wrongdoing and his or her employer's liability. The nurse uses his or her own judgment within the context of the scope and standards of practice (ANA, 2010) and the business relationship with the employer. The insurer of the employer healthcare institution might have reason to focus on itself, rather than fully defending the nurse. Thus, the nurse needs to have his or her own insurer that will pay for the nurse's defense.

Nursing Licensure

■ History of Licensure

Nursing has evolved on a track parallel with other healthcare professions. The education of nurses particularly parallels the education of doctors of medicine. Both disciplines first experienced apprenticeship education followed by gradual evolution to education within educational institutions. Even today, a critical piece of this education remains the opportunity for clinical practice in healthcare facilities. Increasingly, however, understanding of human physiology has been refined to examination at the cellular and molecular levels. Advances in diagnostic and treatment technology have also occurred. These changes have bred the need for an increasing knowledge base at both the foundational and specialization levels of education in both nursing and medicine (Kalisch & Kalisch, 1995).

Licensure was not always a requirement for nursing practice. In fact, the acknowledged founder of modern nursing, Florence Nightingale, did not believe nurses should be recognized by a government body (Kalisch & Kalisch, 1995). Members of the fields of medicine and nursing eventually thought otherwise. An increasing knowledge base led to increasing risk for patients. Evidence of a basic education with recognized components led to nurses first being registered and later being licensed. The term *registered nurse* is of historical vintage and reflects the period of permissive licensure for nurses. Permissive licensure meant anyone could practice nursing, but only a person with a recognized foundation of nursing education could use the title "registered nurse." During this time, which in some states spanned 60 years, from the first to the sixth decade of the 1900s, the education of nurses primarily took place in hospital schools of nursing. Because hospitals were not recognized as institutions of higher learning, state licensure boards set the standards for nursing education. Boards of nursing continue to be involved in program accreditation today—despite the advent of accreditation bodies for nursing education. The advent of practical nursing education (known as vocational nursing in some states) was another reason for the change from permissive to mandatory licensure. Permissive licensure provides for title recognition. Mandatory licensure provides for a scope of practice. Two levels of nursing practice necessitated defining a scope of

KEY COMPETENCY 12-2

Examples of Applicable *Nurse of the Future: Nursing Core Competencies*

Professionalism:

Knowledge (K2) Describes legal and regulatory factors that apply to nursing practice

Skills (S2b) Implements plan of care within legal, ethical, and regulatory framework of nursing practice

Attitudes/Behaviors (A2b) Values and upholds legal and regulatory principles

Source: Massachusetts Department of Higher Education (2010), p. 13.

practice. Today there are also advanced practice nurses who have specified scopes of practice under the titles nurse practitioner, nurse midwife, nurse anesthetist, and clinical specialist.

Nursing licensure boards contrast with medical boards in that they license or certify at multiple levels rather than a single basic level. In medicine, a student of medicine obtains board certification by passing a professional examination that then allows the physician to practice in a specialty area; there is only one level of licensure. Nurse licensure boards require that nurses with a master's degree in a particular area pass a certification exam generated by a recognized nursing professional organization prior to being recognized as advanced practice nurses.

Nurses initially licensed in one state can acquire licensure in another state through a process called endorsement. Endorsement requires verification that the nurse's license has not been disciplined in another state. Previous discipline might or might not preclude licensure by endorsement depending on the circumstances of the discipline. The nurse seeking endorsement also must meet licensure requirements in the endorsing state. Criminal background checks and continuing education requirements are two examples of such requirements.

In the late 1990s, the National Council of State Boards of Nursing developed the Nurse Licensure Compact. The compact is a statutory agreement between and among states to permit nurses who are residents of one state to have the privilege of practice in another state without acquiring a license in the second state. The nurse does become subject to the provisions of the law and rules of the second state. In this respect, compact state nurses enjoy the same privileges provided by a state driver's license. Drivers in one state can travel through others subject to the vehicular laws of other states. If, however, the driver becomes a resident of another state, the driver must obtain a license in that state. In the case of the compact, until all states adopt the compact, the nurse will have to determine whether the state in which he or she seeks to practice requires licensure by endorsement or is a member of the compact along with the nurse's current state of licensure. A major advantage of the compact is the facilitation of practice in border areas of states.

The National Council of State Boards of Nursing (2010) generates the initial licensure exam for both the licensed practical nurse and registered nurse. Initial licensure measures competence at a minimal level to ensure safe practice. Clearly, the changing nature of practice demands acquisition of knowledge consistent with continuing competence. The content of the NCLEX-RN test plan is organized into four major client needs categories: safe and effective care environment, health promotion and maintenance, psychosocial integrity, and physiological integrity. The category that relates to legal aspects of nursing is found primarily under the category of safe and effective care. The related content includes the following:

- Advance directive
- Advocacy
- Client rights
- Collaboration with interdisciplinary team
- Confidentiality and information security
- Delegation
- Ethical practice
- Informed consent
- Legal rights and responsibilities

Although continuing education has never been clearly demonstrated to be evidence of continuing competence in nursing, many states require continuing education for licensure renewal. It is argued that conscientious nurses would undertake continuing education voluntarily, and mandatory continuing education adds only reluctant nurses to program attendance with perhaps little impact on the reluctant nurses' competence (Hall, 1996). Current competence is also of concern for nurses reentering practice. Mandatory refresher courses seem desirable but have the drawback of high cost for persons who might be reentering practice for economic reasons. Ideally, the burden of maintaining competence rests with the nurse and the nurse's workplace. The workplace should provide and support opportunities for gaining new knowledge and determine its application in practice.

■ The Function of Boards of Nursing

Composition and Role of Boards

The statutory law governing nursing practice in all states and territories of the United States is known as the Nurse Practice Act. Boards of nursing are the state or territorial agencies that administer the law. Members of boards of nursing represent various types of nursing expertise and various geographic areas within the state or territory. A recent trend has been for boards to include consumer members to represent the public. Board members are generally appointed by the governor of the state or territory.

The overriding obligation of all board members is to protect the safety of the public by initially and continuously licensing only competent nurses. Board members direct the activities of the agency through providing direction to the executive director of the board, who in turn directs the activities of board staff. Board staffs can be as few as 2 or as many as 50 or more, depending on the number of licensees in the state or territory. Boards set standards of practice and delegation and often standards for nursing education through the rule-making process. Other board rules govern the disciplinary process and programs such as alternative programs for drug and alcohol abuse and practice intervention improvement.

Boards meet at regularly scheduled intervals during the year to act on disciplinary matters, approve nursing education programs, and review and update the nurse practice act and regulations governing practice as nursing practice evolves. A trend among nursing boards has been to assume the legal oversight of other types of healthcare providers as well. These include nursing assistants, dialysis technicians, community health workers, and medication technicians.

Discipline of Nurses

In legal terms, licensure is a privilege not a right. Not surprisingly, a privilege can be withdrawn or withheld from a person if the behavior of the person does not merit the privilege. Thus, a board of nursing holds legal authority to discipline a nurse who holds a license or to act to withhold licensure from a person seeking initial licensure within a state or territory.

In recent years, boards of nursing have moved to bar from initial licensure persons who have been convicted of, who have pled guilty to, or who had a judicial finding of guilt for felonies involving potential or actual physical harm to persons. Examples of such felonies include murder, robbery, kidnapping, rape, sexual battery, or sexual imposition. Because a large proportion of board disciplinary actions is related to alcohol and substance abuse, boards are concerned about previous histories of drug abuse and drug treatment. Uncontrolled psychiatric illness is also often associated with incompetent practice and substance abuse. Persons with a history of drug-related and psychiatric health problems seeking initial licensure in a state may be allowed to practice but are required to enter into an agreement to be monitored for a period of time under a set of prescribed conditions to ensure that they are safe practitioners. The monitoring would not constitute a disciplinary action. However, if monitoring conditions are violated or the person's practice is unsafe, the board can consider the full range of disciplinary actions. According to Clevette and colleagues (2007), common disciplinary categories reviewed by boards of nursing include the following:

- Substandard nursing practice not involving medications including verbal abuse, using force to administer medications, or failing to respond to changes in patient condition
- Destruction or alteration of patient records including fraudulent charting and/or signatures and/or replacement of records with intent to mislead or deceive
- Physical patient abuse, such as when a nurse hits, strikes, or performs similar physical acts of aggression involving physical contact
- Failure to follow policy such as violation of an employer's policy statements
- Medication "errors," including inaccurate documentation, discarding meds and charting them as given, wrong dosages, wrong route, wrong time, and/or incorrect medication technique

- Controlled substance violations or chemical dependency including diversion of drugs from facility or patient for self-use or sale, prescription fraud, doctor-shopping to obtain prescriptions, or practicing under the influence
- Impaired mental or physical competency. For example, practice is negatively affect by mental or physical incapacity
- Inappropriate management decision such as when a supervisor or manager makes a decision contrary to acceptable nursing standards such as permitting practice without a license
- Practice beyond the authorized scope such as administering medications without a physician's order
- Sexual misconduct including nurse and client communication or contact of a sexual nature or convictions related to sexual misconduct not with clients but related to the practice of nursing
- Patient or employer abandonment such as leaving or not arriving for a patient care assignment
- Unethical actions with a rational relationship to nursing practice, including actions not directly related to nursing care such as falsification of licensure or employment applications, diversion of third-party payments, embezzlement, or distribution of a controlled substance
- Actions demonstrating poor judgment, including irrational behavior not described under the other categories

Boards of nursing have a number of disciplinary choices: denying a license, imposing a fine, issuing a reprimand, placing restrictions on a license, and suspending or revoking a license. Boards must follow a designated process before taking action against a license. First, the board must receive a complaint. Complaints are investigated by board staff. If board staff conclude that the evidence merits action against the nurse's license, a consent agreement might be offered. This procedure is a disciplinary action that bypasses the hearing process, and the nurse agrees to conditions placed on his or her license. An example would be a period of suspension with random drug testing and treatment for drug abuse. Compliance with the agreement would lead to returning to practice with a person in the workplace assigned to report on the nurse's practice at regular intervals. The nurse might also be expected to provide evidence of attendance at a support group for persons with addictions. Consent agreements must be approved by the state's board of nursing before being implemented.

In the absence of a consent agreement, the nurse receives a notice of opportunity for a hearing. When a timely response requesting a hearing is not received, the board members decide the disciplinary action at a subsequent board meeting. Hearings might be conducted by a board or a hearing examiner. In both instances, board members must make the final decision with respect to action against a nursing license.

Reasons for disciplinary action are described in the nurse practice act. Some common examples include conviction of a misdemeanor in the course of practice, conviction of any felony, self-administering a prescription medication without a prescription, impairment of ability to practice safely because of habitual or excessive use of drugs or alcohol, and assaulting or causing harm to a patient. Nurses working in long-term care and home health are at risk for violations of the practice act such as theft and crossing professional boundaries, often resulting in sexual offenses (Driscoll, 2004).

■ Alternative Programs for Nurses

In many states, an **alternative program** for persons with drug and alcohol addictions exists. Nurses must qualify for the program. A criterion is likely to be that the nurse turns herself in to the board because the nurse recognizes the addiction and no person or facility has made a complaint to the board. These programs grew as addiction became viewed as a disease resulting in calls for state boards and nurse employers to provide support for the addicted nurse (Caroselli-Karinja & Zboray, 1986; Daniel, 1984). Successful completion of a monitoring program results in no disciplinary action by a board. The nurse's license remains unscathed. Data from these programs are emerging. Haack and Yocom (2002) found similar rates of relapse in a 6-month period after admission to both alternative and disciplinary programs, although disciplinary action was more likely with criminal convictions, and those persons were less likely to be employed or hold an active license. Although not generalizeable, the study does provide support for the rehabilitative approach provided by the alternative program.

Intervention programs as an alternative to discipline are not limited to substance abuse. Practice intervention improvement programs are also emerging as an alternative to discipline.

CRITICAL THINKING QUESTION

What are the differences between nursing disciplinary action by a board of nursing and legal ramifications set forth by state and federal laws?

Professional Accountability: Informed Consent, Privacy and Confidentiality, and Delegation

■ Informed Consent

Informed consent "mandates to the physician or independent healthcare practitioner the separate legal duty to disclose needed material facts in terms that patients can reasonably understand so that they can make an informed choice" (Guido, 2001, p. 129). The practitioner is required to inform the patient who will perform the procedure or treatment, discuss available alternatives to the recommended treatment, and identify possible complications of the procedure in terms that the patient can understand.

The American Medical Association (2007) states that informed consent is more than simply getting a patient to sign a written consent form. It is a process of communication between a patient and physician that results in the patient's authorization or agreement to undergo a specific medical intervention.

In the communications process, the physician providing or performing the treatment and/or procedure (not a delegated representative) should disclose and discuss with the patient the following information:

> **Informed consent is more than simply getting a patient to sign a written consent form.**

- The patient's diagnosis, if known
- The nature and purpose of a proposed treatment or procedure
- The risks and benefits of a proposed treatment or procedure
- Alternatives (regardless of their cost or the extent to which the treatment options are covered by health insurance)
- The risks and benefits of the alternative treatment or procedure
- The risks and benefits of not receiving or undergoing a treatment or procedure

This communication process is both an ethical obligation and a legal requirement spelled out in statutes and case law in all 50 states.

Informed consent cases are a type of malpractice suit. An informed consent case can be brought by a patient when a risk of a procedure occurs that should have been divulged but was not or when alternatives to the procedure were not provided that the patient would have chosen had he or she known the particular risk. Informed consent cases arise with invasive procedures and complicated treatment regimens such as those for cancer. Central to informed consent is ensuring that the patient is capable of comprehending the information; otherwise, the consent is invalid.

Information components of informed consent include explanation by the physician of the nature of the procedure, its risks, its benefits, and alternatives to the procedure, including the risks and benefits of the alternatives. The information to be provided is generally described as what is material to the patient's decision to go forward with the procedure, decline the procedure, or select an alternative to the proposed procedure. Material risks are expected serious risks such as death, hemorrhage, infection, or any other risk that would seriously compromise the functioning of a person, such as a stroke or paralysis. Failure to meet these standards of disclosure puts the physician at risk for a malpractice suit resulting from failure to provide informed consent if the undisclosed risk occurs and the patient is harmed (*Nickell v. Gonzalez*, 1985). In a leading case that helped establish this type of malpractice suit, the physician did not inform the patient of the risk of paralysis with back surgery (*Canterbury v. Spence*, 1972). In an Ohio case, a patient's incapability to express himself because of temporary aphasia led to the signing of a consent form for a procedure that in his individual case put him at high risk for a stroke, and a stroke occurred (*Greynolds v. Kurman*, 1993). In a California case (*Truman v. Thomas*, 1980), a physician was sued for failing to warn the patient of the risks of not consenting to a diagnostic test.

The standards used for determining whether consent information is sufficient vary from state to state. The first is the medical standard—what are regarded as material risks in the medical community. The second is what a reasonable patient would need to know. The third is what a particular patient needs to know. The first errs in favor of the medical community. The second is considered objective because it provides a standard favoring the patient community. The third is clearly subjective and essentially leaves physicians in the dark as to what information to give patients.

Is there a role for nurses when informed consent is required? There is an advocacy role. When a nurse obtains a signature on a hospital or ambulatory facility consent form, that interaction provides an opportunity to ascertain whether the patient has questions about a procedure. When a conversation reveals that the patient has misconceptions about the procedure or its risks and benefits, the nurse should contact the physician so that additional communication regarding the procedure can occur. The advocacy role of the nurse in this situation is not a legally defined role. It falls in the realm of professional performance standards and a code of ethics responsibility to collaborate with other healthcare providers and the patient to ensure appropriate care. The legal role of the nurse in this situation is acting as a witness to the patient's signature.

www. CRITICAL THINKING QUESTIONS ✳

Are there differences in the responsibility related to informed consent for the nurse and physician? If so, what are the differences? ✳

■ Privacy and Confidentiality

Privacy is the right of a person to be free from unwanted intrusion into the person's personal affairs. To receive appropriate health care, however, a person often must disclose very personal information. Sexual activity and acknowledgment of alcohol or drug abuse are examples of such personal information. Because of the stigma attached to mental illness, patients might also be reluctant to disclose a family or personal history of mental illness. To fulfill their social contract to provide nursing care, nurses must often gather such sensitive information from patients. Thus, the nurse, along with other caregivers, has the obligation to keep healthcare information confidential. Privacy is the right of the patient. **Confidentiality** is the obligation of all healthcare providers.

The *Code of Ethics for Nurses with Interpretative Statements* addresses privacy and confidentiality under provision 3, "The nurse promotes, advocates for, and strives to protect the health, safety, and rights of the patient" (ANA, 2001). Rules of boards of nursing can also spell out the nurse's duty of confidentiality.

In 2000, final federal rules protecting patient privacy were issued. The rules affect health plans, healthcare clearinghouses, and healthcare providers who engage in electronic transactions. The rules were a response to concerns that patient privacy would be compromised without legal standards for the scope of information that could be shared. The rules required all of these groups (called entities) to be in compliance with the rules by April 14, 2003, with the exception of small health plans. The small health plan compliance date was April 14, 2004. The rules were promulgated by the Department of Health and Human Services under provisions of the Health Insurance Portability and Accountability Act (HIPAA) of 1996.

The rules assure patients that only necessary information will be shared with groups such as insurers and third-party intermediaries who administer insurance plans by engaging in functions such as claims processing and membership tracking. The rules also ensure access to patient records by patients themselves, although a reasonable period of time might be needed to copy those records, and the patient might be charged for the cost of copying and sending records. The rules prohibit patient information from being shared for marketing purposes without the patient's consent. The rules require employee training on the provisions of the rules for employees of all healthcare employers.

HIPAA protection of patient privacy highlights the traditional value placed on patient privacy by the healthcare professions. Nurses should remember that conversations in healthcare facilities about patients should occur only among healthcare providers. Elevators and cafeterias are not appropriate sites for such discussions. Pictures of patients and specific healthcare information should be shared with family members only with the express permission of the patient. Generally, medical records cannot be sent to anyone without written consent except when the record is subpoenaed.

Each nurse needs to be aware of and follow the policies and procedures related to oral, written, or electronic patient-identifiable data set up by the healthcare organization regarding issues where the nurse practices; however, some key areas are affected by these new privacy regulations:

- Patients must be informed of their privacy rights.
- Patients must be informed as to who will see their records and for what purpose.
- Patients have the right to inspect and obtain a copy of their medical records. (There are some exceptions to this that each organization should make clear to staff.)

- Valid authorization to release health information must contain certain information, such as a copy of the signed authorization given to the patient, in understandable language, and how the patient may revoke authorization.
- Although information might be used for research purposes to assess outbreak of a disease, all individual identifiable data must be removed.
- Personal data may not be used for marketing (for example, pharmacies may not share this information with others for this purpose) (Finkelman, 2006).

■ Delegation

Today, nurses face many work-related issues, such as the nursing shortage, the increasing need for services, and constant changes within the environment and government. "In an effort to reduce labor costs by decreasing registered nurse positions, hospitals have increasingly turned to a new kind of healthcare worker, unlicensed assistive personnel (UAP)" (Kleinman & Saccomano, 2006, p. 164). The use of UAP helps fill the chasm caused by the nursing shortage and helps decrease the cost of patient care. However, in the past, "nurses were educated in practice settings where the model of care was primary nursing or a similar model in which the registered nurses were responsible for most of the direct care needs of the patients" (Kleinman & Saccomano, 2006, p. 166). Therefore, many nurses are not familiar with how to delegate tasks to UAP because they were not taught these skills. Thus, legal **delegation** has become an increasing challenge for registered nurses (RNs).

As licensed professionals, RNs are responsible to the community for providing safe, competent, and effective care for patients in a variety of healthcare settings. In each setting, RNs work beside other licensed professionals and assign and delegate tasks to these other licensed professionals to give efficient care to patients. Additionally, RNs remain accountable or answerable for patient outcomes and are responsible for supervising delegated tasks. The ANA and the National Council of State Boards of Nursing (NCSBN) define delegation as "the process for a nurse to direct another person to perform nursing tasks and activities" (ANA & NCSBN, 2006, p. 1). Delegation can be direct (i.e., verbal instructions) or indirect (i.e., tasks verified by hospital policy) in the healthcare setting (Trappen, Weiss, & Whitehead, 2004). The RN or nurse manager judges which staff member is competent to perform an assigned duty; however, permitted tasks might depend on the organization or institution.

In terms of accountability, nurses must take responsibility for their actions and the actions of others involved in the delegation process. When allegations of unethical,

> **RNs remain accountable or answerable for patient outcomes and are responsible for supervising delegated tasks.**

illegal, and inappropriate conduct occur, nurses "must answer to patients, nursing employers, the board of nursing, and the civil and criminal court system when the quality of patient care provided is compromised" (ANA, 2005, p. 4). Therefore, it is important for RNs and nurse managers to be knowledgeable of the delegation guidelines within each state's nurse practice act, job descriptions, and the scope of practice of all personnel.

Delegation is part of the language of management. Work might be within the job description of a healthcare worker, but this does not automatically make delegation of a particular task appropriate. The nurse making an assignment is acting as a manager of care. The nurse must carefully select the person to whom a task is assigned because ultimately the nurse as manager is accountable for whether the task is accomplished and whether the desired outcome is achieved. Complete independence in caring for a complex critical care patient would not be an appropriate assignment for a newly licensed registered nurse. Licensed practical nurses cannot shoulder complete responsibility for acting on assessment of a newly admitted patient. Unlicensed assistive personnel may take blood pressures, but they should do so with clear parameters established for communicating deviance from those parameters.

Certain activities cannot be delegated. An advanced practice nurse may delegate the drawing of blood to a nursing assistant but cannot delegate the decision for the types of lab tests to be performed (ANA, 2004). Only the advanced practice nurse can make the judgment as to what tests are necessary. Furthermore, the advanced practice nurse could not delegate the blood draw to a nursing assistant if the nursing assistant had not learned the proper technique for drawing blood and had not received sufficient supervision in carrying out the procedure to determine the nursing assistant's competence.

Unlicensed assistive personnel cannot delegate a task delegated to them by a nurse because that would be engaging in the practice of nursing without a license. Similarly, a nurse cannot delegate a task if the nurse does not know how to do the task. That would be delegating beyond the nurse's scope of practice.

The nurse delegating any task must provide supervision to the unlicensed person. This means determining the competence of the person to carry out the task properly. If the unlicensed person does not properly carry out the task, the unlicensed person should not again be delegated the task until further education ensures that the person has reached a level of competence. Demonstrated competence does not eliminate the supervisory role.

The five rights of delegation as outlined by the National Council of State Boards of Nursing in 2006 are as follows:

- The right task: One that is delegable for a specific patient.
- The right circumstances: An appropriate patient setting, available resources, and consideration of other relevant factors.

- The right person: The right person is delegating the right task to the right person to be performed on the right person.
- The right direction and communication: A clear, concise description of the task, including objectives, limits, and expectations.
- The right supervision and evaluation: Appropriate monitoring, intervention, and as needed, feedback.

Keeping this rights mantra in mind helps the nurse to delegate care according to the legal standard of acting as a reasonable prudent nurse would do in similar circumstances. However, authority to delegate varies, so licensed nurses must check the jurisdiction's statutes and regulations. RNs might need to delegate to the LPN the authority to delegate to the UAP.

Barriers to Delegation

Nurses face many challenges when trying to delegate to others. Contributing factors leading to delegation barriers "range from not having had educational opportunities to learn how to work with others effectively to not knowing the skill level and abilities of nursing assistive personnel to simplify the work pace and turnover of patients" (ANA & NCSBN, 2006, p. 4). Also, the scope of the nursing practice is changing and the tasks performed by UAP are increasing in complexity. This can make many nurses apprehensive in delegating tasks because of a fear of endangering their own licensure. Plus, because of the nursing shortage, many inexperienced nurses are being placed at the helm. Thus, many nurses are not knowledgeable of how to communicate effectively and how to use the institution's resources efficiently. Ultimately, barriers that lead to ineffective delegation place a strain on the quality of patient care.

In 2005, Kalisch conducted a qualitative study to examine the care missed on medical-surgical units. By interviewing 107 RNs, 15 LPNs, and 51 nursing assistants (NAs) from two hospitals in the United States, Kalisch (2006) found that the following activities were frequently missed: "ambulation, turning, feedings, patient teaching, discharge planning, emotional support, hygiene, intake and output documentation, and surveillance" (p. 307). Several factors contributed to why hospital employees missed these important measures; ineffective delegation was cited as one of the major factors. Kalisch (2006) discovered that many NAs were not present during routine nursing reports, and neither did the nurses report to the NAs. "Even when NAs received report, there was a lack of collaborative planning for patient care" (Kalisch, 2006, p. 310). Therefore, lack of communication might have been a problem.

Also, many nurses had difficulty retaining accountability. "Many nurses considered the work delegated to NAs as no longer the RN's responsibility"

(Kalisch, 2006, p. 310). This is a major misconception because the nurse remains accountable for the care given to the patient. Another problem was that many staff members did not feel that it was their job to perform a particular task. "Nurses stated that certain tasks such as vital signs were the NA's responsibility, and if the NA did not complete these tasks, it was the 'fault' of the NA, not the RN" (Kalisch, 2006, p. 310). State nurse practice acts define the scope of practice and what nurses can delegate. Also, hospitals and institutions have policies and procedures that help define which tasks can be delegated.

Kalisch (2006) also cites that many nurses had difficulty with conflict management. "Many nurses reported limited authority and influence over the NAs and expressed reluctance to confront NAs who did not 'do their job' " (Kalisch, 2006, p. 310). In several cases, staff members tried to avoid confrontation and had difficulty engaging in conflict management to strive for a solution. "If delegates are resistant, the delegator may simply choose to do the task him or herself to avoid confrontations; instead, the situation should be reevaluated from the UAP's point of view" (Quallich, 2005, p. 122). In some cases, UAP might lack the confidence or knowledge to perform a task; however, if UAP refuse to perform a task as a way to defy authority, guidelines for delegation should be clearly reinstituted. Also, if a nurse lacks confidence and does not trust the abilities of other staff members, delegation is unlikely to occur. "Similarly, delegation will be unsuccessful if the only tasks that are delegated are those that are time-consuming or unpleasant; this approach risks exhausting staff that are otherwise capable" (Quallich, 2005, p. 122).

Regardless of the institution, delegation has a strict chain of command among employees. Nurses sometimes might experience feelings of guilt about those to whom they delegate tasks. The RN also might worry about being labeled as lazy when delegating a task to other employees. "But working in an organizational hierarchy should not result in the delegator taking on disproportionate amounts of responsibility in order to respect the feelings of other delegatees" (Quallich, 2005, p. 122). Some nurses might also feel that they should show loyalty to other nurses and should delegate to student and graduate nurses only. However, this loyalty or discrimination is not cost-efficient and only acts as another delegation barrier. Plus, if a nurse refuses to delegate a task as instructed by the employer, the nurse can face disciplinary actions by the employer (Haslauer & Jones, 2003). If a nurse has concerns regarding the implementation of a task or activity, it is important to document concerns for patient safety and to inform the employer. After the staff become comfortable with their skill at delegation, the next challenge is making sure they have the skills necessary to assess the competence of their UAP for individual tasks.

Delegation Decision-Making Tree

In 1997, the NCSBN developed a delegation decision-making tree that identifies several steps nurses can take to help them make delegation decisions.
In 2006, the ANA and the NCSBN published a joint paper on the topic of
delegation that includes the ANA principles of delegation and the NCSBN
decision-making tree. The decision-making tree is a useful tool or "grid that
may be used by staff education specialists to provide orientation and education
to staff nurses and UAP" (Kleinman & Saccomano, 2006, p. 168). The decision-making tree is available online at www.ncsbn.org/Joint_statement.pdf.

Healthcare Reform

The U.S. Congress passed the Patient Protection and Affordable Care Act
on March 21, 2010, a sweeping healthcare reform law that will expand
healthcare coverage to 32 million Americans. A Gallup poll on behalf of the
Robert Wood Johnson Foundation of 1,500 participants recruited from academia, insurance companies, and healthcare organizations found that nurses
had the least influence on the design of this healthcare reform. Nurses are in
a position to focus on prevention and management of chronic disease as well
as to promote healthy aging and wellness. It is important for nurses to continue to stay abreast of new healthcare laws and to remain politically active.

The first nationwide effort to improve healthcare access for low-income
and elderly Americans was in the 1960s with the creation of Medicare,
Medicaid, and Community Health Centers. Despite these improvements,
50 years later, racial, ethnic, and socioeconomic disparities remain both in
health care as well as health status. The Affordable Care Act addresses racial
and ethnic health care and health status disparities in several important ways.
The act provides access to insurance for all Americans through tax credits
and premium assistance, which should significantly improve access to health
care. This new healthcare legislation is 2,400 pages long and has 10 major
sections (govtrack.us, 2010). Because of the complexity of the legislation, few
people even within the healthcare industry are fully aware of all the intrica-
cies involved. As this law is enacted, drastic changes will be made to the way
health care is financed and delivered in the United States.

Ethical, Legal, and Moral Courage to Confront Bullying in the Workplace

Workplace verbal and physical abuse has many sources; however, it is most
stressful when a coworker is the predator (Center for American Nurses, 2007).

The nurse who bullies others is often using power as a way to control another person. Nurses have an ethical and legal responsibility to support a colleague who is being bullied: The ethical obligation is outlined by ANA (2001) as follows:

> The principle of respect for persons extends to all individuals with whom the nurse interacts. The nurse maintains compassionate and caring relationships with colleagues and others with a commitment to the fair treatment of individuals ... the standard of conduct precludes any form of harassment or threatening behavior, or disregard for the effect of one's behavior on others. (p. 9)

Nurses should support each other and maintain the dignity and integrity of other nurses. Acting legally and morally requires knowledge of professional ethical obligations and the courage to confront the problem assertively.

Preventing Legal Problems

Preventing legal problems intentionally runs as a theme through this chapter. In summary, prevention requires consistently following the nursing process—the decision-making process of nursing in all nursing care situations. Because nurses act as managers of care, following management principles also reduces the risk of legal problems. This is especially true with delegation of care, an activity that predictably will increase as care systems adjust to the nursing shortage.

Communication with patients, families, nursing staff, and other healthcare providers also reduces the risk of legal problems. A once-a-year commitment to reviewing the state nurse practice act and rules as well as professional standards of care and code of ethics will enhance the nurse's appreciation of legal accountability in care. Beyond these general activities the nurse should tailor risk prevention to being aware of the law and rules that affect the nurse's particular practice situation. Hospital and long-term care settings are affected by different law and rules. Nurses holding administrative positions should know the laws and rules affecting their area of practice. In turn, they should educate nursing staff in their responsibilities to carry out the law in their practice setting.

The practice of nursing is never static. Practice is a continuous quest involving adaptation to the current healthcare environment with a commitment to making that environment as safe as possible for the patients for whom nurses care.

Conclusion

Nurses are generally law-abiding citizens who have a positive relationship and respect for their profession. However, nurses must develop a clear understanding of the legal system, sources of law, nurse practice acts, delegation, standards of care, healthcare reform, and strategies for avoiding legal problems. Nurses should make every effort to provide high-quality care for patients that not only helps them recover their health but also avoids lawsuits. Nurses have a legal and ethical duty to be knowledgeable about their scope of practice and legal issues.

---

www CASE STUDY 12-1

As the nurse on the medical-surgical unit, you are responsible for the care of eight acute patients. You have two nursing assistants working with you on this shift. Both of the nursing assistants have worked on the unit for several years. To provide adequate care for all of the patients under your care, it is necessary to delegate some of the nursing care to the nursing assistants working with you. You request that the first nursing assistant check the vital signs for Mr. Martin and you request that the second nursing assistant assess Ms. Smith's level of pain because you have recently administered pain medication.

Case Study Questions

1. Is the delegation of the assignment to the first nursing assistant in the case study appropriate? Why or why not?
2. Is the delegation of the assignment to the second nursing assistant in the case study appropriate? Why or why not? ■

Classroom Activity 1

A mock trial is a fun way to explore some of the concepts in this chapter. Assign roles to students and use a graduation gown for the judge to increase the realism. Make up your own case or use one already prepared such as the excellent mock trial presented in *Nurse Educator* by Haidinyak (2006). www

References

American Medical Association. (2007). *Informed consent*. Chicago, IL: Author.

American Nurses Association. (2001). *Code of ethics for nurses with interpretive statements*. Washington, DC: Author.

American Nurses Association. (2004). *Nursing: Scope and standards of practice*. Washington, DC: Author.

American Nurses Association. (2005). Principles for delegation [Brochure]. Retrieved from http://www.healthsystem.virginia.edu/internet/e-learning/principlesdelegation.pdf

American Nurses Association. (2010). *Nursing: Scope and standards of practice*. Silver Spring, MD: Author.

American Nurses Association & National Council of State Boards of Nursing. (2006). Joint statement on delegation. Retrieved from http://www.ncsbn.org/Joint_statement.pdf

Bolin, J. N. (2005). When nurses are reported to the national practitioner's data bank. *Journal of Nursing Law, 10*(3), 141–148.

Canterbury v. Spence, 464 F.2d 772 (D.C. Cir. 1972).

Caroselli-Karinja, M. F., & Zboray, S. D. (1986). The impaired nurse. *Journal of Psychosocial Nursing and Mental Health Services, 24*(6), 14–19.

Castledine, G. (2006). Nurse whose inexperience and negligence in bladder washout put her patient at risk. *British Journal of Nursing, 15*(3), 141–143.

Center for American Nurses. (2007). Lateral violence and bullying in the workplace. Retrieved from http://www.mc.vanderbilt.edu/root/pdfs/nursing/center_lateral_violence_and_bullying_position_statement_from_center_for_american_nurses.pdf

Clevette, A., Erbin-Rosenmann, M., & Kelly, C. (2007). Nursing licensure: An examination of the relationship between criminal convictions and disciplinary actions. *Journal of Nursing Law, 11*(1), 5–8.

Daniel, I. Q. (1984). Impaired professionals: Responsibilities and roles. *Nursing Economics, 2*, 190–193.

Driscoll, K. (2004). Current issues: Crossing professional boundaries: Ethical, legal, and case perspectives. *Rehabilitation Nursing, 29*(3), 78–79.

Finkelman, A. W. (2006). *Leadership and management in nursing*. Upper Saddle River, NJ: Pearson Prentice Hall.

Fremgen, B. F. (2002). *Medical law and ethics*. University of Notre Dame. Upper Saddle River, NJ: Prentice Hall.

Garner, B. A. (2009). *Black's law dictionary* (9th ed.). St. Paul, MN: West Group.

Govtrack.us. (2010). H.R. (111th) 3590: Patient protection and affordable care act. Retrieved from http://www.govtrack.us/congress/bills/111/hr3590

Greynolds v. Kurman, 91 Ohio App.3d 389 (1993).

Grossman, S. C. (2005). *The new leadership challenge*. Philadelphia, PA: F. A. Davis.

Guido, G. (2001). *Legal and ethical issues in nursing* (3rd ed.). Upper Saddle River, NJ: Prentice Hall.

Haack, M. R., & Yocom, C. J. (2002). State policies and nurses with substance abuse disorders. *Journal of Nursing Scholarship, 34*, 89–94.

Haidinyak, G. (2006). Try a mock trial. *Nurse Educator, 31*(3), 119–123.

Hall, J. K. (1996). *Nursing ethics and law*. Philadelphia, PA: Saunders.

Haslauer, S., & Jones, D. (2003, Winter). Delegation: Concept, art, skill, process. *Arkansas State Board of Nursing Update*, 22–24.

Havinghurst, C. (1998). *Health care law and policy: Readings, notes and questions.* Westbury, NY: Foundation Press.

Institute of Medicine. (2000). *To err is human: Building a safer health system.* Washington, DC: National Academy Press.

Institute of Medicine. (2001). *Crossing the quality chasm: A new health system for the 21st century.* Washington, DC: National Academy Press.

Institute of Medicine. (2004). *Keeping patients safe: Transforming the work environment of nurses.* Washington, DC: National Academy Press.

Institute of Medicine. (2007). *Informing the future: Critical issues in health.* Washington, DC: National Academies Press.

Kalisch, B. J. (2006). Missed nursing care: A qualitative study. *Journal of Nursing Care Quality, 21*(4), 306–313.

Kalisch, P. A., & Kalisch, B. J. (1995). *The advance of American nursing* (3rd ed.). Philadelphia, PA: Lippincott.

Kleinman, C. S., & Saccomano, S. J. (2006). Registered nurses and unlicensed assistive personnel: An uneasy alliance. *Journal of Continuing Education in Nursing, 37*(4), 162–170.

Longest, B. B. (2002). *Health policymaking in the United States* (3rd ed.). Chicago, IL: Health Administration Press.

Massachusetts Department of Higher Education. (2010). *Nurse of the future: Nursing core competencies.* Retrieved from http://www.mass.edu/currentinit/documents/NursingCoreCompetencies.pdf

Montgomery, V. L. (2007). Effect of fatigue, workload, and environment on patient safety in the pediatric intensive care unit. *Pediatric Critical Care Medicine, 8*(Suppl. 2), S11–6.

Murphy, E. K. (2004). Implications for perioperative nurses. *American Operating Room Nurse, 80*(2), 314–317.

National Council of State Boards of Nursing. (2010). *NCLEX-RN test plan.* Chicago, IL: Author.

Nickell v. Gonzalez, 17 Ohio St.3d 136, 477 N.E.2d 1145 (1985).

Quallich, S. A. (2005). A bond of trust: Delegation. *Urologic Nursing, 25*(2), 120–123.

State Office of Administration for the Courts. (1997). *A citizen's guide to Washington courts. The procedure for a civil trial.* Washington, DC: Author.

Trappen, R. M., Weiss, S. A., & Whitehead, D. K. (2004). *Essentials of nursing leadership and management* (3rd ed., pp. 91–103). Philadelphia, PA: F. A. Davis.

Truman v. Thomas, 27 Cal. 3d 285, 611. P2d (1980).

U.S. Department of Health and Human Services. (2003). *Survey of the national practitioner's data bank.* Washington, DC: Author.

The Role of the Professional Nurse in Patient Education

13

Kathleen Masters

Patient education has formally been a part of nursing care since the time of Florence Nightingale (1860/1969). During the 1900s, patient education increasingly became identified as a role of the professional nurse; however, it was not until 1973 that the American Nurses Association (ANA, 1973) defined patient education as a component of the practice of the registered nurse. Beginning in 1976, the Joint Commission on Accreditation of Healthcare Organizations (The Joint Commission, 1995) included patient and family education as a function critical to patient care. The American Association of Colleges of Nursing (AACN, 1998, 2008) also recognized that the implementation of the professional nursing role requires that nurses are prepared to teach patients effectively. Today, patient education is both an expectation and legal obligation of the professional nurse.

Learning Objectives

After completing this chapter, the student should be able to:

1. Differentiate between patient education and patient teaching.
2. Discuss the purposes of patient education.
3. Describe the process of patient education.
4. Identify three domains of learning.
5. Discuss two theoretical frameworks related to the learning process.
6. Demonstrate use of a readability formula to assess reading grade level.
7. Discuss strategies to accommodate for age-related barriers to learning in older adults.
8. Discuss the development of culturally appropriate patient education.

Key Terms and Concepts

» **Patient teaching**
» Patient education
» Learning domains
» Andragogy
» Health Belief Model (HBM)
» Social learning theory
» Self-efficacy
» Readiness to learn
» Health literacy
» Age-related changes

Patient Education: What Is It?

"Patient education is any set of planned, educational activities designed to improve patients' health behaviors, health status, or both" (Lorig, 2001, p. xiii). There is nothing in this definition about improving knowledge, although a change in knowledge might be necessary to reach the goal of changing health status or health behaviors. In contrast, activities aimed at improving knowledge are known as **patient teaching** (Lorig, 2001, p. xiv). The point is that the purpose of **patient education** involves more than a change in knowledge.

The purposes of patient education are to maintain health, to improve health, or to slow deterioration of health. These purposes are met through changes in health-related behaviors and attitudes (Lorig, 2001). These changes are not easily achieved. Effective patient education requires the nurse to have the ability to communicate effectively with patients to assess the individual needs, attitudes, and preferences of the patient that can affect health behaviors before any changes can be expected (Falvo, 2004, 2011).

> The purposes of patient education are to maintain health, to improve health, or to slow deterioration of health. These purposes are met through changes in health-related behaviors and attitudes.

In addition to communication and assessment skills, if the nurse is to be effective as a patient educator, the nurse must also have sufficient knowledge of the information that needs to be taught. If the knowledge base of the nurse is insufficient, the nurse risks providing inadequate or inaccurate information to the patient (Falvo, 2004, 2011).

Finally, to be an effective patient educator, it is important that the nurse have an understanding of how to conduct patient education. The remainder of this chapter provides a foundation for the conduct of patient education.

Theories and Principles of Learning

Many educational theories and principles can be used to guide the patient education process. Some that are most commonly used in the healthcare setting are presented here.

■ Domains of Learning

First, we should examine the nature of learning in relationship to **learning domains**. Identification of the learning domain reflects the type of learning desired as a result of the patient education process. Learning occurs in three domains: the cognitive, the psychomotor, and the affective (Bloom, 1956). Each domain has levels, and each level builds on the previous one in a hierarchical fashion. In the cognitive and psychomotor domains, levels are arranged in the order of increasing complexity. In the affective domain, levels are organized according to the degree of internalization of a value or attitude.

Cognitive learning encompasses the intellectual skills of remembering, understanding, applying, analyzing, evaluating, and creating. Psychomotor learning refers to learning of motor skills and performance of behaviors or skills that require coordination. Affective learning requires a change in feelings, attitudes, or beliefs (Anderson & Krothwohi, 2001).

Understanding which domain is the target of learning helps guide the planning, implementation, and evaluation of learning. For example, if based on assessment you know that a patient is knowledgeable about insulin administration and is committed to administering the injection but has not yet been able to manipulate the syringe correctly to administer the injection, you know that your target domain for learning is the psychomotor domain, and the focus of your objectives, planning, learning activities, and evaluation will be on the performance of the identified behaviors.

■ Andragogy

Andragogy, initially defined as "the art and science of helping adults learn" (Knowles, 1970), has taken on a broader meaning over the past 35 years and is currently used to refer to learner-focused education for people of all ages (Conner, 2004). The andragogic model asserts that four issues be considered and addressed in learning. These include the following (Knowles, Swanson, & Holton, 1998, 2011):

- Letting learners know why something is important to learn
- Showing learners how to direct themselves through information
- Relating the topic to the learners' experiences
- Realizing that people will not learn until they are ready and motivated

Adults learn best when there is immediate opportunity for application. Adults in particular are motivated to learn when they recognize a gap between what they know and what they want to know or what they need to know (Knowles, 1970). Therefore, adult learners are rarely interested in learning detailed anatomy and physiology related to their chronic disease, but they are motivated to learn how to care for themselves after discharge from the hospital. Effective patient education will be based on principles that capitalize on these characteristics of the adult learner.

■ Health Belief Model

The **Health Belief Model (HBM)** is one of the most widely used frameworks in research and programs related to health promotion and patient education. This model was originally developed to predict the likelihood of a person

---

KEY COMPETENCY 13-1

Examples of Applicable *Nurse of the Future: Nursing Core Competencies*

Communication (Teaching/ Learning):

Knowledge (K5d) Is aware of the three domains of learning: cognitive, affective, and psychomotor

Attitudes/Behaviors (A5c) Values the need for teaching in all three domains of learning

Source: Massachusetts Department of Higher Education (2010), p. 29.

following a recommended action and to understand the person's motivation and decision making regarding seeking health services (Hochbaum, 1958). According to the HBM, the likelihood of a person acting in response to a health threat depends on six factors:

- The person's perception of the severity of the illness
- The person's perception of susceptibility to illness and its consequences
- The value of the treatment benefits (i.e., do the cost and side effects of treatment outweigh the consequences of the disease?)
- Barriers to treatment (i.e., expense, complexity of treatment)
- Costs of treatment in physical and emotional terms
- Cues that stimulate taking action toward treatment of illness (i.e., mass media campaigns, pamphlets, advice from family or friends, and postcard reminders from healthcare providers)

The HBM can provide a framework for assessing areas where patients have gaps in knowledge, such as severity of illness or susceptibility to illness, and then address those areas to increase the potential for compliance with the treatment regimen. Through use of the HBM, you can easily categorize and cover the essential components of your educational message, thus providing the patient with a basic understanding of the severity of the illness, the risk and consequences of the illness, the value of treatment, the barriers to treatment, and the costs of treatment.

> **www CRITICAL THINKING QUESTION** *
>
> Think about your own life. Do you act to prevent a disease or accident when you perceive that you are not susceptible to the disease or at risk for the accident? *

■ Social Learning Theory

According to Bandura's **social learning theory**, if a person believes that he or she is capable of performing a behavior (**self-efficacy**) and also believes that the behavior will lead to a desirable outcome, the person will be more likely to perform the behavior (Bandura, 1997). In contrast, if a person does not believe that he or she is capable of performing a behavior, he or she will have no incentive to do so, even if the person is actually capable. Perceptions of self-efficacy are particularly important in relationship to a patient's learning complex activities or long-term changes in behavior (Prohaska & Lorig, 2001, p. 163).

There are four methods for developing or enhancing efficacy expectations if assessment reveals a need for such enhancement. These methods are as follows:

- Performance accomplishments
- Vicarious experience or modeling
- Verbal persuasion
- Interpretation of physiologic state

Performance accomplishment is the most direct and influential way to enhance self-efficacy. In this method, the patient first performs tasks that he or she can easily perform. By succeeding with these first tasks, the patient develops a sense of competence and enhancement of self-efficacy before proceeding to more difficult tasks. Along these same lines, it is also important to set short-term goals that are measurable so that patients can see their success and the impact of the change in their behavior. A patient who can see the benefits of a behavior change within a reasonable time is more likely to continue practicing the behavior.

The second method for enhancing self-efficacy is through modeling, where the patients observe others who appear to be similar and who are successfully performing behaviors. Modeling can also be achieved through the use of illustrations in pamphlets or in programming materials by using illustrations and models that are of various cultures, body shapes, and ages (Prohaska & Lorig, 2001).

Verbal persuasion can also be an effective method of enhancing self-efficacy expectations. The content of the message needs to include basic factual information that emphasizes the importance of performing the behavior. It is usually better to ask for incremental changes or ask the patient to do just slightly more than he or she is currently doing (Prohaska & Lorig, 2001). Encouragement and support not only from the nurse but also from family and friends help the patient to be successful.

Most illnesses present with symptoms, and most new behaviors cause some physiologic changes. Addressing the meaning of symptoms and physiologic states can influence self-efficacy. For example, a patient who is trying to quit smoking can expect withdrawal symptoms. If the patient understands the reasons for the symptoms and the limitation in the duration of the symptoms, the patient might decide that he or she has the ability to make the change. Without that knowledge, the patient might give up because he or she experiences physiologic changes that are not understood.

KEY COMPETENCY 13-2
Examples of Applicable *Nurse of the Future: Nursing Core Competencies*
Communication (Teaching/ Learning):
Knowledge (K5c) Understands the principles of teaching and learning
Skills (S5c) Assists patients and families in accessing and interpreting health information and identifying healthy lifestyle behaviors
Attitudes/Behaviors (A5b) Accepts the role and responsibility for providing health education to patients and families
Source: Massachusetts Department of Higher Education (2010), p. 29.

The Patient Education Process

According to Redman (2001, 2006), the process of patient education can be viewed as parallel to the nursing process. Each of these processes begins with assessment, negotiation of goals and objectives, planning, intervention, and finally evaluation (Rankin, 2005; Rankin & Stallings, 2001).

■ Assessment

The goal of the nurse in the process of patient education is to assist the patient in obtaining the knowledge, skills, or attitude that will help the patient develop behaviors to meet needs and maximize the potential for positive health

> **The process of patient education can be viewed as parallel to the nursing process.**

outcomes (Falvo, 2004, 2011). Because no patient or situation is exactly the same, an assessment is required.

Many available guides are helpful in assessing the learning needs of patients (Redman, 2003). Some nurses construct their own assessment tools to meet specific needs. Observation, interviews, open-ended questions, focus groups, and the patient's medical record are additional ways to gather information for the assessment of learning needs.

Rankin and Stallings (2001, p. 200) suggest some specific questions that must be addressed in the assessment of learning needs. These questions are as follows:

- What information does the patient need?
- What attitudes should be explored?
- What skills does the patient need to be able to perform healthcare behaviors?
- What factors in the patient's environment may be barriers to the performance of desired behaviors?
- Is the patient likely to return home?
- Can the family or caregiver handle the care that will be required?
- Is the home situation adequate or appropriate for the type of care required?
- What kinds of assistance will be required?

■ Learning Styles

To provide the most effective patient teaching the nurse must also assess patient learning style. Although most people learn best when multiple techniques are used in patient teaching, assessment of the patient's learning style is a fundamental step prior to beginning any learning activity. Learning styles are methods of interacting with, taking in, and processing information that allow individuals to learn. Learning styles are generally categorized as visual, auditory, or tactile/kinesthetic.

The patient who is a visual learner prefers written instructions rather than verbal instructions but prefers photographs and illustrations to written instructions. The nurse teaching the patient who is a visual learner should use a variety of interesting visual learning materials, including organized visual presentations, photographs, or computerized materials (Russell, 2006).

The patient who is an auditory learner remembers verbal instructions well and learns through discussion. The nurse teaching a patient who is an auditory learner will want to be sure the patient is positioned to be able to hear and will want to rephrase what is said several different ways to be sure the intended message is communicated. The nurse might also want to use multimedia that incorporate sound in patient teaching (Russell, 2006).

The patient who learns best through getting physically involved is the tactile or kinesthetic learner. The kinesthetic learner learns through doing or experiencing physically. The kinesthetic leaner has difficulty staying in one place for very long and enjoys hands-on activities. The nurse teaching the kinesthetic learner should provide activities during the session and should provide samples or supplies for practicing or demonstrating skills (Russell, 2006).

■ Readiness

An important variable in the patient education process is **readiness to learn.** After a need to learn has been identified, a patient's readiness or evidence of motivation to receive information at that particular time must also be assessed (Falvo, 2004, 2011; The Joint Commission, 1999, 2003; Redman, 2001). A variety of factors such as pain, anxiety, and emotional reactions can affect a patient's readiness to learn. Moderate to severe anxiety has been shown to interfere with a patient's ability to concentrate and understand new information (Stephenson, 2007). If a patient is distracted by physical or emotional pain, attempts at patient teaching will not be successful. The better choice is to wait until the pain has subsided or to address the anxiety that the patient is experiencing, and then when the patient is ready, proceed with patient education activities (Redman, 2001, 2006; Stephenson, 2007).

■ Health Literacy

Health literacy is defined as the ability to read, understand, and act on health information. Today there is more access to healthcare information than at any time in history. The low health literacy problem is not an issue of access to information, but rather, it is a crisis of understanding medical information (Doak & Doak, 2002). It is a crisis. Research studies have demonstrated that patients with low health literacy skills make more errors with their medications and treatments (Baker et al., 1996; Williams, Baker, Honig, Lee, & Nowlan, 1998). They often fail to seek preventive care and are also at higher risk for hospitalization, which results in higher annual healthcare costs (Baker, Parker, Williams, & Clark, 1998; Weiss, 1999).

Currently in the United States, one in five adults and nearly two of five older adults and minorities read at the 5th-grade level or below. The average American reads at the 8th- to 9th-grade level. Most materials used for patient education are written above 10th-grade reading level (Doak & Doak, 2002; Doak, Doak, & Root, 1996). We know that when the reading level of printed materials is beyond the skill of the learner, comprehension is decreased, recall is sketchy and inaccurate, and motivation to learn is decreased (Redman, 2001, 2006).

When information is complex or time is limited, nurses frequently rely on printed materials by instructing patients to read or review the information at home. These materials are helpful when they provide patients who have adequate reading skills with a resource to remind them of the instructions

KEY COMPETENCY 13-3

Examples of Applicable *Nurse of the Future: Nursing Core Competencies*

Communication (Teaching/ Learning):

Knowledge (K5a) Understands the influences of different learning styles on the education of patients and families

Attitudes/Behaviors (A5a) Values different means of communication used by patients and families

Source: Massachusetts Department of Higher Education (2010), p. 29.

given by the nurse, but for those patients with low health literacy skills, the printed materials might be of no use. Patients with low health literacy skills are generally too embarrassed to reveal to the nurse that they cannot read or cannot read well enough to understand the written instructions. It is therefore important that the nurse take the initiative in the assessment of literacy skills of patients if written materials are going to be used in the patient education process.

Direct questioning of patients about reading ability is usually not effective. Thus, how can you determine the reading ability of the patient? One option is to use one of several instruments that have been developed to assess patient literacy quickly. Some of the literacy assessment instruments most commonly used in healthcare settings include the Rapid Estimate of Adult Literacy in Medicine (Davis et al., 1993) and the Wide Range Achievement Test (Jastak & Wilkinson, 1993).

One of the best ways to assess literacy is simply through careful observation of your patient. Clues that might be observed in a patient with low health literacy skills include forms that are filled out incompletely or incorrectly, written materials that are handed to a person accompanying the patient, aloofness or withdrawal during provider explanations, surveillance of the behavior of others in the same situation to copy their actions, and a request for help from staff or other patients. Verbal responses such as "I will read this at home" or "I can't read this now because I forgot my glasses" are also common (Bastable, 2006; Doak & Doak, 2002).

www | CRITICAL THINKING QUESTIONS ✳

Have you ever been assigned to read a book that had so many big words in it that you had to keep the dictionary by your side? If it was assigned for school, you probably struggled through it for the sake of not failing the test; but, what about if you were not being graded? Would you bother to read it? If you did read it because you knew it would help you, would you have enough understanding to actually apply the information? ✳

■ Assessing the Readability of Patient Education Materials

Many health-related teaching materials are written on a level that is above the average patient's literacy level and contain too much medical jargon (National Center for Education Statistics, 2007). Written materials can still be useful supplements for patients with low health literacy skills if the written materials selected are appropriate to the reading level of the patient. Written materials for patients with low health literacy skills should be written at or below fifth-grade reading level (Doak & Doak, 2002).

Several readability formulas are available to determine the grade level of materials (Flesch, 1948; Fry, 1968; McLaughlin, 1969). One of the easiest formulas to use is the SMOG formula, which predicts the reading grade level of materials within 1.5 grades 68% of the time (McLaughlin, 1969). The procedure for using the SMOG readability formula is outlined in **Box 13-1**, and an example of the use of the formula is provided in **Box 13-2**.

BOX 13-1 SMOG READABILITY FORMULA

1. Choose 10 consecutive sentences near the beginning, 10 consecutive sentences from the middle, and 10 consecutive sentences from the end of the material.
2. In these 30 sentences, count the number of words containing three or more syllables, including repetitions. Consider hyphenated words as one word. Proper nouns are also counted. Numerals and abbreviations should be counted as they would if the words were written out. When a colon divides words, each portion of the sentence is considered a separate sentence.
3. Estimate the square root of the number of polysyllabic words counted.
4. Add three to the square root. This gives the SMOG grading, which is the reading grade level that a person must have achieved to fully understand the material.
5. The quickest way to assess reading grade level is to use the SMOG conversion table. Simply compare the total number of words containing three or more syllables in the 30 sentences with the SMOG Conversion Table.

However, not all written patient education materials contain 30 sentences. To assess materials with fewer than 30 sentences:

1. Count all of the polysyllabic words.
2. Count the number of sentences.
3. Find the average number of polysyllabic words per sentence.
4. Multiply that average by the number of sentences short of 30.
5. Add that figure to the total number of polysyllabic words.
6. Find the square root of the number you obtained in step 5 and add the constant of three. This procedure also gives you the SMOG grading.

SMOG Conversion Table

Word Count	Grade Level
0–2	4
3–6	5
7–12	6
13–20	7
21–30	8
31–42	9
43–56	10
57–72	11
73–90	12
91–110	13
111–132	14
133–156	15
157–182	16
183–210	17
211–240	18

Source: Data are from Office of Cancer Communications, National Cancer Institute (1989).

BOX 13-2 USING THE SMOG READABILITY FORMULA (FOR MATERIALS WITH FEWER THAN 30 SENTENCES)

Check Your Weight and Heart Disease IQ

The following statements are either true or false. The statements test your knowledge of overweight and heart disease. The correct answers can be found on the back of this sheet.

1. Being overweight puts you at risk for heart disease.
2. If you are overweight, losing weight helps lower your high blood cholesterol and high blood pressure.
3. Quitting smoking is healthy, but it commonly leads to excessive weight gain, which increases your risk for heart disease.
4. An overweight person with high blood pressure should pay more attention to a low-sodium diet than to weight reduction.
5. A reduced intake of sodium or salt does not always lower high blood pressure to normal.
6. The best way to lose weight is to eat fewer calories and to exercise.
7. Skipping meals is a good way to cut down on calories.
8. Foods that are high in complex carbohydrates (starch and fiber) are good choices when you are trying to lose weight.
9. The single most important change most people can make to lose weight is to avoid sugar.
10. Polyunsaturated fat has the same number of calories as saturated fat.
11. Overweight children are very likely to become overweight adults.

Source: U.S. Department of Health and Human Services (1993).

Low health literacy can be a barrier to effective patient education, but the patient with low health literacy skills is capable of learning if the nurse is willing to invest the extra time that is required. It is important for the nurse to take extra care to present information in terms that the patient is familiar with rather than using medical jargon, to use alternate formats such as pictographs when possible, to restate information using simple words, and to verify the patient's understanding by having him or her convey the information in his or her own words. The dividends for the extra effort include the patient who is able to manage his or her own illness, make informed health decisions, and make health-related behavior changes as a result of a patient education process that has accommodated for his or her weaknesses.

■ Planning

The patient and the nurse share the planning process for patient education, but it is the responsibility of the nurse to guide the process. The nurse guides the process through the use of goals and objectives. Learning goals are derived from the learning assessment, and nursing diagnosis and objectives are developed based on goals in collaboration with the patient. The use of goals and objectives helps the nurse to focus on what is important for the patient to learn and keep patient education focused on outcomes (Rankin & Stallings, 2001).

Patient education is directed toward behavioral change. Therefore, the objectives for patient education are stated as behavioral objectives. There are three components of behavioral objectives that include performance, conditions, and criteria (Mager, 1997). Performance refers to the activity that the patient will engage in and answers this question: "What can the learner do?" The condition refers to special circumstances of the patient's performance and answers this question: "Under what conditions will the learner perform the behavior?" The criteria or evaluation component refers to how long or how well the behavior must be performed to be acceptable and answers this question: "What is the performance standard?" (Rankin & Stallings, 2001).

The learning objectives should be specific, measurable, and attainable (Rankin, 2005; Rankin & Stallings, 2001). Learning objectives are also written in a manner that is learning domain specific. Recognizing the targeted domain of learning as cognitive, psychomotor, or affective helps guide the process of writing behavioral learning objectives and thus guides the selection of learning activities.

■ Implementation

The next stage of the process involves the actual intervention. Whether the teaching will occur in a group or with an individual patient, learning activities need to be consistent with learning objectives.

Using various learning activities can make learning more fun and more effective. Some common learning activities include lectures, demonstrations, practice, games, simulations, role playing, discussions, and self-directed learning through computer-assisted instruction or self-directed workbooks.

Patient education materials are frequently used in the implementation stage of the patient education process. Patient education materials can be designed to be used alone or to supplement other types of patient education activities but should be previewed before use and used only if consistent with learning objectives. There are many types of patient education materials currently on the market, or you might opt to produce your own materials.

Patient education materials generally include audiovisual materials, computer programs, Internet resources, posters, flip charts, charts, graphs, cartoons, slides, overhead transparencies, photographs, drawings, patient education newsletters, or written patient materials such as handouts, brochures, or pamphlets. These materials, even if designed to be used alone, should not be used without some verbal instruction as to why the patient is being instructed to view the videotape or read the brochure (Falvo, 2004, 2011). Additionally, the nurse should keep the door of communication open by inviting questions that the patient might have as a result of exposure to the teaching materials.

You must evaluate a variety of factors as you look at the appropriateness of patient education materials. Three important criteria for judging patient education materials include the following (Doak, Doak, Gordon, & Lorig, 2001, p. 184):

- The material contains the information that the patient wants.
- The material contains the information that the patient needs.
- The patient understands and uses the material as presented.

It is an expectation of the Joint Commission that the right educational materials are used in patient and family education and that the materials are accurate, age specific, easily accessible, and appropriate to patient needs (The Joint Commission, 1999, 2003). To address all of these criteria, the nurse needs to conduct a needs assessment before preparing or choosing patient education materials.

Considerations: Patient Education with Older Adults

When caring for older adults, one of the primary considerations related to the patient education process is accommodation for age-related barriers to learning. The age-related barriers particularly important in the patient education process include **age-related changes** in cognition, vision, and hearing. Research has demonstrated that teaching is not as effective if it does not accommodate for age-related cognitive and sensory changes (Donlon, 1993; Masters, 2001; Weinrich, Weinrich, Boyd, Atwood, & Cervenka, 1994). Gerogogy in patient education has been defined as the transferring of essential information that has been designed, modified, and adapted to accommodate for the physiologic and psychologic changes in elderly persons by taking into account the person's disease process, age-related changes, educational level, and motivation (Pearson, 2012).

> When caring for older adults, one of the primary considerations related to the patient education process is accommodation for age-related barriers to learning.

Age-related changes in cognitive function occur slowly and are thought to begin at approximately 60 years of age in healthy adults (Miller, 2004). Age-related visual changes are the most prevalent physical impairments affecting older adults. Hearing impairment ranks as one of the four most prevalent chronic conditions affecting the older population, occurring in one-third of the U.S. population between the ages of 65 and 74 years and in 47% of the population 75 years of age and older (National Institutes of Health, 2012). Each of these age-related changes can have a profound effect on the teaching and learning process. Specific age-related changes in cognition, vision, and hearing are listed in **Box 13-3**.

Specific strategies can be used during the patient education process to help overcome the age-related learning barriers in cognition, vision, and hearing. Some of these strategies are included in **Box 13-4**.

BOX 13-3 AGE-RELATED BARRIERS TO LEARNING

Category of Age-Related Change	Cognitive and Sensory Changes
Cognitive	<ul><li>Changes in encoding and storage of information</li><li>Changes in the retrieval of information</li><li>Decreases in the speed of processing information*</li></ul>
Visual	<ul><li>Smaller amount of light reaches the retina</li><li>Reduced ability to focus on close objects</li><li>Scattering of light resulting in glare</li><li>Changes in color perception results in difficulty distinguishing colors such as dark green, blue, and violet</li><li>Decrease in depth perception and peripheral vision†</li></ul>
Hearing	Reduced ability to hear sounds as loudly<ul><li>Decrease in hearing acuity</li><li>Decrease in ability to hear high-pitched sounds</li><li>Decrease in the ability to filter background noise†</li></ul>

Sources: *Merriam & Caffarella (1999, 2007); †Miller (2004).

BOX 13-4 STRATEGIES TO ACCOMMODATE FOR AGE-RELATED BARRIERS TO LEARNING

Category of Age-Related Change	Strategies to Accommodate for Cognitive and Sensory Changes
Cognitive	<ul><li>Slow the pace of the presentation.</li><li>Give smaller amounts of information at a time.</li><li>Repeat information frequently.</li><li>Reinforce verbal teaching with audiovisuals, written materials, and practice.</li><li>Reduce distractions.</li><li>Allow more time for self-expression of learner.</li></ul>

(continues)

BOX 13-4 STRATEGIES TO ACCOMMODATE FOR AGE-RELATED BARRIERS TO LEARNING (*continued*)

Category of Age-Related Change	Strategies to Accommodate for Cognitive and Sensory Changes
	• Use analogies and examples from everyday experience to illustrate abstract information. • Increase the meaningfulness of content to the learner. • Teach mnemonic devices and imaging techniques. • Use printed materials and visual aids that are age specific*
Visual	• Make sure patient's glasses are clean and in place. • Use printed materials with 14- to 16-point font and serif letters. • Use bold type on printed materials, and do not mix fonts. • Avoid the use of dark colors with dark backgrounds for teaching materials, but instead use large, distinct configurations with high contrast to help with discrimination. • Avoid blue, green, and violet to differentiate type, illustrations, or graphics. • Use line drawings with high contrast. • Use soft white light to decrease glare. • Light should shine from behind the learner. • Use color and touch to help differentiate depth. • Position materials directly in front of the learner.†
Hearing	• Speak distinctly. • Do not shout. • Speak in a normal voice, or speak in a lower pitch. • Decrease extraneous noise. • Face the person directly while speaking at a distance of 3 to 6 feet. • Reinforce verbal teaching with visual aids or easy-to-read materials.†

Sources: *Weinrich, Boyd, & Nussbaum (1989); †Oldaker (1992) and Weinrich, Boyd, & Nussbaum (1989).

Cultural Considerations

Developing an educational program that is culturally appropriate is not much different from creating any other patient education program. You begin with a needs assessment; then, you write objectives and design the program. The difference is that you must be culturally sensitive and incorporate cultural information that you have learned about the target group into the patient education process (Bastable, 2006; Gonzalez & Lorig, 2001; Lengetti, Ordelt, & Pyle, 2007).

How important is it that you incorporate cultural information in the patient education process? Cultural awareness and sensitivity of nurses can influence the ability of patients to receive and apply information regarding their health care (Campinha-Bacole, Yahle, & Langenkamp, 1996). The way that information is communicated can influence a patient's perception of the healthcare system and affect adherence to prescribed treatments. In a recent study, patients who received care from nurses with cultural sensitivity training not only showed improvement in use of social resources but also improvement in overall functional capacity (Majumdar, Browne, Roberts, & Carpio, 2004).

In addition to the difference that it can make in relationship to patient outcomes, Joint Commission standards require not only that the patient's learning needs, abilities, and readiness to learn are assessed but also that the patient's preferences are assessed. This assessment must consider cultural and religious practices, as well as emotional and language barriers (The Joint Commission, 1999, 2003).

How do you incorporate cultural information into the patient education process? Gonzalez and Lorig (2001, p. 172) suggest the following:

- Change the information into more specific or more relevant terminology.
- Create descriptions or explanations that fit with different people's understanding of key concepts.
- Incorporate a group's cultural beliefs and practices into the program content and process.

In addition, any visual aids that are used should reflect the target group or population. The use of culturally relevant analogies can also help people to understand complex, abstract, or foreign concepts (Gonzalez & Lorig, 2001).

Evaluation

Evaluation determines worth by judging something against a standard. The standard used in the patient education process is the learning objective. Thus, the term *evaluation* as used here implies measuring the outcomes resulting from systematically planned activities implemented as a part of a patient education program or patient education process against the learning objectives to determine whether learning occurred.

Initiation of the patient education evaluation process is the responsibility of the nurse, and according to Rankin and Stallings (2001, p. 326), the evaluation process should include the following:

- Measuring the extent to which the patient has met the learning objectives
- Identifying when there is a need to clarify, correct, or review information
- Noting learning objectives that are unclear
- Pointing out shortcomings in patient teaching interventions
- Identifying barriers that prevented learning

Nurses commonly use several methods to evaluate patient learning. These methods include direct observation, the teach-back method or asking patients to explain something in their own words, situational feedback to determine if the patient selects appropriate behavior, records of health-related behaviors that patients report, patient interviews and questionnaires, and critical incidents such as readmission, emergency room visits, and mortality (McNeill, 2012).

Documentation of Patient Education

It is essential that the process of patient education be documented. Documentation functions to promote communication among members of the healthcare team, to provide a legal record, to support quality assurance efforts, to promote continuity of care, to promote reimbursement, and to meet Joint Commission standards.

Documentation of patient education should be concise, organized, and focused on patient outcomes. Documentation systems vary by setting, but the following elements of the patient education process should be included in documentation (Rankin & Stallings, 2001, p. 336):

- Initial assessments and reassessments
- Nursing diagnoses, patient needs, and priorities
- Interventions planned and interventions provided
- Patient's response and outcomes of care
- Patient and family ability to manage needs after discharge

Conclusion

This chapter provides an introduction to some of the major concepts related to the process of patient education. There is no recipe for patient education that will fit everyone, but if you mix the basic principles discussed in this chapter with some practice, you will be on your way to providing your patients with effective education.

CASE STUDY 13-1 ▪

Mr. Martin, an 82-year-old African American patient, is ready for discharge from the medical unit after a 3-day hospitalization resulting from exacerbation of heart failure. Prior to discharge from the hospital, the student nurse reviews the medication orders and provides Mr. Martin with standard patient education materials related to control of heart failure symptoms.

Case Study Questions

1. What else could the student nurse in the case study do to enhance the effectiveness of the patient education process for Mr. Martin?
2. Do you have any suggestions for the student nurse related to accommodating for age-related changes of this patient?
3. Do you have any suggestions for the student nurse related to cultural considerations as she educates this patient? ▪

Classroom Activity 1

Provide students with a copy of printed patient education materials. These can be obtained from a local healthcare organization or from online sources such as the American Heart Association. Ask students to evaluate the materials for readability using the SMOG formula in Box 13-1. Next ask students to evaluate the materials for use with older adults using the information presented in Box 13-3 and Box 13-4. Finally, have students evaluate the materials for use with a population of a different culture. Ask students to share findings during informal presentations to classmates. www

Classroom Activity 2

Divide the class into small groups and ask students to create a patient education brochure that conforms to recommended reading levels, considers age-related learning barriers, and accommodates cultural differences. The group may choose a fictitious case scenario or an actual scenario from a recent clinical experience.

For this activity, several students will need to bring laptops to class, the class will need to have access to a computer lab, or the students will need colored pencils and paper. Alternately, this activity could be assigned to students to complete outside of class to be shared with the class or submitted for a grade. www

References

American Association of Colleges of Nursing. (1998). *The essentials of baccalaureate education for professional nursing practice.* Washington, DC: Author.

American Association of Colleges of Nursing. (2008). *The essentials of baccalaureate education for professional nursing practice.* Washington, DC: Author.

American Nurses Association. (1973). *Standards of nursing practice.* Kansas City, MO: Author.

Anderson, L. W., & Krothwohi, D. R. (2001). *A taxonomy for learning, teaching and assessing: A revision of Bloom's taxonomy of educational objectives.* New York, NY: Addison-Wesley.

Baker, D. W., Parker, R. M., Williams, M. V., & Clark, W. S. (1998). Health literacy and the risk of hospital admission. *Journal of General Internal Medicine, 13,* 791–798.

Baker, D. W., Parker, R. M., Williams, M. V., Pitkin, K., Parikh, N. S., Coates, W., & Imara, M. (1996). The health care experience of patients with low literacy. *Archives of Family Medicine, 5,* 329–334.

Bandura, A. (1997). *Self-efficacy: The exercise of control.* New York, NY: W. H. Freeman.

Bastable, S. B. (2006). *Essentials of patient education.* Sudbury, MA: Jones and Bartlett.

Bloom, B. (1956). *Taxonomy of educational objectives.* New York, NY: Addison-Wesley.

Campinha-Bacole, J., Yahle, T., & Langenkamp, M. (1996). The challenge of cultural diversity for nurse educators. *Journal of Continuing Education in Nursing, 27*(2), 59–64.

Conner, M. (2004). Andragogy and pedagogy. *Ageless Learner.* Retrieved from http://www.agelesslearner.com/intros/andragogy.html

Davis, T. C., Long, S. W., Jackson, R. H., Mayeaux, E. J., George, R. B., & Murphy, P. W. (1993). Rapid estimate of adult literacy in medicine: A shortened screening instrument. *Family Medicine, 25,* 391.

Doak, C., Doak, L., Gordon, L., & Lorig, K. (2001). Selecting, preparing, and using materials. In K. Lorig (Ed.), *Patient education: A practical approach* (3rd ed., pp. 183–197). Thousand Oaks, CA: Sage.

Doak, C. C., Doak, L. G., & Root, J. H. (1996). *Teaching patients with low literacy skills.* Philadelphia, PA: Lippincott.

Doak, L. G., & Doak, C. C. (Eds.). (2002). Pfizer health literacy principles. Retrieved from http://www.pfizerhealthliteracy.com

Donlon, B. C. (1993). *The effect of practical education programming for the elderly (PEPE) on the rehospitalization rate of older congestive heart failure patients: A quasi-experimental study.* Unpublished doctoral dissertation. University of Southern Mississippi.

Falvo, D. (2004). *Effective patient education: A guide to increased compliance* (3rd ed.). Sudbury, MA: Jones and Bartlett.

Falvo, D. R. (2011). Effective patient education: A guide to increased adherence (4th ed.). Sudbury, MA: Jones & Bartlett Learning.

Flesch, R. (1948). A new readability yardstick. *Journal of Applied Psychology, 32*(3), 221–233.

Fry, E. (1968). A readability formula that saves time. *Journal of Reading, 11*, 513–577.

Gonzalez, V. M., & Lorig, K. (2001). Working cross-culturally. In K. Lorig (Ed.), *Patient education: A practical approach* (3rd ed., pp. 163–182). Thousand Oaks, CA: Sage.

Hochbaum, G. M. (1958). *Public participation in medical screening programs: A socio-psychological study*. Public Health Service Publication No. 572. Washington, DC: U.S. Government Printing Office.

Jastak, S., & Wilkinson, G. S. (1993). *Wide range achievement test: Review 3*. Wilmington, DE: Jastak Associates.

The Joint Commission. (1995). *Comprehensive accreditation manual for hospitals* (Vols. 1 and 2). Oakbrook Terrace, IL: Author.

The Joint Commission. (1999). *Hospital accreditation standards*. Oakbrook Terrace, IL: Author.

The Joint Commission. (2003). *Joint Commission guide to patient and family education*. Oakbrook Terrace, IL: Author.

Knowles, M. (1970). *The modern practice of adult education: Andragogy versus pedagogy*. New York, NY: Association Press.

Knowles, M., Swanson, R., & Holton, E. (1998). *The adult learner: The definitive classic in adult education and human resource development*. Houston, TX: Gulf.

Knowles, M., Swanson, R., & Holton, E. (2011). *The adult learner: The definitive classic in adult education and human resource development* (7th ed.). New York, NY: Elsevier.

Lengetti, E., Ordelt, K., & Pyle, N. (2007, November). Patient teaching competency for staff. *Patient Education Management*, 123–124.

Lorig, K. (2001). *Patient education: A practical approach* (3rd ed.). Thousand Oaks, CA: Sage.

Mager, R. (1997). *Preparing instructional objectives* (3rd ed.). Atlanta, GA: Center for Effective Performance.

Majumdar, B., Browne, G., Roberts, J., & Carpio, B. (2004). Effects of cultural sensitivity training on health care provider attitudes and patient outcomes. *Journal of Nursing Scholarship, 36*(2), 161–166.

Massachusetts Department of Higher Education. (2010). *Nurse of the future: Nursing core competencies*. Retrieved from http://www.mass.edu/currentinit/documents/NursingCoreCompetencies.pdf

Masters, K. (2001). *The effect of education that is modified to accommodate for age-related barriers to learning in older adult home health patients with congestive heart failure*. Unpublished doctoral dissertation. Louisiana State University Health Sciences Center.

McLaughlin, G. H. (1969). SMOG grading—a new readability formula. *Journal of Reading, 12*, 639–646.

McNeill, B. E. (2012, January–March). You "teach" but does your patient really learn?: Basic principles to promote safer outcomes. *Tar Heel Nurse*, 9–16.

Merriam, S. B., & Caffarella, R. S. (1999). *Learning in adulthood: A comprehensive guide*. San Francisco, CA: Jossey-Bass.

Merriam, S. B., & Caffarella, R. S. (2007). *Learning in adulthood: A comprehensive guide*. San Francisco, CA: Jossey-Bass.

Miller, C. A. (2004). *Nursing for wellness in older adults: Theory and practice* (4th ed.). Philadelphia, PA: Lippincott.

National Center for Education Statistics. (2007). Literacy in everyday life: Results from the 2003 National Assessment of Adult Literacy. Retrieved from http://nces.ed.gov/pubsearch/pubsinfo.asp?pubid=2007480

National Institutes of Health. (2012). NIHSeniorHealth: Hearing loss. Retrieved from http://nihseniorhealth.gov/hearingloss/hearinglossdefined/01.html

Nightingale, F. (1969). *Notes on nursing: What it is and what it is not*. New York, NY: Dover. (Original work published 1860)

Office of Cancer Communications, National Cancer Institute. (1989). *Making health communications work*. Rockville, MD: Author.

Oldaker, S. M. (1992). Live and learn: Patient education for the elderly orthopaedic client. *Orthopaedic Nursing, 11*(3), 51–56.

Pearson, M. (2012, June–August). Gerogogy in patient education—revisited. *Oklahoma Nurse*, 12–17.

Prohaska, T. R., & Lorig, K. (2001). What do we know about what works: The role of theory in patient education. In K. Lorig (Ed.), *Patient education: A practical approach* (3rd ed., pp. 163–182). Thousand Oaks, CA: Sage.

Rankin, S. H. (2005). *Patient education in health and illness*. Philadelphia, PA: Lippincott.

Rankin, S. H., & Stallings, K. D. (2001). *Patient education: Principles and practice* (4th ed.). Philadelphia, PA: Lippincott.

Redman, B. K. (2001). *The practice of patient education* (9th ed.). St. Louis, MO: Mosby.

Redman, B. K. (2003). *Measurement tools in patient education* (2nd ed.). New York, NY: Springer.

Redman, B. K. (2006). *The practice of patient education: A case study approach* (10th ed.). St. Louis, MO: Mosby.

Russell, S. S. (2006). An overview of adult-learning processes. *Urologic Nursing, 26*(5), 349–352, 370.

Stephenson, P. L. (2007). Before teaching begins: Managing patient anxiety prior to providing education. *Clinical Journal of Oncology Nursing, 10*(2), 241–246.

U.S. Department of Health and Human Services. (1993). *Check your weight and heart disease I.Q.* Publication No. 93-3034. Washington, DC: U.S. Government Printing Office.

Weinrich, S. P., Boyd, M., & Nussbaum, J. (1989). Continuing education: Adapting strategies to teach the elderly. *Journal of Gerontological Nursing, 15*(11), 17–21.

Weinrich, S. P., Weinrich, M. C., Boyd, M. D., Atwood, J., & Cervenka, B. (1994). Teaching older adults by adapting for aging changes. *Cancer Nursing, 17*(6), 494–500.

Weiss, B. D. (1999). *Twenty common problems in primary care*. New York, NY: McGraw-Hill.

Williams, M. V., Baker, D. W., Honig, E. G., Lee, T. M., & Nowlan, A. (1998). Inadequate literacy is a barrier to asthma knowledge and self-care. *Chest, 114*, 1008–1015.

Informatics and Technology in Professional Nursing Practice

14

Cathy K. Hughes

Healthcare delivery largely depends on information for effective decision making. Every nursing action relies on knowledge based on information. The nursing process begins with obtaining and communicating information in the initial and ongoing assessment. Nursing informatics (NI) is the management of data, information, knowledge, and wisdom relevant to nursing (American Nurses Association [ANA], 2008). As we enter the era of the electronic health record (EHR), NI has become an indispensable element in the practice of nursing. All nurses utilize informatics skills in their practice.

> As we enter the era of the electronic health record (EHR), NI has become an indispensable element in the practice of nursing.

Nursing Informatics Defined

Nursing informatics (NI) is together a field of study and an area of specialization. In the mid-1900s, NI was first identified as the use of information technology

Learning Objectives

After completing this chapter, the student should be able to:

1. Define nursing informatics (NI).
2. Discuss influences and direction of the future of NI practice.
3. Discuss levels of nurse informatics competencies for professional nursing practice.
4. Discuss principles to evaluate information on the Internet and websites.
5. Describe the use of electronic databases to obtain information.
6. Describe factors to consider when accessing and evaluating health information online.
7. Discuss and apply the privacy regulations of the Health Insurance Portability and Accountability Act (HIPAA) to NI.
8. Explain security and privacy issues for electronic health records.
9. Discuss social media, telehealth, and handheld devices with applications to nursing and NI.
10. Envision future trends in healthcare technology.

Key Terms and Concepts

» **Nursing informatics (NI)**
» HIPAA
» Search engines
» Databases
» EBSCO Publishing
» CINAHL
» ERIC
» Health Source
» MEDLINE
» PsycINFO
» Electronic health record
» Email
» Listservs
» Asynchronous
» Social media
» Telehealth
» PDAs

www.

KEY COMPETENCY 14-1

Examples of Applicable *Nurse of the Future: Nursing Core Competencies*

Informatics and Technology:

Knowledge (K7) Describes the rationale for involving the interdisciplinary team in the design, selection, implementation, and evaluation of applications and systems in health care

Skills (S7a) Provides input to the design, selection, and application of information technologies to support patient care

Attitudes/Behaviors (A7) Values nurses' involvement in design, selection, implementation, and evaluation of information technologies to support patient care

Source: Massachusetts Department of Higher Education (2010), p. 24.

---

in nursing practice (Hannah, 1985). In 1992, the American Nurses Association (ANA) recognized NI as a nursing specialty. The original ANA *Scope and Standards of Nursing Informatics Practice* published in 2001 was revised in 2008 and defines NI as

> a specialty that integrates nursing science, computer science, and information science to manage and communicate data, information, and knowledge in nursing practice. Nursing informatics facilitates the integration of data, information, knowledge, and wisdom to support patients, nurses, and other providers in their decision making in all roles and settings. This support is accomplished through the use of information structures, information processes, and information technology. (ANA, 2008, p. 92)

Informatics contributes to the discipline of nursing by connecting the art of nursing to the science of nursing (Saba, 2001). The specialty of NI is focused on developing and implementing solutions for the management and communication of health information pertinent to providing better quality patient/client care (Zykowski, 2003).

The definition of NI continues to evolve as technology is incorporated into health care. The updated ANA *Scope and Standards* (2008) for nursing informatics includes "redirecting the discussion on roles from job titles to functions that may be integrated into various NI roles and subspecializations" (p. 2). The roles or functions of an informatics nurse can include project manager, consultant, educator, researcher, budget manager, or distance learning developer. Instruction or management of telenursing, telehealth education, electronic health, the computerized patient record, and application of new or evolving technology are also integral roles. The informatics nurse contributes to selection, testing, and implementation of healthcare systems as well as maintenance and evaluation of the systems.

NI provides the support for information management for all of the nursing specialties. The American Nurses Association at www.nursingworld.org has a webpage focused on Health Information Technology (Health IT) Initiatives with current participation in listed initiatives and Health IT resources. The American Nursing Informatics Association website (www.ania.org) and the Alliance for Nursing Informatics website (www.allianceni.org) both offer information related to nursing in the digital world, including membership, conferences, and online resources.

Nursing Informatics: Direction for the Future

Can patient care be improved with information technology (IT)? Many forces are a part of reform of nursing education and nursing practice that include the integration of nursing informatics and health information technology for improved outcomes in healthcare delivery. Some of these are as follows:

- American Association of Colleges of Nursing BSN Essentials, www.aacn.nche.edu
- American Nurses Association (ANA) *Scope and Standards*, www.nursingworld.org
- Carnegie Foundation Report *Educating Nurses: A Call for Radical Transformation*, www.carnegiefoundation.org/elibrary/educating-nurses-highlights
- Institute of Medicine (IOM) reports
- Joint Commission, Robert Wood Johnson Foundation Initiative on the Future of Nursing at the Institute of Medicine, www.jointcommission.org/assets/1/18/RWJ_Future_of_Nursing.pdf
- National League for Nursing (NLN) Position Statements, www.nln.org
- Quality and Safety Education for Nurses (QSEN), www.qsen.org
- Robert Wood Johnson Foundation Future of Nursing Campaign for Action IOM recommendations, thefutureofnursing.org/recommendations
- Technology Informatics Guiding Education Reform (TIGER) Initiative, www.tigersummit.com

■ American Association of Colleges of Nursing

Some of the informatics and technology-related outcomes suggested by the AACN for baccalaureate nursing graduates are the following:

- Demonstrate skills in using patient care technologies, information systems, and communication devices that support safe nursing practice.
- Apply safeguards and decision-making support tools embedded in patient care technologies and information systems to support a safe practice environment for both patients and healthcare workers.
- Understand the issues of Clinical Information Systems (CIS) to document interventions related to achieving nurse-sensitive outcomes.
- Use standardized terminology in a care environment that reflects nursing's unique contribution to patient outcomes.
- Uphold ethical standards related to data security, regulatory requirements, confidentiality, and clients' right to privacy.
- Recognize that redesign of workflow and care processes should precede implementation of care technology to facilitate nursing practice (American Association of Colleges of Nursing [AACN], 2008, pp. 18–19).

■ National League for Nursing

The National League for Nursing (NLN, 2008) position paper supports the "reform of nursing education to promote quality education that prepares a workforce capable of practicing in a health care environment where technology continues to increase in amount and sophistication" (p. 2). With the charge to "prepare the next generation of nurses with the necessary informatics competencies to provide safe and quality care" (p. 2), the NLN recommends actions for faculty, administrator, members, and the NLN.

■ Quality and Safety Education for Nurses

Sponsored by the Robert Wood Johnson Foundation, Quality and Safety Education for Nurses (QSEN) has the overall goal of "preparing future nurses who will have the knowledge, skills and attitudes (KSAs) necessary to continuously improve the quality and safety of the healthcare systems within which they work" (Quality and Safety Education for Nurses [QSEN], 2012). This initiative is directed to develop competencies of future nursing graduates in six key areas including patient-centered care, evidence-based practice, quality improvement, teamwork and collaboration, safety, and informatics. Phases I and II have been completed by a distinguished team. In Phases I and II, the competencies were defined and piloted in six nursing schools to develop strategies for implementation. Some of the goals of Phase III in 2009–2012 are innovative development of methods for assessment of student learning of KSAs of the six IOM/QSEN competencies and faculty expertise development in the QSEN competencies. Five of these competencies are from the IOM competencies (IOM, 2011). The application of informatics in nursing practice will be a vital component in the mastery of the defined KSAs.

■ Technology Informatics Guiding Education Reform Initiative

With key aspects of NI the focus, hundreds of practicing nurses and nursing students volunteered their time to work in nine collaborative teams on aspects of the Technology Informatics Guiding Education Reform (TIGER) Initiative. Forty nursing professional organizations also were a part of the input process. "The teams identified resources, references, gaps, and areas that need further development, and provide recommendations for the industry to accelerate the adoption of IT for nursing" (Technology Informatics Guiding Education Reform, 2008, p. 2). Awareness raising with nursing stakeholders focused on three key areas:

- Develop a U.S. nursing workforce capable of using electronic health records to improve the delivery of health care.
- Engage more nurses in the development of a national healthcare information technology (NHIT) infrastructure.
- Accelerate adoption of smart, standards-based, interoperable technology that will make healthcare delivery safer, more efficient, timely, accessible,

and patient-centered (Technology Informatics Guiding Education Reform, 2008, pp. 3–5).

Some of the recommendations for nursing practice include the development of the minimum set of nursing informatics competencies and standards with tutorials for nurses. A priority is to address the educational needs of the existing workforce and develop education programs with learners with different levels of computer use comfort. The ultimate focus involves the development of innovative ways to use technology to improve healthcare delivery. One example is development of virtual learning platforms for nurses to explore technologies. See www.tigersummit.com for more information. With the federal mandate for the adoption of all electronic health records by 2014 (White House Archives, 2004), the overall goals of the TIGER Initiative are timely and important.

Informatics Competencies

All nurses need competencies in informatics. Defined levels of competencies vary from beginning nurse, experienced nurse, informatics specialist, to informatics innovator (Hebda & Czar, 2009; McGonigle & Mastrian, 2009; Staggers, Gassert, & Curran, 2001). The beginning nurse entering practice is expected to have computer literacy and basic information management skills. Computer literacy skills include skills in use of word processing, healthcare database and spreadsheet applications, presentation software, and email. Information literacy skills enable a nurse to locate, access, and evaluate clinical data. Access includes the ability to perform bibliographic retrievals using the Internet and library-based resources (McNeil et al., 2003).

Important technology skills of the entry-level nurse include knowing how to use nursing-specific software such as computerized documentation; use of patient care technologies such as monitors, pumps, and medication dispensing; and information management for patient safety (AACN, 2008, pp. 19–20). The constructs of implementing and maintaining health policies focus on privacy, security, and confidentiality of client information such as mandated by the Health Information Privacy and Portability Act (**HIPAA**) and influence of all facets of NI.

Experienced nurses should be skilled in information management and computer technology to sustain their specific area of practice. These skills include making judgments based on trends of data in addition to collaboration with informatics nurses (IN) in the development of nursing systems.

An informatics nurse specialist (INS) has advanced informatics preparation at the graduate level and assists the practicing nurse in meeting his or her needs for information (ANA, 2008). The informatics innovator also has advanced informatics preparation and possesses skills for conducting informatics research along with theory development (Thede, 2003). Certification for NI became available in 1995 through the American Nurses Credentialing Center (2007). Information on eligibility and test content is available at www.nursecredentialing.org/Certification/NurseSpecialties/Informatics.aspx.

Internet Resources

Not since the invention of the printing press has the speed with which new information can be obtained changed so much as with the development of the Web. Search tools and **search engines** assist users in finding specific topics on the Web by compiling a database of Internet sites. Popular search engines are AltaVista, InfoSeek, WebCrawler, Yahoo, Northernlight, and Hotbot. All have different search features and produce somewhat differing results. In addition to search engines, there are metasearch engines. A metasearch engine conducts a search of a variety of search engines. Metacrawler (www.metacrawler.com), Google (www.google.com), and Dogpile (www.dogpile.com) are examples of metasearch engines. Each search engine queries different databases using different search techniques (Bliss & DeYoung, 2002) and uses a range of engines for retrieval of information. Although a popular web source, Wikipedia.com is not considered an acceptable source for nursing reference.

www CRITICAL THINKING QUESTION

How can you locate online sources for more information on a new treatment or medication for a health condition you discussed in a nursing class or clinical this week?

Website Evaluation

The Web has grown rapidly since its beginning, and information can be published easily and inexpensively. An Internet site can be created by anyone with the ability to create a webpage. Many sites are for commercial purposes, and others simply publish the opinions of the website owner. Websites are under no guidelines or standards. Additionally, no official organization is responsible for site evaluation. As a result, a vast amount of information is available on the Web, but not all information is reliable.

www CRITICAL THINKING QUESTION

What is your role as a nurse in the evaluation of information on the Internet?

Applying these guidelines can assist you in evaluating a resource on the Web (Thede, 2003; Thede & Sewell, 2010) and acquiring reliable information from the Web:

- Accuracy: Is the information accurate, reliable, and free from error? Spelling and punctuation errors can indicate an untrustworthy site.
- Authority or source: Look for the credentials of the author or the reputation of the hosting organization. A good indication of authority is peer review.

- Objectivity: What are the goals and objectives of the site? What biases are present? Is the site trying to present a specific or neutral point of view?
- Currency or timeliness: Look for publication and updated dates to determine if the information is current. Dead links can indicate old information.
- Coverage or quality: Is the subject matter presented on the site of appropriate quality for the intended audience?
- Intended purpose: Does the site have choices for users such as the public, healthcare providers, students, or educators (Hebda & Czar, 2009; Thede, 2003)?
- Usability: Is the site designed for easy navigation? Are there excessive graphics that require long download times? Are all links current and do they load easily?

Some websites that feature webinars and online programs have closed captioning (CC) and copies of the scripts available on demand for these programs. Language options are available on some websites for print and audible programs. If the website is a health resource, privacy considerations with easily understandable statements and meeting of accepted privacy standards should also be evaluated (Thede & Sewell, 2010). Nurses can consider assisting clients by educating them on how to evaluate web-based information.

In addition, site users can gain insight into domain ownership to verify the domain registration. Is the authorship or sponsor identified? One domain registration verification source is easywhois.com.

Electronic Databases

An increasing number of **databases** are available on the Internet and can be accessed through local libraries or by subscription from a vendor such as **EBSCO Publishing**, which provides access to online databases and e-journals. Most of the databases allow keyword searches and are capable of limited or advanced searching as well as limited to full text. Some of the most beneficial databases to nursing include the following:

- **CINAHL** (Cumulative Index of Nursing and Allied Health Literature) is the authoritative resource for nursing and allied health professionals, students, educators, and researchers. This database provides indexing and abstracting for more than 1,700 current nursing and allied health journals and publications dating back to 1982, totaling more than 880,000 records.
- Cochrane Library is an online collection of six databases with "independent high-quality evidence for healthcare decision making" (The Cochrane Collaboration, 2012). This is available at academic institutions and is also funded for free access in many countries and regions of the world.

- **ERIC**, the Educational Resource Information Center, is a national information system supported by the U.S. Department of Education, the National Library of Education, and the Office of Educational Research and Improvement. It provides access to information from journals included in the Current Index of Journals in Education and Resources in Education Index. ERIC provides full text of more than 2,200 digests along with references for additional information and citations and abstracts from more than 1,000 educational and education-related journals.

- Google Scholar (googlescholar.com), launched in 2004, contains some full-text peer-reviewed journals, abstracts, links to subscription journals, and articles for purchase as well as technical reports, theses, and books.
- **Health Source**, the Nursing/Academic Edition, provides more than 550 scholarly full-text journals, including more than 450 peer-reviewed journals focusing on many medical disciplines, including nursing and allied health.
- **MEDLINE**, created by the National Library of Medicine, is the largest biomedical literature database that provides authoritative medical information on medicine, nursing, dentistry, veterinary medicine, the health-care system, and preclinical sciences. In MEDLINE, users can search abstracts from more than 4,600 current biomedical journals. Included are citations from Index Medicus, International Nursing Index, Index to Dental Literature, PREMEDLINE, AIDSLINE, BIOETHICSLINE, and HealthSTAR.
- **PsycINFO** contains nearly 2 million citations and summaries of journal articles, book chapters, books, dissertations, and technical reports, all in the field of psychology. It also includes information about the psychological aspects of related disciplines such as medicine, psychiatry, nursing, sociology, education, pharmacology, physiology, linguistics, anthropology, business, and law.

Web access to government organizations and nonprofit organizations is also available. The U.S. National Library of Medicine (www.nlm.nih.gov/hinfo.html) offers a wealth of health information websites. PubMed and MedlinePlus permit searches of multiple retrieval systems and provide excellent information. The evaluation guidelines discussed earlier should be applied to all Internet sites before using the information in patient teaching (Thede, 2003; Thede & Sewell, 2010).

Health Information Online

The number of people accessing health information online continues to grow. This increase in numbers demonstrates the critical importance that healthcare websites provide reliable and credible information. Nurses are responsible for assisting the public in evaluating health information available on the Web. Additionally, nurses are in the ideal position to provide health promotion education to their patients and to the public at large.

Whether nurses are developing online materials or using existing online information, it is important for them to understand what makes the information accessible to all people (Thede, 2003) and to be able to make informed recommendations about websites to individuals with disabilities (Carmona, 2005; Smeltzer, Simmerman, Frain, DeSiltes, & Duffin, 2003). Contents of sites should be presented in a way that people with disabilities and with low-end technology are able to navigate and use. Websites displaying the "Bobby Approved" icon (www.accessible.org/bobby-approved.html) have been screened for accessibility by individuals with disabilities, and the icon is an indication of the site's appropriateness for patient use.

Vulnerable populations and underserved populations, which include persons with lower socioeconomic status, with lower reading levels, in rural areas, or with disabilities, have issues with access to care and access to information about health care. For persons in these populations, the term *digital divide* has typically been used to describe decreased access to information technologies, particularly the via the Internet (Chang et al., 2004, p. 449).

> **www CRITICAL THINKING QUESTION ✳**
>
> Discuss issues of the digital divide. Explore resources in your city and county for the general public to have free Internet access and assistance. What other technology-type resources are available for underserved populations? ✳

As the Internet continues to gain in popularity, more people are using the Web for finding health information. Web-knowledgeable nurses need to assist patients and their families in evaluating the quality of Web resources. The Health on the Net Foundation (HON), founded in 1995, is a nonprofit organization dedicated to assisting people in obtaining reliable health information on the Web. The HON Code of Conduct (HONcode) is available at www.hon.ch/HONcode/Conduct.html (Health on the Net Foundation, 2009). To obtain certification, a website applies for registration. The site is evaluated and, if approved, qualifies to display the HONcode seal. The site is randomly checked for compliance. From the HON website, the HON toolbar can be downloaded and added to your Web browser. The seal is illuminated when a certified site is accessed.

Another organization that can be used as a resource is the Hardin MD (Hardin Meta Directory) at www.lib.uiowa.edu/hardin/md. The site is maintained by Hardin Library for the Health Sciences at the University of Iowa and lists several directors for health and medicine. MedlinePlus (available at www.nlm.nih.gov/medlineplus) is a consumer-oriented site that combines information from the National Library of Medicine (NLM), the National Institutes of Health (NIH), and other government agencies and health-related organizations. The site is maintained by the National Library of Medicine.

Several sites with the Office of the National Coordinator for Health Information Technology (ONC, 2011a) of HIT such as HealthIT.gov at www.healthit.gov/patients-families/types-e-health-tools have information on e-health tools for the public to review and use. Sites such as Health 2.0 Developer Challenge (2012) at www.health2con.com/devchallenge hold innovation competitions and community action programs to address solutions for key challenges in health information technology.

Confidentiality, Security, and Privacy of Healthcare Information

Protecting an individual's personal and private information from others has historically been a significant issue for nursing. Healthcare information is a collection of data relating to acutely personal aspects of an individual's life. Improper disclosure can cause devastating consequences. Many people depend on the understanding that information provided to a healthcare provider will not be disclosed. It is possible for patients not to disclose certain types of information essential to their care if they believe the information would not continue to be confidential. The introduction of electronic documentation and communication has increased the difficulty of maintaining privacy. Improved access to healthcare information can and does increase efficiency and improve patient care, but accompanying the benefits are greater difficulties in maintaining privacy and confidentiality. Preserving security of the information system becomes critical because unauthorized access to the computerized healthcare information system compromises the privacy and confidentiality of personal records.

Protection against unauthorized access can be achieved by implementing a login process that verifies that the user has permission to use the system. The majority of systems rely on a user ID and password for verification. Passwords must be changed frequently to protect against breach of security. Users should never divulge or share passwords. Healthcare agencies have written policies regarding the penalties of misuse of the system. Consequences are usually severe and can result in termination of the employee (Thede, 2003).

▪ Health Insurance Portability and Accountability Act

In 1996, Congress passed the Health Insurance Portability and Accountability Act (HIPAA) to improve the efficiency and effectiveness of the healthcare system by encouraging the development of a health information system. Several areas are addressed by the act, including simplifying healthcare claims, developing standards for data transmission, and implementing privacy regulations. The privacy regulations protect clients by limiting the ways that health plans, pharmacies, hospitals, and other entities can use clients' personal medical information. The regulations protect medical records and other individually identifiable health information, whether it is communicated orally, on paper, or electronically.

Accompanying the privacy regulations are specific security rules that protect health information in electronic form. To be in compliance, agencies must ensure the confidentiality and integrity of all electronic health information that is created, received, transmitted, or stored; protect against threats to security; protect against disclosures of information; and ensure compliance of its employees (Garner, 2003). HIPAA, when fully implemented, will contribute to a "fully integrated healthcare system" (Thede, 2003, p. 327).

> **www. CRITICAL THINKING QUESTION** *
>
> What is your role as a nurse in protecting patient healthcare information? *

Electronic Health Records

In 2004, President George Bush, as part of the National Health Information Infrastructure, established a technology agenda authorizing the development of an **electronic health record** for all Americans by 2014 (Healthcare IT, 2004). Information on this agenda can be found at the U.S. Department of Health and Human Services website: georgewbush-whitehouse.archives.gov/news/releases/2004/05/print/20040527-2.html.

Electronic information systems contribute to more effective communication and collection of patient information, resulting in more effective patient care (Thede, 2003). The electronic information system can maximize the time nurses spend on direct patient care, improve the accuracy of documentation, decrease medication errors, and promote patient safety. Why automate nursing and healthcare documentation? Up-to-date, accurate information of each step of the nursing process is the power behind safe, high-quality patient-centered care.

"The goal of nursing informatics (NI) is to improve the health of populations, communities, families, and individuals by optimizing information management and communication" (ANA, 2001, p. 17). Information management is integral to providing high-quality health care cost-effectively. To provide this level of care, it is important to have accurate clinical information. The health information system or electronic health record (EHR) represents multiple systems that interface to share data and are networked to support information management and communication within a healthcare organization.

EHRs have numerous advantages compared with traditional paper records. They can store large amounts of data that are accessible from remote sites by many people at the same time. Information can be accessed more easily and quickly, allowing more time for patient care. The EHR can provide clinical alerts and reminders, identify abnormal parameters of laboratory and assessment data, and prompt clinicians on important tasks and protocols (Hebda & Czar, 2009; Young, 2000).

> **KEY COMPETENCY 14-4**
>
> Examples of Applicable *Nurse of the Future: Nursing Core Competencies*
>
> Informatics and Technology:
>
> Knowledge (K6) Describes patients' rights as they pertain to computerized information management
>
> Skills (S6ba) Discusses the principles of data integrity, professional ethics, and legal requirements; (S6c) Describes ways to protect data
>
> Attitudes/Behaviors (A6) Values the privacy and confidentiality of protected health information in electronic health records
>
> *Source:* Massachusetts Department of Higher Education (2010), p. 24.

Thede (2003) identifies the following types of information systems used within healthcare organizations:

- Admission, discharge, and transfer: This system collects and tracks patient information, such as demographics, hospital number, relatives, and primary physician. All patient contacts are connected to the information in this system.
- Financial systems: This system is responsible for the fiscal operations of an organization.
- Order entry: From a computer screen, a clinician places an order for a specific service. The system is capable of scheduling, reporting, and billing. The system might have the potential of programmed patient safety functions that identify and report potential errors.
- Ancillary systems: Ancillary applications permit sharing of information among multiple systems and specialty areas such as those of radiology, laboratory, physical therapy, and pharmacy.
- Clinical documentation: This system enables the EHR, or chart, to be accessed at any time.
- Scheduling applications are used for staff, patients, supplies, and procedures.
- Acuity applications attempt to predict the resources necessary for patient care. They are integrated with other systems such as staffing to create adequate staffing.
- Specialty systems are found in specialized units within the healthcare setting. Examples include monitoring equipment in intensive care units that automatically measure and record physiologic data, generate trends, sound alarms for abnormalities, and interact with other information systems within the patient environment.
- Communication systems such as email and Internet accessibility facilitate communication among various disciplines within the organization.
- Critical pathways, generated by information systems, identify specific patient outcomes and make documentation by different disciplines possible. This promotes cost-effective care through effective communication.

Thede (2012) reports a "cardinal rule in informatics is one entry of a piece of data, many uses" (p. 2). As data are entered into the system, the application can prompt the clinician for additional information that might be missed. The same data can be used in a variety of reports, leading to decreased redundancy of charting. Data such as pulse rate or blood pressure can be collected directly from monitors attached to the client and fed into the system (Hunter, 2002). Clinical documentation systems have the advantage of collecting data to use in planning and research.

Sensmeier (2008) offers ways to improve nursing practice with technology, including seeking nursing input related to workflow, investing in IT training, promoting IT excellence, and working for a staged approach to adopting a paperless EHR. Thede (2008) suggests that nursing professionals must engage in discussion to decide how documentation data will be utilized. The profession must consider which data are to be included in the EHR and the acceptable terminology used when recording the data. Nursing informatics provides the tools and skills to assist health care to move ahead in the ever-changing world.

Communication Online

■ Email

Email (electronic mail) can be sent to anyone in the world who has an email address. This allows many healthcare providers to be able to communicate with patients. In moments, messages can be sent across time zones, allowing instant communication. For several reasons, attention must be paid to the content of messages sent by email. Someone other than the intended recipient can access a message while it is transmitted over the Internet. Also, messages containing sensitive information can accidentally or purposefully be forwarded. Protected health information (PHI) is covered under HIPAA. Privacy of email is a legal and ethical issue (Thede, 2003). Although email can be a way of facilitating direct communication between consumers of health care and healthcare providers, precautions must be taken to ensure that only the intended recipient receives health-related email messages.

To send and receive email, a person must have an individual address that consists of two main parts separated by an at (@) sign. The first part is called a login name or a user ID. The part after the @ is the name of the computer used to access the Internet. The characters after the last dot in an email address indicate the domain or main subdivision of the Internet to which the computer belongs. Addresses must be accurate for the message to be sent. Appropriateness of address must be considered when selecting your login name. Professionals should not use suggestive or insensitive wording for their login names.

Email is a special form of communication and carries its own form of etiquette. Pagana (2007) suggests nurses follow these guidelines when sending a business or professional message:

- Don't use all uppercase letters. Typing in all caps is deemed shouting.
- Include a specific subject line.
- Sign your messages with text that includes your email address and contact information.
- Use the "reply to all" function appropriately because not everyone is interested in receiving your comments.
- Avoid forwarding chain letters, and delete all unnecessary information from forwarded messages.

KEY COMPETENCY 14-5

Examples of Applicable *Nurse of the Future: Nursing Core Competencies*

Informatics and Technology:

Knowledge (K5) Describes the computerized systems presently utilized to facilitate patient care

Skills (S5a) Applies technology and information management tools to support safe processes of care and evaluate impact on patient outcomes; (S5b) Accesses, enters, retrieves data used locally for patient care

Attitudes/Behaviors (A5) Values the importance of technology on patient care

Source: Massachusetts Department of Higher Education (2010), p. 23.

- Do not send confidential information, and check for correct recipients before sending.
- Use the spell-check and grammar functions.
- Do not use email for thank-you correspondence.

Listserv Groups and Mailing Lists

Mailing lists and **listservs** are forms of group email that provide an opportunity for people with similar interests to share information. Subscribing to a list is usually free. Once subscribed, you can send and receive messages to and from the list. The communication is **asynchronous**, meaning it does not occur in real time. Someone posts a question or comment to the list, and other members reply in time. List groups are usually layperson oriented or professional oriented. There are numerous groups devoted to the topic of nursing. To find a list, ask friends and colleagues or visit L-Soft, a searchable database that can be accessed at www.lsoft.com/catalist.html.

Most listservs provide specific instructions on subscribing. Every listserv has two addresses. One address is used to join, and the second is used to send messages that can be read by the group. Listserv groups can be open to anyone, or you might have to have permission to join.

It is important to remember that messages sent to the listserv are read by everyone subscribed to that listserv. Posting a personal message to an individual on a listserv is generally not considered appropriate. Do not send attachments to the list. The list might have hundreds of members, and some will not have computers that support sophisticated graphics or large files. Additionally, viruses can be transmitted in attachments.

The ability for multiple people to send and receive messages in multiple places is having a direct impact on health care. For example, through the use of email, nurses can easily and efficiently facilitate a virtual support group for families and patients with chronic conditions or limitations in accessing health care. The lists connect the participants to individuals with similar health concerns so that they can share experiences, receive advice on difficulties, and alleviate the feeling of isolation (Mendelson, 2003).

Social Media

Social media are "Internet-based applications that enable people to communicate and share resources and information" (Lindsay, 2011). Examples of social media are YouTube, Facebook, LinkedIn, and Twitter, as well as blogs, wikis, and chat rooms. The many choices of how users can "share" information can be found on the American Nurses Association website (www.nursingworld.com). The drop-down menu on the Share button lists the various options available for users.

Growing participation in social networking sites poses challenges for nursing. Although social networking aids with personal and professional knowledge exchange and prompts interaction with others, it comes with risks. Personal and patient privacy issues (i.e., HIPAA requirements) can be raised. Some networking discussions might be viewed as "fact" and not validated. ANA has adopted the Principles for Social Networking, which include the following:

- Nurses must not transmit or place online individually identifiable patient information.
- Nurses must observe ethically prescribed professional patient–nurse boundaries.
- Nurses should understand that patients, colleagues, institutions, and employers might view postings.
- Nurses should take advantage of privacy settings and seek to separate personal and professional information online.
- Nurses should bring content that could harm a patient's privacy, rights, or welfare to the attention of appropriate authorities.
- Nurses should participate in developing institutional policies governing online contact (ANA, 2011a, 2011b).

The National Council of State Boards of Nursing has also adopted guidelines related to the responsible use of social media and has endorsed the principles adopted by ANA. The guidelines from the NCSBN (National Council of State Boards of Nursing [NCSBN], 2011) are available at www.ncsbn.org/Social_Media.pdf and address issues of confidentiality and privacy, common myths and misunderstandings related to social media, possible consequences in the use of social media including consequences with board of nursing implications, and how to avoid problems. The guidelines also include seven scenarios related to social media use by nurses with board of nursing implications.

According to the NCSBN (2011) white paper, depending on the jurisdiction, the board of nursing might investigate reports of inappropriate disclosures related to the use of social media on the grounds of the following: unprofessional conduct, unethical conduct, moral turpitude, mismanagement of patient records, revealing a privileged communication, and breach of confidentiality. If allegations are found to be true, the nurse could face disciplinary action by the board of nursing that can include a reprimand, sanction, assessment of a fine, or the temporary or permanent loss of licensure. In addition, improper use of social media might violate state and federal laws, resulting in civil or criminal penalties that carry with them fines or jail time.

Social networking can have both positive and negative consequences. Negative consequences can affect not only nurses' personal reputations but also their professional standing. Nurses should consider that current or future employers might view their personal social media pages.

KEY COMPETENCY 14-6

Examples of Applicable *Nurse of the Future: Nursing Core Competencies*

Informatics and Technology:

Skills (S6b) Maintains privacy and confidentiality of patient information

Source: Massachusetts Department of Higher Education (2010), p. 24.

On the other hand, social media can be used in disasters as a means of disseminating information and as an emergency management tool. Social media can be a source of information in a crisis situation as well as part of a plan to mobilize responders. In disaster preparation, social media sites can be used to publicize training events and dates (Lindsay, 2011).

Future challenges of social media include the use of the technology for the delivery of accurate and pertinent information by experts and healthcare providers and by peers and the lay public. Healthcare provider's uses of social media technology may include public education related to sources of information and monitoring the impact of social media on health outcomes.

www **CRITICAL THINKING QUESTIONS** *

What needs of populations in your region or state could be addressed by telehealth? What ideas can you envision to assist in the access to and delivery of healthcare services where you live or work? *

Telehealth

Telehealth is defined as "using electronic communication for transmitting healthcare information such as health promotion, disease prevention, professional or lay education, diagnosis, or actual treatments to people located at different geographical locations" (Thede, 2003, p. 129). Hardware and software such as personal digital assistants, pagers, cellular phones, laptop computers, and mobile hardware peripherals are being used by clinicians in increasing numbers. Healthcare providers can monitor and send messages to patients in their homes regarding changes in health status. Information and images can be communicated digitally for consultation with other healthcare providers. This form of healthcare promises to provide many solutions for patient care in the future (Newbold, 2003).

Almost a decade ago, Nelson (2003) proposed the following ideas for the future of health care: The traditional office visit will be replaced with the virtual appointment through the use of videophones and monitoring equipment. Shopping malls will have ambulatory surgery centers and health booths providing access to healthcare providers. Treatment information obtained by email will be common practice for patients and caregivers. Online communities and support groups will assist patients in self-care and disease management. Patients will be able to download personal physiologic data from any site. Wearable technology will monitor, detect, and send data wirelessly to healthcare facilities. It will be possible to predict disease as a result of technology installed in the home or worn on the person. Think of how many of these predictions today are a part of the everyday healthcare environment:

- Home health, hospice, and primary care NPs in the home setting use tablets or notebook computers to document and communicate information to main or branch offices. Supplies can be ordered online immediately following the visit.

- Computers on Wheels (COWs) are used in clinical settings for point-of-use documentation.
- Webcams in computers are used for two-way communication with patients in home settings.
- For pay home alert services are available to aid with safety in the home setting.
- Practitioners in remote areas can connect to large hospital emergency department staff or referral content experts for consultations and second opinions.
- From a motor vehicle crash site, the emergency medical system (EMS) response field team can transmit information and documentation to the emergency department for care direction and in preparation for arrival.
- Mobile disaster response units dispatched at the site of a disaster can bring computer-based registration and tracking systems and an information reference database. This disaster response system can include a two-way linkup with consultation applications to discuss specific patient needs with other HCPs at another site.
- Patients with home use of continuous positive airway pressure (CPAP) machines can bring in the unit's memory file to the HCP for review of effectiveness of the intervention of sleep apnea episodes since the last visit.
- The monitoring of maternal preterm contractions has advanced in the home setting.
- The use of interactive conferencing by interdisciplinary health professional teams is expanding.
- Patients can maintain and carry a personal copy of their personal health records (PHRs) on a flash drive.

Patient privacy is protected by HIPAA regulations, and variances in state regulations also exist. Considerations for the future include discussion of HIPAA privacy protection if the patient's primary care location and the telehealth practitioner are in different states.

Handheld Devices

Personal digital assistants (**PDAs**) are handheld devices that have wireless connectivity and can synchronize data and information between the PDA and a computer. Use of the PDA is becoming widely popular in health care and nursing. The devices can be used as a digital reference for obtaining drug information, dosage calculations, and diagnostic test results, as well as decision protocols for administration. They are useful tools for data collection and management of patient outcomes. PDAs can be interfaced with the electronic medical record to obtain and update vital patient information. Immediate access to the Internet allows the healthcare provider to obtain valuable information through national and international resources.

HIPAA regulations must be strictly followed when using PDAs and other wireless technology (Thompson, 2005). The use of PDAs in the clinical setting must be compliant with HIPAA rules and regulations. Faculty and nursing students must be advised and taught about security and storage of patient information (Mastrian, McGonigle, Mahan, & Bixler, 2011).

Hybrid devices have a combination of capabilities, such as a cell phone that is also an Internet-enabled PDA with an MP3 player and camera that includes text messaging capabilities, maps and directions assistance, and interactive voice assistance. Available options can vary with different service plans, coverage areas, and memory size. Upon employment and when there are any corporate policy changes, nurses must review the healthcare facility policies on the use of handheld devices while at work.

Present and Future Trends

Beginning in 2012, an initiative of the Centers for Medicare & Medicaid Services (CMS), the Hospital Value-Based Purchasing (VBP) Program, affected performance and quality of care in determining how much the hospital is paid for services. Many specific measures of patient care by nurses will need to be reported. Some process measures include discharge instructions, serum glucose levels for postoperative cardiac patients, and several other specific measures for the patient undergoing surgery. Some measures of patient experiences of care have benchmarks for communication with nurses, communication about medicines, responsiveness of the hospital staff, and discharge information (CMS, 2012). Education, surveillance, reporting, and communication of VBP measures for the nursing and hospital staff will be a priority role for informatics nurses.

> **www CRITICAL THINKING QUESTIONS** ✳
>
> What is your nursing role in early detection, reporting, and surveillance of emerging threats in your geographical area? What sources are available and how current are they? ✳

The Office of the National Coordinator for Health Information Technology (ONC) at www.HealthIT.gov is a source of information for healthcare providers, patients and families, as well as policy researchers (Murphy, 2011; ONC, 2011a). The Medicare and Medicaid EHR Incentive Programs have the focus of the "meaningful use" of certified EHR technology in achieving health goals. Financial incentives are attached to these goals. There are five patient-driven domains: to "improve quality, safety, efficiency; engage patients & families; improve care coordination; improve public and population health; ensure privacy and security for personal health information" (ONC, 2011b). Fifteen core objectives are described and linked to the domains. Resources about questions to explore and measures are linked for each objective. The use of HIT presently and in the future will be vital in evolving healthcare programs and delivery systems. It is essential to have a qualified workforce to meet the demands of these programs.

Clearly, computerized technology will shape the future of health care. Recognizing this fact, the former Healthy People 2010 objectives (U.S. Department of Health and Human Services [DHHS], 2000) call for increasing the number of households with access to the Internet. Health communication and health information technology is noted as objectives of Healthy People 2020 with the goal to improve healthcare quality and safety (U.S. DHHS, 2012). Many healthcare organizations and public service agencies use the Internet as the main avenue for information delivery. Thus, having access to the Internet will be essential to acquiring health information and services. Changes in delivery of patient care are common in clinical facilities in many areas of the country. Nurses and healthcare providers have become accustomed to computerized order entry for medical directives and point-of-care technology for patient care, automated medication dispensing, physiologic monitoring systems, and "smart" infusion pump delivery systems (Saba & McCormick, 2006).

Advances in technology might make vaccines for cancer and medications to prevent vascular disease available someday. New organs and body parts that correct or improve function might be commonly accessible. It is conceivable that bloodless surgery will be performed and drugs without side effects will be developed. Computer programs and clinical simulators will be used universally for practice in health education. Robotics will perform nursing support services for patient care through providing medication administration and physiologic monitoring.

Informatics technologies will have roles in protection and response for bioterrorism and national security. These capabilities will include emergency response systems, health alert networks, automated access to governmental support networks, and enlistment of workforce solutions. Informatics nurses will be called upon to establish, implement, and evaluate these initiatives.

> **www] CRITICAL THINKING QUESTIONS** ∗
>
> Explore online sources and discuss: What services utilizing robotics are available in a 1-hour radius from your home? Which populations can benefit from these services? How many persons by age groups potentially could need these services in the next 10 years? ∗

In the future, work must be done to refine and implement standardized nursing terminologies (SNTs) that better express nursing care. As SNTs become unique to nursing, some benefits include better communication, improved patient care, and uniform style for nursing data collection to aid in evaluation of nursing care outcomes (Thede & Schwiran, 2011).

Conclusion

Nursing informatics provides the solution to many of the challenges that health care is facing—from easing the strain of the nursing shortage to improving patient safety. "Between the health care we have and the care we could have lies not just a gap, but a chasm" was reported in the IOM (2001) landmark report. Nurses must embrace technology and integrate it into their nursing practice. Technology will not go away. It will continue to transform healthcare delivery systems. Because of technology, individuals and groups communicate in new ways, the methods with which we teach and learn have changed, and the way health care is delivered and acquired has changed. Nursing must continue to take a leadership role in the incorporation of technology in health care. Nursing informatics will provide the tools and skills to assist health care to move ahead in the ever-changing world. The baccalaureate-prepared nurse should continue to strive to explore and practice the constructs of NI competencies to improve population health outcomes and healthcare quality.

> **Nursing informatics provides the solution to many of the challenges that health care is facing—from easing the strain of the nursing shortage to improving patient safety.**

Classroom Activity 1

Explore key words a nurse would use to locate more information about aspects of a health issue topic or a population of interest of your choice. Report what single or combination of key words yielded the best results for your topic or population.

Classroom Activity 2

Explore possible Web sources to locate support groups available for individuals needing services in your area, county or parish region, and state.

Classroom Activity 3

Locate two consumer-focused listservs that you can suggest as resources for the healthcare consumer.

Classroom Activity 4

On the Internet locate a support group for a specific need that is available for individuals in your area or state.

Classroom Activity 5

View the NCSBN Social Media Guidelines video that is available at www.ncsbn.org/2930.htm

References

American Association of Colleges of Nursing. (2008, October 20). *The essentials of baccalaureate education for professional nursing practice.* Retrieved from http://www.aacn.nche.edu/education-resources/BaccEssentials08.pdf

American Nurses Association. (2001). *Scope and standards of nursing informatics practice.* Washington, DC: Author.

American Nurses Association. (2008). *Nursing informatics: Scope and standards of practice.* Washington, DC: Author.

American Nurses Association. (2011a). *Fact sheet. Navigating the world of social media.* Silver Springs, MD: Author.

American Nurses Association. (2011b). *6 tips for nurses using social media.* Silver Springs, MD: Author.

American Nurses Credentialing Center. (2007). Informatics nurse certification exam. Retrieved from www.nursecredentialing.org/Certification/NurseSpecialties/Informatics.aspx

Bliss, J. B., & DeYoung, S. (2002). *Working the Web: A guide for nurses.* Upper Saddle River, NJ: Prentice Hall.

Carmona, R. H. (2005, July 26). A call to caring: Remarks at press conference to launch. *The Surgeon General's Call to Action to Improve the Health and Wellness of Persons with Disabilities.* Retrieved from http://www.surgeongeneral.gov/news/speeches/07262005.html

Centers for Medicare & Medicaid. (2012). Hospital value-based purchasing. Retrieved from http://www.cms.gov/Medicare/Quality-Initiatives-Patient-Assessment-Instruments/hospital-value-based-purchasing/index.html?redirect=/Hospital-Value-Based-Purchasing/

Chang, B. L., Bakken, S., Brown, S. S., Houston, T. K., Kreps, G. L., Kukafka, R., ... Stavri, P. Z. (2004). Bridging the digital divide: Reaching vulnerable populations. *Journal of the American Medical Informatics Association, 11*(6), 448–457.

Garner, J. C. (2003). Final HIPAA security regulations: A review. *Managed Care Quarterly, 3*(11), 15–27.

Hannah, K. (1985). Current trends in nursing informatics: Implications for curriculum planning. In K. Hannah, E. J. Builenmin, & D. N. Corkin (Eds.), *Nursing uses of computer and information science*. Amsterdam, Netherlands: North-Holland.

Health on the Net Foundation. (2009). HON code of conduct. Retrieved from http://www.hon.ch/HONcode/Pro/intro.html

Health 2.0 Developer Challenge. (2012). Developer challenge. Retrieved from http://www.health2con/devchallenge/

Healthcare IT. (2004). President Bush continues HER push, sets national goals. Retrieved from http://www.healthcareitnews.com/news/president-bush-continues-ehr-push-sets-national-goals

Hebda, T., & Czar, P. (2009). *Handbook of informatics for nurses and healthcare professionals* (4th ed.). Upper Saddle River, NJ: Pearson Prentice Hall.

Hunter, K. M. (2002). Electronic health records. In S. Englebardt & R. Nelson (Eds.), *Health care informatics: An interdisciplinary approach* (pp. 209–230). St. Louis, MO: Mosby.

Institute of Medicine. (2001). *Crossing the quality chasm: A new health system for the 21st century*. Retrieved from http://www.nap.edu/catalog/10027.html

Institute of Medicine. (2011). *Future of nursing: Leading change, advancing health*. Washington, DC: National Academies Press. Retrieved from http://www.nap.edu/catalog.php?record_id=12956

Lindsay, R. (2011). *Social media and disasters: Current uses, and future options, and policy considerations*. Congressional Research Service, 7-5700. CRS Report R41987. Retrieved from www.crs.gov

Massachusetts Department of Higher Education. (2010). *Nurse of the future: Nursing core competencies*. Retrieved from http://www.mass.edu/currentinit/documents/NursingCoreCompetencies.pdf

Mastrian, K.G., McGonigle, D., Mahan, W. L., & Bixler, B. (2011). *Integrating technology in nursing education. Tools for the knowledge era*. Sudbury, MA: Jones & Bartlett Learning.

McGonigle, D., & Mastrian, K. (2009). Nursing informatics and the foundation of knowledge. Sudbury, MA: Jones and Bartlett.

McNeil, B. J., Elfrink, V. L., Bickford, C. J., Pierce, S. T., Beyea, S. C., Averill, C., & Klappenbach, C. (2003). Nursing information technology knowledge, skills, and preparation of student nurses, nursing faculty, and clinicians: A US survey. *Journal of Nursing Education, 42*(8), 341–349.

Mendelson, C. (2003). Gentle hugs: Internet listservs as source of support for women with lupus. *Advances in Nursing Science, 26*(4), 299–306.

Murphy, J. (2011). Engaging patients and families in eHealth. *Nurse Informatics, 29*(6), 339–341.

National Council of State Boards of Nursing. (2011). *White paper: A nurse's guide to the use of social media.* Retrieved from https://www.ncsbn.org/Social_Media.pdf

National League for Nursing. (2008). Position statement. Preparing the next generation of nurses to practice in a technology-rich environment: An informatics agenda. Retrieved from http://www.nln.org/aboutnln/PositionStatements/informatics_052808.pdf

Nelson, A. (2003). Using simulation to design and integrate technology for safer and more efficient practice environments. *Nursing Outlook, 51*(3), S27–S29.

Newbold, S. K. (2003). New uses for wireless technology. *Nursing Management, 34*(Suppl. 10), 22–23, 32.

Office of the National Coordinator for Health Information Technology. (2011a). Health IT. Retrieved from http://www.healthit.gov

Office of the National Coordinator for Health Information Technology. (2011b). How to implement EHRs. Retrieved from http://www.healthit.gov/providers-professionals/ehr-implementation-steps/step-5-achieve-meaningful-use

Pagana, K. D. (2007). E-mail etiquette. *American Nurse Today, 2*(7), 45.

Quality and Safety Education for Nurses. (2012). About QSEN. Retrieved from http://www.qsen.org/about_qsen.php

Saba, V. K. (2001). Nursing informatics: Yesterday, today and tomorrow. *International Nursing Review, 48,* 177–187.

Saba, V. K., & McCormick, K. A. (2006). *Essentials of nursing informatics* (4th ed.). New York, NY: McGraw-Hill.

Sensmeier, J. (2008, September). Deep impact: Informatics and nursing practice. *Nursing Management,* 2, 4, 6. Retrieved from http://journals.lww.com/nursingmanagement/Fulltext/2008/09001/Deep_impact__Informatics_and_nursing_practice.1.aspx?WT.mc_id=HPxADx20100319xMP. doi:10.1097/01.NUMA.0000357564.51644.42

Smeltzer, S., Simmerman, V., Frain, M., DeSiltes, L., & Duffin, J. (2003). Accessible online health promotion information for persons with disabilities. *OJIN: The Online Journal of Issues in Nursing.* Retrieved from http://nursingworld.org/MainMenuCategories/ANAMarketplace/ANAPeriodicals/OJIN/TableofContents/Volume92004/No1Jan04/ArticlePreviousTopic/AccessibleInformation.html

Staggers, N., Gassert, C. A., & Curran, C. (2001). Informatics competencies for nurses at four levels of practice. *Journal of Nursing Education, 40*(7), 303–316.

Technology Informatics Guiding Education Reform. (2008). The TIGER initiative. Collaborating to integrate evidence and informatics into nursing practice and education: An executive summary. Retrieved from http://www.tigersummit.com

The Cochran Collaboration. (2012). The Cochrane Library. Retrieved from http://www.thecochranelibrary.com/view/0/index.html

Thede, L. (2008, August 18). The electronic health record: Will nursing be on board when the ship leaves? *OJIN: The Online Journal of Issues in Nursing, 13*(3). doi:10.3912/OJIN.Vol13No03InfoCol01

Thede, L. (2012, January 23). Informatics: Where is it? *OJIN: The Online Journal of Issues in Nursing, 17*(1). doi:10.3612/OJIN.Vol17No1InfoCol01

Thede, L., & Schwiran, P. (2011, February 25). Informatics: The standardized nursing terminologies: A national survey of nurses' experiences and attitudes—survey I. *OJIN: The Online Journal of Issues in Nursing, 16*(2). doi:10.3912/OJIN.Vol16No02InfoCol01

Thede, L. Q. (2003). *Informatics and nursing: Opportunities and challenges* (2nd ed.). Philadelphia, PA: Lippincott Williams & Wilkins.

Thede, L.Q., & Sewell, J. P. (2010). *Informatics and nursing competencies and applications*. Philadelphia, PA: Wolters Kluwer Lippincott Williams & Wilkins.

Thompson, B. W. (2005). HIPAA guideline for using PDAs. *Nursing, 99*(35), 24.

U.S. Department of Health and Human Services. (2000, November). *Healthy People 2010*, With understanding and improving health and objectives for improving health (2nd ed., 2 vols.). Washington, DC: U.S. Government Printing Office.

U.S. Department of Health and Human Services. (2012). *Healthy People 2020*. Retrieved from http://healthypeople.gov/2020/topicsobjectives2020/overview.aspx?topicid=18

White House Archives. (2004). *Fact sheet: Transforming health care for all Americans*. Retrieved from http://georgewbush-whitehouse.archives.gov/news/releases/2004/05/20040527-2.html

Young, K. M. (2000). *Informatics for healthcare professionals*. Philadelphia, PA: F. A. Davis.

Zykowski, M. E. (2003). Nursing informatics: The key to unlocking contemporary nursing practice. *AACN Clinical Issues, 14*(3), 271–281.

Future Directions in Professional Nursing Practice

15

Katherine Elizabeth Nugent

> The hardest thing is not to get people to accept new ideas; it is to get them to forget old ones.
>
> —John Maynard Keyes

A discussion of future directions in nursing practice must be considered within the context of the immense changes that have occurred in health care. In the past decade, health care has experienced dramatic changes in technology, reimbursement of services, increased aging population needing chronic illness management, increased demand for access to care and increased consumer awareness demanding high-quality, cost-effective care. These changes, although providing the U.S. healthcare system with the opportunity to transform itself and delivery of care, are placing a tremendous strain on the traditional hierarchical, organizational structures of healthcare agencies that are struggling to adapt to the new business model in health care. Successfully transitioning will require the transformation of organizational systems and entities providing health care and especially the profession of nursing, which has the largest number of healthcare providers.

Peter Drucker stated that the best way to predict the future is to create it. Since the publication of the first edition of this book, several important trends have emerged that affect the future directions of health care and professional

Key Terms and Concepts

- » **Nursing shortage**
- » Nursing faculty shortage
- » Cultural competence
- » Clinical nurse leader (CNL)
- » Doctor of Nursing Practice (DNP)
- » Gap between education and practice

Learning Objectives

After completing this chapter, the student should be able to:

1. Identify present trends associated with the profession of nursing that affect the transition of professional nursing practice for the future.

2. Articulate the vision for the future of nursing practice.

3. Reflect on the appropriate response of nursing leadership concerning issues affecting the future of nursing practice.

nursing practice. Several organizations such as the Institute of Medicine, Robert Wood Johnson Foundation, and the Tri Council for Nursing (which includes the American Association of Colleges of Nursing, the American Nurses Association, the American Organization of Nurse Executives), and the National League for Nursing have promoted change in nursing through publications and position statements reflecting issues associated with nursing practice, education, and research. The Agency for Healthcare Research and Quality (AHRQ), which has a mission to improve the quality, safety, efficiency, and effectiveness of health care for all Americans, has positioned quality health care as a priority.

In 2008, the Robert Wood Johnson Foundation (RWJF) and the Institute of Medicine (IOM) formed a partnership to assess and respond to the needed transformation in health care. The premise of their partnership was that transformation in health care could not occur without the leadership and transformation of the nursing profession. Therefore, they conducted a 2-year study on transformation needed in the nursing profession to realize the vision of a new healthcare system that provided access to quality, efficient patient care. The product of this study was the publication of *The Future of Nursing: Leading Change, Advancing Health* (IOM, 2011), which contains key recommendations discussed later in this chapter.

In 2010, Congress passed and President Obama signed into law comprehensive healthcare legislation. The Patient Protection and Affordable Care Act (Public Law 111-148) and the Health Care and Education Affordability Reconciliation Act (Public Law 111-152) propose the broadest changes to the healthcare system since the conception of the Medicare and Medicaid programs.

It is important to note that in the midst of these significant changes, the profession of nursing is facing some daunting challenges that will affect its response to transformation, such as a nursing shortage, workplace issues, the education–practice gap, unclear practice roles, and changes in population demographics. Although it is true that each of these issues is not a new challenge to nursing practice, it is critical to now acknowledge the collective impact of all of these together in the contemplation of future directions in professional nursing practice.

Inherent in these challenges is the acknowledgment of the chaotic, complex context of healthcare systems and the emerging use of complexity science in the business, organization, and management of health care. The convergence of chaos and complexity signals a transition between the past, present, and the future. This phenomenon is true of healthcare institutions, educational institutions, and the practice of nursing. Evidence, as reflected in quality outcomes, exists daily, signaling that the healthcare system and the practice of nursing are straining to adapt to the forces of change (Harris, 2012). It is critical for nursing to analyze existing evidence and control nursing's transition for future success.

Nursing is rich in history, resilient in its journey to develop as a profession and a discipline, and adaptive in its practice to meet the healthcare needs of the patient. Throughout the history of nursing, there are identifiable periods of time in which the practice and education of nurses responded to the evolving changes in health care and in society. Today, nursing is again at the crossroads of a major transition in its education and practice. An awareness of the merging of these issues creates urgency when contemplating the role, practice, and education of nurses.

> **Nursing is at the crossroads of a major transition in its education and practice.**

This chapter explores the phenomenon of the nursing shortage, workforce issues and changes in population demographics, cost and access to care, the education–practice gap, and their cumulative effect on the practice of nursing and future directions.

Nurse Shortage

The shortage of nurses is not a new issue; the predicted shortage has been prominent in the media for most of nursing's history and more recently in the past several years. Data from the Health Resources and Services Administration, Bureau of Health Professions, National Center for Health Workforce Analysis ("the center") establish that the most recent **nursing shortage** began in the year 2000 when there was an estimated supply of 1.89 million nurses and a projected demand of 2 million, or 6% more than what existed. The center further projected the anticipated demand for nurses should continue to exceed the supply until 2010 when the shortage would reach 12%. "At that point demand will begin to exceed supply at an accelerated rate and by 2015 the shortage, a relatively modest 6% in the year 2000, will have almost quadrupled to 20%. If not addressed, and if current trends continue, the shortage is projected to grow to 29% by 2020" (Health Resources and Services Administration [HRSA], 2002).

More recently, the U.S. Bureau of Labor Statistics estimated that more than 1 million new and replacement nurses would be needed by 2016 (Dohm & Shniper, 2007). Buerhaus, Auerback, and Staiger (2009) project shortage of nurses in the United States could be as high as 500,000 in 2025. These projections are based on the following trends: increase in population, a larger proportion of elderly persons, increases in technology, and advances in medical science (HRSA, 2002). Other issues affecting the projected supply of nurses include declines in the number of nursing school graduates, aging of the RN workforce, declines in relative earning, and emergence of alternative job opportunities, especially for women, who are the prominent gender in nursing.

History documents a cyclic pattern of nursing shortages, making it difficult to comprehend the seriousness of this shortage, especially viewed through the lens of history, the current economic slowdown, the decreased vacancies in healthcare agencies, especially hospitals, and the uncertainty of the consequences of healthcare reform given the Affordable Care Act (2010). In 2009, schools of nursing began documenting that significant numbers—54,000—of qualified nursing school applicants were denied admission to nursing schools (American Association of Colleges of Nursing [AACN], 2010). In recent years, employers in various parts of the United States have reported a decrease in the demand for RNs, and nursing students report that it is more challenging after graduation to find employment, when sometimes it takes 6 months to a year.

These findings led many people to question whether the nursing shortage still exists. Experts claim that the recession might have given some hospitals a temporary reprieve from chronic shortages, but it isn't curing the longer-term problem and might be making it worse (Robert Wood Johnson Foundation [RWJF], 2009). The Tri-Council for Nursing (2010) released a joint statement cautioning stakeholders about declaring an end to the nursing shortage. The statement says, "The downturn in the economy has led to an easing of the shortage in many parts of the country, a recent development most analysts believe to be temporary." The council raises serious concerns about slowing the production of RNs given the projected demand for nursing services, particularly as the country considers healthcare reform. It further states that diminishing the pipeline of future nurses can put the health of many Americans at risk, particularly those from rural and underserved communities, and leave our healthcare delivery system unprepared to meet the demand for essential nursing services.

Where do we stand today? A report from the Bureau of Labor Statistics on employment projections identifies registered nursing workforce as the top occupation in terms of job growth through 2020 (Bureau of Labor Statistics, 2012). The number of employed nurses is expected to grow from 2.74 million in 2010 to 3.45 million in 2020 and a need for 495,500 replacements in the nursing workforce is projected for 2020.

Data collected in the 2008 National Sample Survey of Registered Nurses (HRSA, 2010) document that the average age of the RN population is 46.8 years. It is significant to note that the average age of the RN population did not increase from the 2004 survey. The plateau in the average age reflects an increase in employed RNs younger than 30 years of age. Between 1988 and 2004, the percentage of employed nurses younger than 30 years fell from 18.3% to 9.1%. The trend of increasing enrollments in schools of nursing, especially baccalaureate programs, is credited for the increased employment of younger nurses (HRSA, 2010).

A recent report from the American Association of Colleges of Nursing shows the enrollment of generic baccalaureate students documented an increase of 5.1% in 2011–2012 and by 17% in the past 5 years (AACN, 2012b). Yet, the following statement is included with the documentation of increased enrollment: "Although the dramatic rise in enrollments and the increase in graduations over the past five years are encouraging, many more baccalaureate-prepared nurses will be needed to meet the health care needs of the population" (AACN, 2012b, p. 3).

A national nurse shortage still exists. Although nursing school enrollments and graduations are increasing and the statistics on younger nurses in the workforce are encouraging, the following factors must be considered in addressing the future of professional nursing practice: Baccalaureate and graduate programs in nursing report that 75,587 qualified applicants were not admitted into nursing programs because of lack of clinical space and faculty shortage; there is a prediction that more than 32 million Americans will soon gain access to healthcare services; the aging population is increasing and needs management of their chronic illnesses, and insufficient nurse staffing results in high nurse turnover (AACN, 2012b).

Nurse Faculty Shortage

In previous cycles of nursing shortage, the primary solution was to increase the enrollment in nursing programs. However, ample evidence supports the conclusion that a national **nursing faculty shortage** also exists. In a survey conducted by the AACN in June 2008, a total of 1,088 faculty vacancies were identified at 603 nursing schools across the nation. In the 2011–2012 survey, AACN reported that the professoriate continues to age. The mean age of doctoral faculty holding the rank of professor is 61 years and the mean age of faculty holding the rank of associate professor is 57.5 years. The national faculty vacancy rate is reported at 7.7% (603 vacancies). Ninety-one percent of the reported vacancies involve doctoral-prepared faculty. This shortage is limiting student capacity in nursing programs across the nation (AACN, 2012a).

The number of nurses employed in nursing education has changed little since 1980, with 31,065 nurses working as faculty. When the number of nurse educators is compared to the increase in number of RNs, the result is actually a decline (2.4%) in the percentage of nurses working in education (HRSA, 2010). The statistics associated with nursing faculty are concerning, especially in consideration of the nursing shortage and healthcare projections of nurse demand in the future.

Nursing Practice and Workplace Environment

Given the anticipated nursing shortage and the increased demand for nurses in the transformed healthcare system, it is important to address the issues associated with the practice of nursing and the environment where nurses work. It is understandable how the shortage of nurses affects the practicing nurse, especially in staff and patient ratios and workload and the resulting influences on nurse turnover rate. However, other issues associated with the nurse practice setting result in problematic quality outcomes, such as nurse job dissatisfaction, unsafe patient care, unhealthy workplace environment, and unclear role expectations.

It is evident that health care and healthcare delivery have changed significantly in the past two decades. Most of these changes have been associated with response to the increasing cost of care, the decreasing cost of reimbursement to healthcare providers, increased use of technology in practice, and the knowledge explosion concerning disease management. A full discussion of each of these issues is beyond the scope of this chapter. However, it is important to note that most of the changes result from a focus on reducing the cost of health care. Cost containment strategies aim to determine the setting of the delivery of care, the length of stay in the hospital, the cost reimbursed to providers of care, and the designation of the appropriate provider of care. To date, it is fair to say that the changes in health care have resulted in chaos and complexity for both the provider and the recipient of care. Evidence indicates that this chaos and complexity has created an environment that decreases access to care, quality of care, and patient safety (Adams & Corrigan, 2003; Hallin & Danielson, 2007; IOM, 2000, 2004) and nurse job satisfaction (HRSA, 2010).

Hospitals remain the most common employment setting for RNs in the United States, with 62.2% of employed RNs reporting hospitals as their primary place of employment (HRSA, 2010). Contrary to earlier predictions, the percentage of nurses working in hospitals increased from 2004 to 2008 (HRSA, 2010). However, also note that the percentage of nurses working in home health services has also increased. Data from the national survey of registered nurses reflect that the percentage of nurses working in hospitals decreases with age of nurse. Only 50% of RNs age 55 years and older work in hospital settings.

Most hospitals are still maintain a hierarchical organizational structure, resulting in nursing work environments being controlled by someone other than the nurses who work in it. This phenomenon creates systematic obstacles that prevent optimal performance in nursing practice. Data from surveys identify the systematic barriers as routine and prevalent (Ulrich, Buerhaus, Donelan, Norman, & Dittus, 2005). Examples include searching for supplies, waiting on medical equipment to be delivered, delays in scheduling tests and receiving results, delays associated with medication administration, lack of staff support, receiving orders, and timely communication with other healthcare providers (Gurses & Carayon, 2007; Lin & Liang, 2007; Storfjell, Omnike, & Ohlson, 2008; Zuzelo, Gettis, Hansell, & Thomas, 2008).

Nurses in hospitals provide care for patients who are sicker, older, and have more complex physical, psychosocial, and economic needs (Brown, 2004;

Clark, 2004). The combination of older patients with higher acuity, sophisticated technology, and shorter hospital stays creates a chaotic environment and demands that nurses assume greater responsibility (Grando, 2006). This chaos increases not only the risk of errors in patient care but the risk of health concerns for the nurse, such as the threat of infection, needle sticks, ever-increasing sensitivity to latex, back injuries, and stress-related health problems. In addition to these health risks, nurses are susceptible to workplace violence (e.g., physical violence, horizontal violence) and sexual harassment (Longo & Sherman, 2006; Ray & Ream, 2007; Smith-Pittman & McKoy, 1999; Valente & Bullough, 2004).

The issues associated with the hospital work environment have been shown to dominate problems and outcomes associated with nursing practice. Because of this environment, the profession of nursing has been challenged to evaluate its practice and outcomes. In fact, a majority of nurses completing surveys stated that they perceived that the unsafe working environment interfered with their ability to provide quality patient care (Houle, 2001; Pellico, Djukic, Kovner, & Brewer, 2009). Staff nurses strongly desire a practice setting in which they feel that they have the ability to provide quality patient care (Schmalenberg & Kramer, 2008) and a work environment that facilitates clinical decision making.

Confounding the chaos of the workplace environment is the shortage of qualified nonnurse healthcare workers, the supervision of unlicensed personnel, the appropriate delegation of care, mandatory overtime, and staffing ratios. The debate over the use of unlicensed personnel and the use of other licensed personnel in providing patient care is well documented in the literature (ANA, 1992, 1997, 1999; Barter & Furmidge, 1994; Manuel & Alster, 1994; Zimmerman, 2006). Research studies indicate that a decrease in RN staff increases patient care errors, infection rates, readmission, and morbidity (Aiken, Clarke, Sloane, Sochalski, & Silber, 2002; Aiken, Smith, & Lake, 1994; Needleman, Buerhaus, Mattke, Stewart, & Zelevinsky, 2002; Sofer, 2005; Stanton & Rutherford, 2004).

Given that research indicates that a decrease in RN staff or use of unlicensed personnel and other licensed personnel influence patient quality outcomes, what is a rationale for this practice? One answer that is quickly provided is the increased costs of a higher RN–patient ratio. Nurses represent about 23% or more of the hospital workforce. The salary of a licensed RN is higher compared to other nonphysician healthcare providers. Thus, the basic assumption is that to employ more unlicensed personnel or other licensed personnel (LVN) reduces the cost of care.

This assumption is not necessarily true when costs other than salary, such as costs of hiring, benefits, training, staff turnover, and responsibilities that must be assumed by a licensed care provider, are considered. Aiken et al. (2002) find that nurses in hospitals with low nurse–patient ratios are more than twice as likely to experience job-related burnout and dissatisfaction with their jobs when compared to nurses in hospitals with the highest nurse–patient ratios. Cooper (2004) and Kalisch and Kyung (2011) note that lower nursing staff ratios also indicate higher costs in a plethora of areas that reflect the actual reality of nursing practice. McCue, Mark, and Harless (2003) find that a 1% increase in nonnurse personnel increases the operating costs by 0.18% and diminishes profits by 0.021%. Are these data significant in the overall budget, considering the rising costs of health care? Zimmerman (2006) suggests that the concept of healthcare organizations competing on value, which includes cost and quality dimensions, has become a reality. In the end, the question that might drive the debate concerning the use of non-RN personnel is what the spending priorities of a hospital should be (p. 325).

Retention

There is a connection among nurse satisfaction, work environment, and nurse retention. The strongest predictor of nurse job dissatisfaction and intent to leave a job is personal stress related to the practice environment. The various causes of job stress include patient acuity, work schedules, poor physician–nurse interactions, new technology, staff shortages, unpredictable work flow or workload, and the perception that the care provided is unsafe (Groff-Paris & Terhaar, 2010). Surveys of practicing nurses document that job dissatisfaction, patient safety concerns, decreases in quality care, inadequate staffing, patient care delays, and mandated overtime are issues that negatively affect nursing practice (Aiken et al., 2002; ANA, 2006; Cooper, 2004; IOM, 1996; Pellico et al., 2009). Nurses have also reported their concern about their own health and safety issues, with job stress the most frequent health problem reported. Other reported health problems include back injuries, HIV, and hepatitis (Houle, 2001).

Despite the effort to address the issues of the chaotic and potentially harmful work environment, strategies to address these issues have fallen short of the target, and the dissatisfaction of hospital nurses persists. In national studies, 41% of nurses currently working report being dissatisfied with their jobs; 43% score high in a range of burnout measures; and 22% are planning to leave their jobs in the next year. Of the latter group, 33% are younger than age 30 years (Beecroft, Dorey, & Wentin, 2008; The Joint Commission, 2002; Laschinger, Finegan, & Welk, 2009). These factors help to fuel the shortage of nurses.

In 2008, 29.3% of RNs reported that they were extremely satisfied with their principal nursing positions, 50.5% were moderately satisfied, and 11.1% were dissatisfied (HRSA, 2010). Nurses working in academic education, ambulatory care, and home health settings reported the highest rate of job satisfaction (86.6%, 85.5%, and 82.8%, respectively). Almost 12%

of RNs employed in hospitals reported moderate or extreme dissatisfaction (HRSA, 2010).

The retention of competent professional nurses in jobs is a major problem of the U.S. healthcare industry, particularly in hospitals and long-term care facilities. An average yearly nurse turnover rate is reported as 5–21% (PricewaterhouseCooper's Health Research Institute, 2007). Other research has found that during the first year of professional practice new registered nurses experience turnover rates around 35–61% (Almada, Carafoli, Flattery, Franch, & McNamara, 2004). Kovner and colleagues (2007) found that 13% of newly licensed RNs had changed principal jobs after 1 year, and 37% reported that they felt ready to change jobs (Huntington et al., 2012; Pellico et al., 2009). In a comprehensive report initiated by the Agency for Healthcare Research and Quality (2007), the authors found that the shortage of registered nurses, in combination with an increased workload, poses a potential threat to the quality of care. In addition, every 1% increase in nurse turnover costs a hospital about $300,000 a year.

Workplace Environment

The healthcare workplace has been transformed over the past 20 years in response to economic and service pressures. However, some of these reforms have had undesirable consequences for nurses' work in hospitals and the use of their time and skills. As the pace and complexity of hospital care increases, nursing work is expanding at both ends of the complexity continuum. Nurses often undertake tasks that less qualified staff could do, while at the other end of the spectrum they are unable to use their high-level skills and expertise. This inefficiency in the use of nursing time can also negatively affect patient outcomes. Nurses' work that does not directly contribute to patient care, engage higher-order cognitive skills, or provide opportunity for role expansion can decrease retention of well-qualified and highly skilled nurses in the health workforce (Duffield, Gardner, & Catling-Paull, 2008).

The major barrier to making progress in patient safety and quality is the failure to appreciate the complexity of the work in healthcare today. Current research focusing on work complexity and related issues enables an increased understanding of RN decision making (the invisible, cognitive work of nursing) in actual care situations and demonstrates how both the knowledge and competencies of RNs as well as the complex environments in which RNs provide care contribute to patient safety, quality of care, and healthy work environments or lack thereof (Ebright, 2010).

Krichbaum et al. (2007) identify a nurse care-delivery experience they term "complexity compression" and note this experience occurs when nurses are expected to assume, in a condensed time frame, additional, unplanned responsibilities while simultaneously conducting their other multiple responsibilities. Nurses report that personal, environmental, practice, administrative, system, and technology factors, as well as autonomy and control factors, all contribute to this experience. Associated with complexity compression is the phenomenon of stacking. Stacking is the invisible, decision-making work of RNs about the what, how, and when of delivering nursing care to an assigned group of patients (Ebright, Patterson, Chalko, & Render, 2003). This process results in decisions about what care is needed, what care is possible, and when and how to deliver this care.

> **The major barrier to making progress in patient safety and quality is the failure to appreciate the complexity of the work in healthcare today.**

A commitment to understanding and appreciating the complexity involved in RN work is needed to guide the more substantive and sustained improvements required to achieve safety and quality. Attention to and action based on an understanding of the complexity of RN work and the value of safe, quality care, desired patient outcomes, and nurse recruitment and retention have the potential to achieve the goals of healthy work environments. Using complexity science to understand the work of nursing is becoming increasingly accepted as a very fitting approach to explaining healthcare organizational dynamics and the work of nursing (Lindberg & Lindberg, 2008).

KEY COMPETENCY 15-1

Examples of Applicable *Nurse of the Future: Nursing Core Competencies*

Systems-Based Practice

Knowledge (K2a) Understands the impact of macrosystem changes on planning, organizing, and delivering patient care at the work unit level

Attitudes/Behaviors (A2a) Appreciates the complexity of the work unit environment

Source: Massachusetts Department of Higher Education (2010), p. 19.

Role Clarity

With the introduction of new nursing models of care to fill perceived gaps in healthcare provision or improve access, it is important that the public, other healthcare providers, and indeed nurses themselves have a clear understanding of the various nursing roles (Gardner, Chang, & Duffield, 2007). The confusion over the naming of nursing roles and their various functions or scopes of practice has confounded nursing and other healthcare professionals for some time and serves to feed role dissonance (Bryant-Lukosius, Dicenso, & Browne, 2004; Gardner et al., 2007; Lowe, Plummer, O'Brien, & Boyd, 2012). For nurse practitioners to have an impact on the provision of health services, a clear understanding of their practice is also imperative. Clarity is required for regulation that provides consistency in the approach to health care, ensuring a consistent, efficient, and effective approach to access to care and quality of care.

Changing Demographics

Despite national trends of increasing diversity, with ethnic and racial minorities reaching almost one-third of the U.S. population, minorities are overall underrepresented in the healthcare profession. The 2010 U.S.

Census reports that 63.7% of the population is white and non-Hispanic and 16.3% are nonwhite or Hispanic. In contrast, the registered nurse population remains predominantly female (94.2%) and 83.2% white, non-Hispanic (HRSA, 2010). The Sullivan Commission (2004) highlights the diversity gap in its hallmark report *Missing Persons: Minorities in the Health Professions*. Together, African Americans, Hispanic Americans, and American Indians make up more than 25% of the U.S. population but only 9% of the nation's nurses, 6% of its physicians, and 5% of dentists. Similar disparities show up in the faculties of health professional schools. For example, minorities make up less than 10% of baccalaureate nursing faculties, 8.6% of dental school faculties, and only 4.2% of medical school faculties. If the trends continue, the health workforce of the future will resemble the population even less than it does today. If these data are viewed in the context of the prediction that no racial or ethnic group will compose a majority by the year 2050, such a decline in a diverse workforce could be catastrophic.

In 2003, the IOM warned of the "unequal treatment" minorities face when encountering the health system. Cultural differences, a lack of access to health care, high rates of poverty, and unemployment contribute to the substantial ethnic and racial disparities in health status and health outcomes (IOM, 2003b). Health services research shows that minority health professionals are more likely to serve minority and medically underserved populations. Increasing the number of underrepresented minorities in the health professions as well as improving the cultural competency of providers are key strategies of reducing health disparities (Betancourt, Green, Carrillo, & Ananeh-Firempong, 2003; IOM, 2003b).

Cultural competence in multicultural societies continues as a major initiative for health care and nursing, specifically. The mass media, healthcare policymakers, the Office of Minority Health and other governmental organizations, professional organizations, the workplace, and health insurance payers are addressing the need for individuals to understand and become culturally competent as one strategy to improve quality and eliminate racial, ethnic, and gender disparities in health care (Purnell & Paulanka, 2008).

Culturally competent healthcare providers reduce patient care error and increase access to and satisfaction with health care. The beginning of cultural competence is self-awareness. Culture has a powerful unconscious impact on health professionals and the care they provide. Purnell and Paulanka (2008) believe that self-knowledge and understanding promote strong professional perceptions that free healthcare providers from prejudice and facilitate culturally competent care.

Nursing has a long history of incorporating culture into nursing practice (DeSantis & Lipson, 2007). In 2008, AACN released a publication identifying cultural competency in baccalaureate nursing education (AACN, 2008a). Yet, some maintain, no matter how culturally competent the nurse might be, the patient's experience remains structured in the nurse's culture (Dean, 2005). Despite nurses' best efforts to understand the culture of the patient, nurses often fail to understand that the patient might be experiencing health care for the first time, not in his or her own culture, but in the nurse's culture of healthcare delivery. The understanding of this concept associated with cultural competence increases the reality of the urgency of increasing the diversity in the nursing workforce.

Nursing Education

The healthcare system of the 21st century is complex, technologically rich, ethically challenging, and ever changing. The roles of all healthcare providers evolve continually, and boundaries of practice shift regularly. Knowledge explodes at unprecedented rates, and although the evidence base for practice grows stronger every day, healthcare providers must repeatedly make decisions and take action in situations that are characterized by ambiguity and uncertainty (Cowan & Moorhead, 2011).

Throughout the years, nursing education has made an effort to transition its curriculum and programs to accommodate the knowledge explosion and the advanced technology associated with health care. However, the transition within the programs of nursing has assumed a patchwork approach instead of significant reform. This is in part the result of the tradition associated with the history of nursing education, the inability to resolve the differences in prelicensure programs, and faculty propensity to be reluctant to "leave behind" what is no longer successful in a changing practice arena. In addition, nurse educators are caught in the "perfect storm" composed of a changing healthcare delivery system, changing practice models, nursing shortage, faculty shortage, changes in external standards of care and educational accreditation, university budget cuts, and changes in external funding that support new nursing programs.

In 2003, the IOM issued a report titled *Health Professions Education: A Bridge to Quality* (IOM, 2003a). This report, which focuses on knowledge that healthcare professionals need to provide quality care, states that students in the health professions are not prepared to address the shifts in the country's demographics nor are they educated to work in interdisciplinary teams. It further states that students were not able to access evidence for use in practice, determine the reasons for or prevent patient care errors, or access technology to acquire the latest information. Specifically, the report expresses concern with the adequacy of nursing education at all levels, yet focuses intensely on education at the prelicensure level. The report identifies five core competencies that all clinicians should possess: (1) provide patient-centered care; (2) work in interdisciplinary teams; (3) use evidence-based practice; (4) apply quality improvement and identify errors and hazards in care; and (5) utilize informatics (IOM, 2003a).

KEY COMPETENCY 15-2

Examples of Applicable *Nurse of the Future: Nursing Core Competencies*

Leadership

Knowledge (K1) Identifies leadership skills essential to the practice of nursing

Attitudes/Behaviors (A1) Recognizes the role of the nurse as a leader

Source: Massachusetts Department of Higher Education (2010), p. 17.

In 2005, the National Council of State Boards of Nursing (NCSBN) released five recommendations regarding prelicensure clinical instruction. These recommendations address the appropriate or desired setting of clinical experience, the scope of clinical experience, the qualifications of clinical faculty, the role of nursing faculty in clinical education, and the need for research. The NCSBN board has also done work associated with postgraduate nurse competence that includes clinical reasoning and judgment, patient care delivery and management skills, communication and interpersonal relationships, and recognizing limits and seeking help (Li, 2007).

Despite these unprecedented changes, new standards of instruction, and new competencies for postgraduates, the educational preparation of nurses has remained virtually unchanged for more than 50 years. Nursing education remains content focused and teacher centered. Faculty feel pressured to cover the content through lectures rather than innovative modalities that focus on inquiry, deep understanding, and development of new skills sets needed for today's practice arena (Benner, Stutphen, Leonard, & Day, 2010; Valiga & Champagne, 2011).

Recently the results of two national studies reinforced the belief that nursing education must be reformed. The two reports, *Educating Nurses: A Call for Radical Transformation* (Benner et al., 2010) and *The Future of Nursing: Leading Change, Advancing Health* (IOM, 2011), explore the issue of whether nurses are entering practice equipped with the knowledge and skills for today's practice and prepared to continue clinical learning for tomorrow's nursing, given the enormous changes in and complexity of current nursing practice and practice settings. In both reports the response is that nurses are not prepared for future healthcare change. Both reports challenge nursing education to make reforms in preparation of new graduates in terms of establishing new competencies and outcomes for graduates, new curriculum designs, new pedagogy, better evaluation models, and new models for clinical education, such as residency programs.

> **Landmark reports challenge nursing education to make reforms in preparation of new graduates in terms of establishing new competencies and outcomes for graduates, new curricula designs, new pedagogy, better evaluation models, and new models for clinical education.**

The Carnegie report on educating nurses identifies four shifts in faculty thinking and approach to nursing education that need to occur. The shifts in faculty thinking are (1) from a focus on covering decontextualized knowledge to an emphasis on teaching for a sense of salience, situated cognition, and action in particular clinical situations; (2) from a sharp separation of classroom and clinical teaching to integrative teaching in all settings; (3) from an emphasis on critical thinking to an emphasis on clinical reasoning and multiple ways of thinking that include critical thinking; and (4) from an emphasis on socialization and role taking to an emphasis on formation (Benner et al., 2010, p. 89). Other recommendations address entry and pathways, student population, student experience, teaching, entry to practice, and national oversight (pp. 215–230).

In response to the changes in healthcare delivery and the call for new roles in nursing, the American Association of Colleges of Nursing proposes two new educational programs for nursing. The first is the **clinical nurse leader (CNL)**, an advanced generalist role prepared at the master's level of education. The CNL oversees the coordination of care for a group of patients, assesses cohort risk, provides direct patient care in complex situations, and functions as a part of an interdisciplinary team (AACN, 2007). The lateral integration of care has been what is missing in the delivery of care to patients with complex needs. No single person oversees patient care laterally and over time and is able to intervene, facilitate, or coordinate care for the entire patient experience. The CNL will be instrumental in helping all disciplines see the interdependencies that exist between and among them (Begun, Hamilton, Tornabeni, & White, 2006).

What makes the CNL movement different from past efforts within nursing? There has been thoughtful and broad engagement in looking at both the educational and competency needs of nursing to function in an environment that has changed dramatically and become extremely complex. This change requires advanced knowledge, new skills, and interdependent relationships. The uniqueness of the inception and implementation of the CNL is the approach that is: (1) being advanced as a partnership with education and practice, (2) occurring at a broad national level of activity, (3) being structured with milestones for the partnerships to attain, and (4) being facilitated by nurses and administrators at the highest levels within healthcare organizations (Begun et al., 2006).

Another new program within nursing is the **Doctor of Nursing Practice (DNP)**. The need for this terminal practice degree is based on the series of reports from the IOM that address quality of health care, patient safety, and educational reform, as well as following the movement of other healthcare professions to the practice doctorate. In 2002, the AACN established a task force to examine the current status of existing advanced practice programs, current existing practice doctorates, and future need for such a program. The AACN, in collaboration with the National Organization of Nurse Practitioner Faculties, met with other constituencies and held regional meetings to discuss the nature of this terminal degree and the need for a terminal degree in practice. After much national discussion and debate, it was determined that a practice doctorate was needed that encompasses any form of nursing intervention that influences healthcare outcomes for individual patients, management of care for individuals and populations, administration of nursing and health organization, and the development and implementation of health policy (AACN, 2004). It is clearly stated that this practice degree is not the same as the research doctoral degree and that graduates would be prepared to blend clinical, economic, organizational, and leadership skills and to use science in improving the direct care of patients, care of patient populations, and practice that supports patient care (Champagne, 2006).

The development of the DNP and the CNL programs of study represent a bold effort by the profession of nursing to address new roles of nursing and educational reform needed to prepare graduates to meet the healthcare needs of the future. Although questions and concerns related to the implementation of these two new programs still exist, the evaluation of the implementation of these programs is mostly positive. One must applaud the spirit of evidence-based educational innovation.

Conclusion

This chapter supports the concept that the challenges of the nursing shortage, workforce issues, cost and access to care, the education–practice gap, and changes in population demographics have merged to create a crisis point for the profession of nursing, especially in light of the constant change in health care. Individually, each identified challenge in itself would create a need for some degree of change in the practice of nursing, and considered individually, nursing would have continued to patch together a response. Together, the compounding consequences of these challenges signal the need for major transformation in nursing. The culminating results of these issues have been connected to a decline in quality care, dissatisfaction in the achieved outcomes of practice, and a wider gap between education preparation and performance in the practice setting.

The issue of the employment of non-RN personnel for patient care is not one that will disappear in the future, given the predicted increase in patient population and the nurse shortage. Currently, 97% of hospitals employ UAP (Zimmerman, 2006). The issue might indeed be how will nursing practice transition? Will the move continue to be from the hospital to other healthcare settings? Will nurses redefine who they are and what constitutes their practice?

The **gap between education and practice** looms larger as the healthcare setting continually changes as a result of advanced technology, knowledge explosion, shorter hospital stays, and rapid changes in disease management. Emphasis is now placed on evidence-based medicine and evidence-based practice. In general, curriculums in nursing programs have not evolved to keep pace with changes in the practice setting. The reasons are varied and include limited funding sources, confinement of higher education boundaries and standards, past success in educational outcomes, inability to differentiate between levels of nursing practice, multiple entry into practice and licensure, and pedagogical methods that emphasize receiving content rather than discovery of evidence. The current emphasis on integrating clinical simulation as a teaching and evaluation strategy and the development of the clinical nurse leader (MSN generalist) and Doctor of Nursing Practice are steps in the right direction.

KEY COMPETENCY 15-3

Examples of Applicable *Nurse of the Future: Nursing Core Competencies*

Leadership

Knowledge (K5) Explains the importance, necessity, and process of change

Skills (S5b) Anticipates consequences, plans ahead, and changes approaches to get best results

Attitudes/Behaviors (A5b) Values new idea and interventions to improve patient care

Source: Massachusetts Department of Higher Education (2010), p. 18.

Evidence supports that a better educated nurse is needed in practice. The initial educational preparation for the largest proportion of RNs is the associate degree. In 2008, the initial educational level of registered nurses indicated that 20.4% were diploma, 45.4% were associate degree, and 34.2% were baccalaureate (HRSA, 2010). In 2004, 33.7% of nurses (981,238) reported the associate degree as their highest level of nursing education, 34.2% (994,276) reported the baccalaureate degree as their highest level, and 13% (376,901) reported a master's or doctoral degree as their highest level of education. Leaders in nursing education must identify a way to move younger students to the desired graduate level of education more expediently.

Clearer roles in practice must be developed, answering the question about what nurses do. The answer will probably be different from the traditional role of nursing practiced by those who are nearing retirement. As the future evolves, an increase in the movement of nurses from the hospitals into other settings of care will be realized. Entrepreneurial opportunities will be available for nurses, and nurses will be able to implement their theory-based practice in providing quality health care to the population.

The theme of promoting cultural competence in health care will be explored from two perspectives: creating practice environments that support culturally competent care and developing educational programs that foster cultural awareness and sensitivity among students in the healthcare professions. As the population continues to become more diverse, culturally competent care will be the basis for quality care, access to care, and alleviation of health disparities, thus promoting healthier population outcomes.

The nursing profession must be able to navigate the high-speed, convoluted pace of the current healthcare delivery system. Nurses must be competent to meet the demands of the current patient population, the complex technology, more responsibility, and cost-contained care. In reality, the changes in advanced technology, the updates in pharmacological interventions, the knowledge explosion, and the advancements in gene therapy will significantly change not only the practice of the nurse but that of all healthcare providers. The innovation in technology, the culture of violence, terrorism, and the increase in natural disasters resulting from global warming will change the practice of nursing.

Where do we go from here? The IOM report *The Future of Nursing: Leading Change, Advancing Health* provides us with a blueprint. The IOM and Robert Wood Johnson Foundation partnered to access and respond to the need to transform nursing to ensure that the nursing workforce has the capacity, in terms of numbers, skills, and competence, to meet the present and future healthcare needs of the public. This transformation would enable nurses to be partners and leaders in the advancing health for the future. The key messages and recommendations of the study are: (1) Nurses should practice to the full extent of their education and training; (2) nurses should achieve higher levels of education and training through an improved education system that promotes seamless academic progression; (3) nurses should be full partners, with physicians and other health professions, in redesigning health care in the United States; (4) effective workforce planning and policy making require better data collection and an improved information infrastructure (IOM, 2011, p. 4). Recommendations from the study are: (1) remove scope-of-practice barriers; (2) expand opportunities for nurses to lead and diffuse collaborative improvement efforts; (3) implement nurse residency programs; (4) increase the proportion of nurses with a baccalaureate degree to 80% by 2010; (5) double the number of nurses with a doctorate by 2010; (6) ensure that nurses engage in lifelong learning; (7) Prepare and enable nurses to lead change to advance health; and (8) build an infrastructure for the collection and analysis of interprofessional healthcare workforce data.

It is imperative that professional nurses control their future and redefine their roles in practice. Noel Tichy (1997) states, "In the future, the real core competence of organizations will be the ability to continuously and creatively destroy and remake themselves." The same might be applied to the profession of nursing. Are you ready to be a part of transforming professional nursing practice as we transition our profession into the future?

> **www CRITICAL THINKING QUESTIONS** ✳
>
> Based on the trends and recommendations presented in this chapter, what do you think nursing education will look like in 2025? What do you think the profession of nursing will look like in the year 2025? ✳

References

Adams, K., & Corrigan, J. (Eds.). (2003). *Priority areas for national action: Transforming health care quality*. Quality Chasm Series. Washington, DC: National Academies Press.

Affordable Care Act. (2010). Retrieved from http://www.healthcare.gov/law/full/

Agency for Healthcare Research and Quality. (2007). *Research news*. Washington, DC: Author.

Aiken, L., Clarke, S., Sloane, D., Sochalski, J., & Silber, J. (2002). Hospital nurse staffing and patient mortality, nurse burnout, and job dissatisfaction. *Journal of the American Medical Association, 288*(16), 1987–1993.

Aiken, L., Smith, H., & Lake, E. (1994). Lower Medicare mortality among a set of hospitals known for good nursing care. *Medical Care, 32*, 771–787.

Almada, P., Carafoli, K., Flattery, J., French, D., & McNamara, M. (2004). Improving the retention rate of newly graduated nurses. *Journal for Nurses in Staff Development, 20*(6), 268–273.

American Association of Colleges of Nursing. (2003). *Special survey on vacant faculty positions*. Washington, DC: Author.

American Association of Colleges of Nursing. (2004). AACN position statement on the practice doctorate in nursing. Press Release. Retrieved from http://www.aacn.nche.edu/DNP/index.htm

American Association of Colleges of Nursing. (2006). Essentials of doctoral education for advanced nursing practice. Retrieved from http://www.aacn.nche.edu/ DNP/index.htm

American Association of Colleges of Nursing. (2007, February). *White paper on the education and role of the clinical nurse leader*. Washington, DC: Author.

American Association of Colleges of Nursing. (2008a). Cultural competency in baccalaureate nursing education. Retrieved from http://www.aacn.nche.edu/leading-initiatives/education-resources/competency.pdf

American Association of Colleges of Nursing. (2008b). List of programs offering the DNP. Retrieved from http://www.aacn.nche.edu/DNP/index.htm

American Association of Colleges of Nursing. (2010). *Nursing faculty shortage fact sheet*. Washington, DC: Author.

American Association of Colleges of Nursing. (2012a). *Nursing faculty shortage fact sheet*. Washington, DC: Author. Retrieved from http://www.aacn.nche.edu/media-relations/fact-sheets/nursing-faculty-shortage

American Association of Colleges of Nursing. (2012b). Enrollment and graduations in baccalaureate and graduate programs in nursing. Author.

American Nurses Association. (1992). *Position statement on registered nurse utilization of unlicensed assistive personnel*. Washington, DC: Author.

American Nurses Association. (1997). *Implementing nursing's report card: Study of RN staffing, length of stay, and patient outcomes*. Washington, DC: Author.

American Nurses Association. (1999). *Principles for nurse staffing*. Washington, DC: Author.

American Nurses Association. (2006). Analysis of American Nurses staffing survey. Retrieved from http://www.nursingworld.org/FunctionalMenuCategories/MediaResources/PressReleases/2001/ANAPressRelease.html

Barter, M., & Furmidge, M. (1994). Unlicensed assistive personnel: Issues related to delegation and supervision. *Journal of Nursing Administration, 24*(4), 36–40.

Beecroft, P., Dorey, F., & Wentin, M. (2008). Turnover intention in new graduate nurses: A multivariate analysis. *Journal of Advanced Nursing, 62*(11), 41–52.

Begun, J., Hamilton, J., Tornabeni, J., & White, K. (2006). Opportunities for improving patient care through lateral integration: The clinical nurse leader. *Journal of Healthcare Management, 51*(1), 19–25.

Benner, P., Sutphen, M., Leonard, V., & Day, L. (2010). *Educating nurses: A call for radical transformation*. San Francisco, CA: Jossey-Bass.

Berlin, L. (2002). The shortage of doctorally prepared nursing faculty: A dire situation. *Nursing Outlook, 50*(2), 50–56.

Betancourt, J. R., Green, A. R., Carrillo, J. E., & Ananeh-Firempong, O. (2003). Defining cultural competence: A practical framework for addressing racial/ethnic disparities in health and health care. *Public Health Report, 118*(4), 293–302.

Brown, B. (2004). From the editor: Restoring caring back into nursing. *Nursing Administration Quarterly, 28*, 237–238.

Bryant-Lukosius, D., Dicenso, A., & Browne, G. (2004). Advanced practice roles: Development, implementation, and evaluation. *Journal of Advanced Nursing, 48*(5), 519–529.

Buerhaus, P., Auerbach, D., & Staiger, D. (2009, June 12). The recent surge in nurse employment: Causes and implications. *Health Affairs*, 657–668.

Bureau of Labor Statistics. (2012, January). *Employment outlook, 2010–2020*. Retrieved from http://www.bls.gov/opub/mlr/2012/01/mlr201201.pdf

Champagne, M. (2006). The future of nursing education: Educational models for future care. In P. Cowen & S. Moorhead (Eds.), *Current issues in nursing* (7th ed.). St. Louis, MO: Mosby Elsevier.

Clark, J. (2004). An aging population with chronic disease compels new delivery systems focused on new structures and practice. *Nursing Administration Quarterly, 28,* 105–115.

Cooper, P. (2004). Nurse–patient ratios revisited. (Editorial). *Nursing Forum, 39*(2), 3–4.

Cowan, P., & Moorhead, S. (2011). Nursing education in transition. In P. S. Cowen & S. Moorhead (Eds.), *Current issues in nursing* (pp. 72–74). St. Louis, MO: Mosby Elsevier.

Dean, P. (2005). Transforming ethnocentricity in nursing: A culturally relevant experience of reciprocal visits between Malta and the Midwest. *Journal of Continuing Education in Nursing, 36*(4), 163, 167.

DeSantis, L., & Lipson, J. (2007). Brief history of inclusion of content on culture in nursing education. *Journal of Transcultural Nursing, 18*(7), 7s–9s.

Dohm, A., & Shniper, L. (2007). Occupational employment projections to 2016: Employment outlook: 2006-16. *Monthly Labor Review*, November, 86–125, U.S. Government Printing Office.

Duffield, C., Gardner, G., & Catling-Paull, C. (2008). Nursing work and the use of time. *Journal of Clinical Nursing, 17,* 3269–3274.

Ebright, P. (2010, January 31). The complex work of RNs: Implications for healthy work environments. *OJIN: The Online Journal of Issues in Nursing, 15*(1).

Ebright, P., Patterson, E., Chalko, B., & Render, M. (2003). Understanding the complexity of registered nurse work in acute care settings. *Journal of Nursing Administration, 33*(12), 630–638.

Gardner, G., Chang, A., & Duffield, C. (2007). Making nurses work: Breaking through the role confusion of advanced practice nursing. *Journal of Advanced Practice Nursing, 57*(4), 382–391.

Grando, V. (2006). Staff nurses working in hospitals: Who they are, what they do, and what are their challenges? In P. Cowen and S. Moorhead (Eds.), *Current issues in nursing* (7th ed.). St. Louis, MO: Mosby Elsevier.

Groff-Paris, L., & Terhaar, M. (2010). Using Maslow's pyramid and the National Database of Nursing Quality Indicators to attain a healthier work environment. *OJIN: The Online Journal of Issues in Nursing, 16*(1), 1–8.

Gurses, A. P., & Carayon, P. (2007). Performance obstacle of intensive care nurses. *Nursing Research, 56*(3), 185–194.

Hallin, K., & Danielson, E. (2007). Registered nurses' experiences of daily work, a balance between strain and stimulation: A qualitative study. *International Journal of Nursing Studies, 44*(7), 1221–1230.

Harris, J. (2012). Forces shaping nursing leadership. In L. Roussell (Ed.). *Management and leadership for nurse administrators* (6th ed.). Burlington, MA: Jones & Bartlett Learning.

Health Resources and Services Administration. (2002). *Projected supply, demand, and shortages of registered nurses: 2000–2020.* Washington, DC: Health Resources and Services Administration, Bureau of Health Professions, National Center for Health Workforce Analysis.

Health Resources and Services Administration. (2010, September). *The registered nurse population: Findings from the 2008 National Sample Survey of Registered Nurses*. Washington, DC: Health Resources and Services Administration, Bureau of Health Professions.

Houle, J. (2001, September). *NursingWorld.org health and safety survey*. Retrieved from http://ana.nursingworld.org/MainMenuCategories/OccupationalandEnvironmental/occupationalhealth/HealthSafetySurvey.aspx

Huntington, A., Gilmour, J., Tuckett, A., Neville, S., Wilson, D., & Turner, D. (2012). Is anybody listening? A qualitative study of nurses' reflections on practice. *Journal of Clinical Nursing, 20*, 1413–1422.

Institute of Medicine. (1996). *Nursing staff in hospitals and nursing homes: Is it adequate?* Washington, DC: National Academy Press.

Institute of Medicine. (2000). *To err is human: Building a safer health system*. Washington, DC: National Academy Press.

Institute of Medicine. (2003a). *Health professions education: A bridge to quality*. Washington, DC: National Academy Press.

Institute of Medicine. (2003b). *Unequal treatment: Confronting racial and ethnic disparities in health care*. Washington, DC: National Academy Press.

Institute of Medicine. (2004). *Keeping patients safe: Transforming the work environment of nurses*. Washington, DC: National Academies Press.

Institute of Medicine. (2011). *The future of nursing: Leading change, advancing health*. Washington, DC: National Academies Press.

The Joint Commission. (2002). *Healthcare at the crossroads: Strategies for addressing the evolving nurse crisis*. Retrieved from http://www.jointcommission.org/assets/1/18/health_care_at_the_crossroads.pdf

Kalisch, B., & Kyung, H. (2011). Nurse staffing levels and teamwork: A cross-sectional study of patient care units in acute care hospitals. *Journal of Nursing Scholarship, 43*(1), 82–88.

Kovner, C., Brewer, C., Fairchild, S., Poornima, S., Hongsoo, K., & Djukic, M. (2007). Newly licensed RNs' characteristics, work attitudes, and intentions to work. *American Journal of Nursing, 107*(9), 58–70.

Krichbaum, K., Diemart, C., Jacox, L., Jones, A., Koenig, P., Mueller, C., & Disch, J. (2007). Complexity compression: Nurses under fire. *Nursing Forum, 42*(2), 86–95.

Laschinger, H., Finegan, J., & Welk, P. (2009, November–December). New graduate burnout: The impact of professional practice environment, workplace civility, and empowerment. *Nursing Economic$, 27*(6).

Li, S. (2007). Assessing clinical competence and practice errors of newly licensed registered nurses. In P. Cowen & S. Moorhead (Eds.), *Current issues in nursing* (p. 93). St. Louis, MO: Mosby Elsevier.

Lin, L., & Liang, B. (2007). Addressing the nursing work environment to promote patient safety. *Nursing Forum, 42*(1), 22–29.

Lindberg, C., & Lindberg, C. (2008). Nurses take note: A primer on complexity science. In C. Lindberg, S. Nash, & C. Lindberg (Eds.), *On the edge: Nursing in the age of complexity* (pp. 23–47). Bordentown, NJ: Plexus.

Longo, J., & Sherman, R. (2006). Leveling horizontal violence. *Nursing Management, 38*(3), 34–37, 50–51.

Lowe, G., Plummer, V., O'Brien, A. P., & Boyd, L. (2012). Time to clarify—the value of advanced practice nursing roles in health care. *Journal of Advanced Nursing, 68*(3), 677–685.

Manuel, P., & Alster, L. (1994). Unlicensed personnel no cure for an ailing health care system. *Nursing & Health Care, 15*(1), 18–21.

Massachusetts Department of Higher Education. (2010). *Nurse of the future: Nursing core competencies.* Retrieved from http://www.mass.edu/currentinit/documents/NursingCoreCompetencies.pdf

McCue, M., Mark, B., & Harless, D. (2003). Nurse staffing, quality, and financial performance. *Journal of Healthcare Finance, 29*(4), 54–76.

National Council of State Boards of Nursing. (2005). Clinical instruction in prelicensure programs. Retrieved from https://www.ncsbn.org/2822.htm?iframe=true&width=500&height=270

Needleman, J., Buerhaus, P., Mattke, S., Stewart, M., & Zelevinsky, K. (2002). Nurse staffing levels and the quality of care in hospitals. *New England Journal of Medicine, 346,* 1715–1722.

Pellico, L., Djukic, M., Kovner, C., & Brewer, C. (2009). Moving on, up, or out: Changing work needs of new RNs at different stages of their beginning nursing practice. *OJIN: The Online Journal of Issues in Nursing, 15*(1).

PricewaterhouseCooper's Health Research Institute. (2007, July). What works: Healing the healthcare staffing shortage. Retrieved from http://www.pwc.com/extweb/pwcpublications.nsf/docid/674D1E79A678A0428525730D006B74A9

Purnell, L., & Paulanka, B. (2008). *Transcultural health care: A culturally competent approach* (3rd ed.). Philadelphia, PA: F. A. Davis.

Ray, M., & Ream, K. (2007). The dark side of the job: Violence in the emergency department. *Journal of Emergency Nursing, 33*(3), 257–261.

Robert Wood Johnson Foundation. (2009, April 17). Has the recession solved the nursing shortage? Experts say no. Robert Wood Johnson Foundation. Retrieved from http://www.rwjf.org/newsroom/product.jsp?id=41728

Schmalenberg, C., & Kramer, M. (2008). Essentials of a productive nurse work environment. *Nursing Research, 57*(1), 2–13.

Smith-Pittman, M., & McKoy, Y. (1999). Workplace violence in healthcare environments. *Nursing Forum, 34*(3), 5–13.

Sofer, D. (2005). You get what you pay for: News flash: Higher nurse–patient ratios still saves lives. *American Journal of Nursing, 105*(11), 20.

Stanton, M., & Rutherford, M. (2004). How many nurses are enough? Hospital staff nursing and quality care research. *Accidents and Emergency Nursing, 15*(1), 1–2.

Storfjell, J. L, Omnike, O., & Ohlson, S. (2008). The balancing act: Patient care time versus cost. *Journal of Nursing Administration, 38*(5), 244–249.

Sullivan Commission. (2004). *Missing persons: Minorities in the health professions. A report of the Sullivan Commission on diversity in the health care workforce.* Retrieved from http://health-equity.pitt.edu/40/

Tichy, N. (1997). *The leadership engine: How winning companies create leaders at all levels.* New York, NY: HarperCollins.

Tri-Council for Nursing. (2010). *Joint statement from the Tri-Council for Nursing on recent registered nurse supply and demand projections.* Retrieved from http://www.tricouncilfornursing.org/documents/JointStatementRecentRNSupplyDemandProjections.pdf

Ulrich, B., Buerhaus, P., Donelan, K., Norman, L., & Dittus, R. (2005). How RNs view the work environment: Results of a national survey of registered nurses. *Journal of Nursing Administration, 35*(9), 389–396.

Valiga, T., & Champagne, M. (2011). Creating the future of nursing education: Challenges and opportunities. In P. Cowen & S. Moorhead (Eds.), *Current issues in nursing* (pp. 75–83). St. Louis, MO: Mosby Elsevier.

Valente, S., & Bullough, V. (2004). Sexual harassment of nurses in the workplace. *Journal of Nursing Care Quality, 19*(3), 234–241.

Zimmerman, P. (2006). Who should provide nursing care? In P. Cowen & S. Moorhead (Eds.), *Current issues in nursing* (7th ed., pp. 324–331). St. Louis, MO: Mosby Elsevier.

Zuzelo, P. R., Gettis, C., Hansell, A. W., & Thomas, L. (2008). Describing the influence of technologies on registered nurses' work. *Clinical Nurse Specialist, 22*(3), 132–140.

Appendix A

American Nurses Association
Standards of Nursing Practice

Standards of Care (Use of the Nursing Process)

Standard 1 Assessment: The registered nurse collects comprehensive data pertinent to the healthcare consumer's health and/or the situation.

Standard 2 Diagnosis: The registered nurse analyzes the assessment data to determine the diagnoses or issues.

Standard 3 Outcomes identification: The registered nurse identifies expected outcomes for a plan individualized to the healthcare consumer or the situation.

Standard 4 Planning: The registered nurse develops a plan that prescribes strategies and alternatives to attain expected outcomes.

Standard 5 Implementation: The registered nurse implements the identified plan of care.

Standard 6 Evaluation: The registered nurse evaluates progress toward attainment of outcomes.

Standards of Professional Performance (Professional Behavior)

Standard 7 Ethics: The registered nurse practices ethically.

Standard 8 Education: The registered nurse attains knowledge and competence that reflects current nursing practice.

Standard 9 Evidence-based practice and research: The registered nurse integrates evidence and research findings into practice.

Standard 10 Quality of practice: The registered nurse contributes to quality nursing practice.

Standard 11 Communication: The registered nurse communicates effectively in all areas of practice.

Standard 12   Leadership: The registered nurse demonstrates leadership in the professional practice setting and profession.

Standard 13   Collaboration: The registered nurse collaborates with healthcare consumer, family, and others in the conduct of nursing practice.

Standard 14   Professional practice evaluation: The registered nurse evaluates her or his own nursing practice in relation to professional practice standards and guidelines, relevant statutes, rules, and regulations.

Standard 15   Resource utilization: The registered nurse utilizes appropriate resources to plan and provide nursing services that are safe, effective, and financially responsible.

Standard 16   Environmental health: The registered nurse practices in an environmentally safe and healthy manner.

Appendix B

American Nurses Association *Code of Ethics*

Provision 1   The nurse, in all professional relationships, practices with compassion and respect for the inherent dignity, worth, and uniqueness of every individual, unrestricted by conditions of social or economic status, personal attributes, or the nature of health problems.

Provision 2   The nurse's primary commitment is to the patient, whether an individual, family, group, or community.

Provision 3   The nurse promotes, advocates for, and strives to protect the health, safety, and rights of the patient.

Provision 4   The nurse is accountable and responsible for individual nursing practice and determines the appropriate delegation of tasks consistent with the nurse's obligation to provide optimum patient care.

Provision 5   The nurse owes the same duties to self as to others, including the responsibility to preserve integrity and safety, to maintain competence, and to continue personal and professional growth.

Provision 6   The nurse participates in establishing, maintaining, and improving healthcare environments and conditions of employment conducive to the provision of quality healthcare and consistent with the values of the profession through individual and collective action.

Provision 7   The nurse participates in the advancement of the profession through contributions to practice, education, administration, and knowledge development.

Provision 8   The nurse collaborates with other health professionals and the public in promoting community, national, and international efforts to meet health needs.

Provision 9　The profession of nursing, as represented by associations and their members, is responsible for articulating nursing values, for maintaining the integrity of the profession and its practice, and for shaping social policy.

The ANA *Code of Ethics with Interpretive Statements* is available in its entirety in print from the American Nurses Association and is also available in its entirety at www.nursingworld.org/MainMenuCategories/EthicsStandards/CodeofEthicsforNurses/Code-of-Ethics.pdf.

Glossary

5-year plan: A plan that has clear objectives and follows specific steps to meet those objectives while allowing for flexibility in adjusting to changing life circumstances.

Academic Center for Evidence-Based Nursing (ACE) Star Model of Knowledge Transformation: This model involves five steps: discovery, summary, translation, implementation, and evaluation.

Access to care: Living in rural areas has unique concerns regarding access to care. As finances influence the closing of many rural hospitals, more communities find themselves struggling to find primary care providers who will work in those areas.

Active euthanasia: Active euthanasia occurs when a person takes an action to end a life (including one's own life). Active euthanasia can include a lethal dose of medication, such as in physician-assisted suicide.

Administrative or regulatory law: The regulatory process is itself governed by statutory law called administrative procedure acts at both federal and state levels. These acts provide that before regulations can be adopted a published notice of the proposed rules and where they are available must occur. The published notice and availability of the proposed rules provide concerned persons with the opportunity to comment on and suggest changes to the rules before final adoption. When rules are adopted, they become administrative law within a set period of time. Thus, the process has three steps: (1) proposal of regulations, (2) consideration of proposed regulations, and (3) adoption of regulations with or without changes.

Advance directive: A written expression of a person's wishes about medical care, especially care during a terminal or critical illness.

Advanced beginner: In Benner's stage 2, the advanced beginner, the student is able to formulate principles that dictate action. For example, the advanced beginner would grasp the rationale behind why different medications require different injection techniques.

Advocacy: The nurse speaks for the patient or maintains the patient's rights in the face of the healthcare system. As the nurse–client relationship develops, the nurse needs professional knowledge to assist clients in their decision making. The nurse fills the role of advocate in the delivery of health care, intervening in crises of AIDS, homelessness, drug and alcohol abuse, teenage pregnancy, child and spouse abuse, and increasing health-care costs. A client advocate is a person who pleads the cause for clients' rights.

Age-related changes: Changes in cognition, vision, and hearing that occur as one ages. Research has demonstrated that teaching is not as effective if it does not accommodate for age-related cognitive and sensory changes.

AGREE instrument: A framework for determining the quality of guidelines for diagnoses, health promotion, treatments, or clinical interventions.

Alternative program: Alternative programs for nurses with drug and alcohol addictions exist. Nurses must qualify for the program.

***American Journal of Nursing* (AJN):** Mary Adelaide Nutting, Lavinia L. Dock, Sophia Palmer, and Mary E. Davis were instrumental in developing the first nursing journal, the *American Journal of Nursing* (*AJN*) in October of 1900. Through the ANA and the *AJN*, nurses then had a professional organization and a national journal with which to communicate with each other.

American Nurses Association (ANA): The ANA is the only full-service professional organization representing the nation's 2.9 million registered nurses (RNs) through its 54 constituent member associations. The ANA advances the nursing profession by fostering high standards of nursing practice, promoting the rights of nurses in the workplace, projecting a positive and realistic view of nursing, and lobbying the Congress and regulatory agencies on healthcare issues affecting nurses and the public.

Andragogy: Initially defined as "the art and science of helping adults learn," andragogy has taken on a broader meaning over the past 35 years and is currently used to refer to learner-focused education for people of all ages.

Assumptions: Assumptions describe concepts or connect two concepts and represent values, beliefs, or goals. When assumptions are challenged, they become propositions.

Asynchronous: Not occurring in real time.

Autonomy: Involves one's ability to self-rule and to generate personal decisions independently.

Barton, Clara: In 1882, Barton was able to convince Congress to ratify the Treaty of Geneva, thus becoming the founder of the American Red Cross.

Basic dignity: Intrinsic, or inherent, and dwells within all humans, with all humans being ascribed this moral worth.

Beliefs: Beliefs indicate what we value and often have a faith component. Three categories of beliefs include: existential, evaluative, and prescriptive/proscriptive beliefs.

Beneficence: Implies that nurses take actions to benefit patients and to facilitate their well-being.

Best interest standard: Based on the goal of the surrogate's doing what is best for the patient or what is in the best interest of the patient.

Bioethics: A specific domain of ethics that is focused on moral issues in the field of health care.

Black Death: During the Middle Ages, a series of horrible epidemics, including the Black Death or bubonic plague, ravaged the civilized world. In the 1300s, Europe, Asia, and Africa saw nearly half their populations lost to the bubonic plague.

Bolton, Frances Payne: This congressional representative from Ohio is credited with the founding of the Cadet Nurse Corps through the Bolton Act of 1945. By the end of World War II, more than 180,000 nursing students had been trained through this act, while advanced practice graduate nurses in psychiatry and public health nursing had received graduate education to increase the numbers of nurse educators.

Boundaries: In nursing, boundaries can be thought of in terms of appropriate professional behavior that serves to maintain trust between patients and nurses and to maintain nurses' good standing within their profession.

Breckenridge, Mary: Founder of the Frontier Nursing Service.

Brewster, Mary: A colleague of Lillian Wald, Brewster established the Henry Street Settlement in the same neighborhood in 1893. She quit medical school and devoted the remainder of her life to "visions of a better world" for the public's health.

Brown Report: *Nursing for the Future* or the Brown Report, authored by Esther Lucille Brown in 1948 and sponsored by the Russell Sage Foundation, was critical of the quality and structure of nursing schools in the United States. The Brown Report became the catalyst for the implementation of educational nursing program accreditation through the National League for Nursing.

Burnout: Occurs when nurses can no longer cope with the stresses and strains of professional nursing and choose to leave the profession to seek employment elsewhere.

Cadet Nurse Corps: World War II and the resulting severe shortage of nurses on the home front resulted in the development of the Cadet Nurse Corps.

Capitalistic society: Profit motivated. Even though we live in a capitalistic society, nursing in the United States has been protected against the details of healthcare finance.

Career management: A planned logical progression of one's professional life that includes clearly defined goals and objectives and a plan for achievement.

Case law: Established from court decisions, which might explain or interpret the other sources of law.

Case management: A current nursing model of nursing care delivery, case management relies on clinical pathways to evaluate care. The critical pathway refers to expected outcomes and interventions that the collaborative practice team establishes. The professional nurse is responsible for initiating and updating the plan of care, care map, or clinical pathway used to consistently guide and evaluate client care.

Case manager: Organizes patient care by major diagnoses or DRGs and focuses on specific time frames to achieve predetermined patient outcomes and contain costs. The case manager makes referrals to other healthcare providers and manages the quality of care.

Chadwick Report: Edwin Chadwick became a major figure in the development of the field of public health in Great Britain by drawing attention to the cost of the unsanitary conditions that shortened the life span of the laboring class and the threats to the wealth of Britain. One consequence of the report was the establishment of the first board of health, the General Board of Health for England, in 1848.

CINAHL: The authoritative resource for nursing and allied health professionals, students, educators, and researchers.

Civil law: The law of civil or private rights, as opposed to criminal law.

Clinical judgment: Use of the clinician's experience and knowledge in assessment, diagnosis, planning, intervention, and evaluation.

Clinical nurse leader (CNL): An advanced generalist role prepared at the master's level of education.

Clinical practice guidelines: Developed to guide clinical practice and represent an effort to put a large body of evidence into a manageable form.

Cochrane Library: The Cochrane Library is a collection of databases that contain high-quality, independent evidence to inform healthcare decision making.

Collaboration: To work jointly with others.

Collaborative critical pathway: Refers to expected outcomes and interventions that the collaborative practice team establishes, emphasizing the interdisciplinary collaboration of the critical pathway.

Collaborative practice: The purpose of collaboration is to achieve high-quality client care and client satisfaction. A collaborative framework with an interdisciplinary team can also limit costs as well as improve quality of care.

Comanagement: Comanagement and referral represent the highest level of collaboration, in which providers are responsible and accountable for their own aspects of care, and then patients are directed to other providers when the problem is beyond their expertise.

Communication, *Nurse of the Future Nursing Core Competencies*: The Nurse of the Future will interact effectively with patients, families, and colleagues, fostering mutual respect and shared decision making, to enhance patient satisfaction and health outcomes.

Competent: Benner's stage 3, competent, is characterized by the ability to analyze problems and prioritize. The nurse has a solid grasp of the rules and principles. The nurse at this stage has had experience in a variety of clinical situations and is able to draw on prior knowledge and experience.

Complementary and alternative medicine: Complementary medicine refers to an approach that combines conventional medicine with less conventional options, whereas alternative medicine is an approach used instead of conventional medicine.

Complex adaptive systems (CASs): A collection of individual agents that are free to act in ways not totally predictable and whose actions are interconnected so that one action changes the context for other agents or units.

Concept: A concept is a term or label that describes a phenomenon. The phenomenon described by a concept might be either empirical or abstract.

Concept mapping: In nursing, concept mapping is used to organize and link information about a patient's health problems so that the nurse can see relationships among a patient's problems and plan interventions that can address more than one problem.

Conceptual model: Defined as a set of concepts and statements that integrate the concepts into a meaningful configuration.

Confidentiality: To fulfill their social contract to provide nursing care, nurses must often gather sensitive information from patients. Thus, the nurse, along with other caregivers, has the obligation to keep healthcare information confidential. Privacy is the right of the patient. Confidentiality is the obligation of all healthcare providers.

Consultations: Obtaining the opinion of a specialist or other caregiver.

Consumerism: The concept of consumers having more control of their healthcare experiences.

Continuous quality improvement (CQI): A structured organizational process that involves personnel in planning and implementing the continuous flow of improvements in the provision of quality health care that meets or exceeds expectations.

Core values: Those values that are most important to us; the values that define who we are as human beings. In 1998, the American Association of Colleges of Nursing developed five core values to facilitate the development of professional nursing values. The core values embraced by the AACN are human dignity, integrity, autonomy, altruism, and social justice.

Critical pathway: Refers to expected outcomes and interventions that the collaborative practice team establishes.

Critical thinking: The ability to think in a systematic and logical manner, solve problems, make decisions, and establish priorities in the clinical setting. Critical thinking is the competent use of thinking skills and abilities to make sound clinical judgments and safe decisions.

Cultural competence: The ability to interact effectively with people of different cultures. Cultural competence comprises awareness of one's own worldviews, attitude toward cultural differences, knowledge of different cultural practices, and cross-cultural skills.

Databases: A collection of electronic data of individual records that are systematically organized, indexed, and cross-referenced. A database allows for the rapid collection, organization, manipulation, and analysis of data.

Deaconesses: Nursing was most influenced by Christianity with the beginning of deaconesses, or female servants, doing the work of God by ministering to the needs of others. This role of the deaconess in the church was considered a forward step in the development of nursing, and in the 1800s would strongly influence the young Florence Nightingale.

Delano, Jane A.: Director of nursing in the American Red Cross, she initiated a national publicity campaign to recruit young women to enter nurses' training.

Delegation: The process by which responsibility and authority for performing a certain task are transferred to another individual.

Deontology: Refers to actions that are duty based, not based on their rewards, happiness, or consequences. One of the most influential philosophers for the deontologic way of thinking was Immanuel Kant, a German philosopher from the 1700s.

Dignity: In general terms, a person has dignity if he or she is in a situation where his or her capabilities can be effectively applied.

Disaster preparedness: Plans designating response during an emergency and often coordinated by local, state, and federal groups. Firefighters, police officers, and healthcare professionals are part of response teams.

Dix, Dorothea Linde: A Boston schoolteacher, Dix became aware of the horrendous conditions in prisons and mental institutions. For the rest of her life, Dorothea Dix stood out as a tireless zealot for the humane treatment of the insane and imprisoned. She had exceptional savvy in dealing with legislators.

Dock, Lavinia Lloyd: Became a militant suffragist, linking women's roles as nurses to the emerging women's movement in the United States.

Doctor of Nursing Practice (DNP): This practice degree encompasses any form of nursing intervention that influences healthcare outcomes for individual patients, management of care for individuals and populations, administration of nursing and health organization, and the development and implementation of health policy. This practice degree is not the same as the research doctoral degree, and graduates are prepared to blend clinical, economic, organizational, and leadership skills and to use science in improving the direct care of patients, care of patient populations, and practice that supports patient care.

Durable power of attorney: The legal document with the most strength, this is a written directive in which a designated person is allowed to make either general or healthcare decisions for a patient.

EBSCO Publishing: An electronic journals service available to both academic and corporate subscribers. It aggregates access to electronic journals from various publishers.

Electronic health record: Represents multiple systems that are interfaced to share data and networked to support information management and communication within a healthcare organization.

Email: A method of composing, sending, receiving, and storing messages over electronic communication systems; the most common use of the Internet.

Environment: One of the four concepts of the metaparadigm of nursing; the environment within which the person exists.

ERIC: The Educational Resource Information Center is a national information system supported by the U.S. Department of Education, the National Library of Education, and the Office of Educational Research and Improvement. It provides access to information from journals included in the Current Index of Journals in Education and Resources in Education Index.

Ethic of care: Personal relationships and relationship responsibilities are emphasized in this ethic. Important concepts in this approach are compassion, empathy, sympathy, concern for others, and caring for others.

Ethical dilemma: An ethical dilemma is a situation in which an individual is compelled to make a choice between two actions that will affect the well-being of a sentient being and both actions can be reasonably justified as being good, neither action is readily justifiable as good, or the goodness of the actions is uncertain. One action must be chosen, thereby generating a quandary for the person or group who must make the choice.

Ethical principlism: A popular approach to ethics in health care. Involves using a set of ethical principles that are drawn from the common or widely shared conception of morality. The four principles that are most commonly used in bioethics are autonomy, beneficence, nonmaleficence, and justice.

Ethics: The study of ideal human behavior and ideal ways of being. The approaches to ethics and the meanings of ethically related concepts have varied over time among philosophers and ethicists. As a philosophical discipline of study, ethics is a systematic approach to understanding, analyzing, and distinguishing matters of right and wrong, good and bad, and admirable and deplorable as they exist along a continuum and as they relate to the well-being of and the relationships among sentient beings.

Evidence-based practice: Allows nurses to provide high-quality patient care based on research evidence and knowledge rather than tradition, myths, hunches, advice from peers, outdated textbooks, or even what the nurse learned in school 5, 10, or 15 years ago.

Evidence-based practice, *Nurse of the Future Nursing Core Competencies*: The Nurse of the Future will identify, evaluate, and use the best current evidence coupled with clinical expertise and consideration of patient's preferences, experience, and values to make practice decisions.

Expert: Benner's final stage, expert, has moved beyond a fixed set of rules. There is an internalized understanding grounded in a wealth of experience as well as depth of knowledge. The expert is always learning and always questioning using subjective and objective knowing.

Expert witness: Someone who has complex knowledge beyond the general knowledge of most people in the court or on the jury.

Feedback: Information that we receive from others about the impact of our behavior on them; it allows us to view ourselves from another's perspective.

Formation: A process that occurs over time that denotes the development of perceptual abilities, the ability to draw on knowledge and skilled know-how, and a way of being and acting in practice and in the world.

Frontier Nursing Service: The first organized midwifery service in the United States was the Frontier Nursing Service. It served isolated Appalachian communities on horseback until World War II.

Functional nursing: In the functional nursing system, client needs are divided into tasks, and each task is assigned to RNs, LPNs, or UAPs. This system is advantageous because each assigned caregiver becomes highly efficient in performing the assigned tasks.

Futile care: When a treatment has no physiologic benefit for a terminally ill person.

Gap between education and practice: Gap that looms larger as the healthcare setting continually changes as a result of advanced technology, knowledge explosion, shorter hospital stays, and rapid changes in disease management.

Gerogogy: The transferring of essential information that has been designed, modified, and adapted to accommodate for the physiologic and psychologic changes in elderly persons by taking into account the person's disease process, age-related changes, educational level, and motivation.

Global aging: In the post–World War II era, fertility rates have increased as death rates decreased in both developed and developing countries, leading to the aging of the global population at an unprecedented rate.

Goldmark Report: A significant report, known simply as The Goldmark Report, *Nursing and Nursing Education in the United States,* was released in 1922 and advocated the establishment of university schools of nursing to train nursing leaders.

Goodrich, Annie: First dean of the Army School of Nursing.

Greek era: The periods of Greek history in classical antiquity, lasting ca. 750 B.C. (the archaic period) to 146 B.C. (the Roman conquest). It is generally considered to be the seminal culture that provided the foundation of Western civilization. Time of Hippocrates, father of medicine. In Greek society, health was considered to result from a balance between mind and body.

Group discussions: Group discussions can assist nursing students in connecting clinical events or decisions with information obtained in the classroom. This form of cooperative learning occurs when groups work together to maximize their own and each other's learning.

Health: One of the four concepts of the metaparadigm of nursing; the health–illness continuum within which the person falls at the time of the interaction with the nurse.

Health Belief Model (HBM): This model was originally developed to predict the likelihood of a person following a recommended action and to understand the person's motivation and decision making regarding seeking health services.

Health literacy: The ability to read, understand, and act on health information.

Health Source: The Nursing/Academic Edition provides more than 550 scholarly full-text journals, including more than 450 peer-reviewed journals focusing on many medical disciplines, including nursing and allied health.

Healthcare delivery system: The healthcare delivery system has changed profoundly over the past several decades for several reasons. Population shifts (demographic changes), cultural diversity, the patterns of diseases, advances in technology, and economic changes have all affected the delivery of health care.

Henry Street Settlement: The Henry Street Settlement was an independent nursing service where Wald lived and worked. This later became the Visiting Nurse Association of New York City, which laid the foundation for the establishment of public health nursing in the United States.

HIPAA: The Health Insurance Portability and Accountability Act (HIPAA) was enacted by the U.S. Congress in 1996. It was intended to improve the efficiency and effectiveness of the healthcare system by encouraging the development of a health information system. Several areas are addressed by the act, including simplifying healthcare claims, developing standards for data transmission, and implementing privacy regulations.

Holistic care: Holistic care is a philosophical approach that emphasizes the uniqueness of the individual, in which interacting wholes are more important than the sum of each part. That is, the whole person is greater than merely each component part of the client: biophysical, psychological, social, and spiritual parts.

Idealism: Idealism contains these assumptions: The world is evolving. There is more than meets the eye. The social world is created. Reality is a conception perceived in the mind. Thinking is dynamic and constructive.

Incivility: Bullying that can include behaviors such as criticism, humiliation in front of others, undervalued efforts, and teasing.

Informatics and technology, *Nurse of the Future Nursing Core Competencies*: The Nurse of the Future will use information and technology to communicate, manage knowledge, mitigate error, and support decision making.

Informed consent: Mandates to the physician or independent healthcare practitioner the separate legal duty to disclose needed material facts in terms that patients can reasonably understand so that they can make an informed choice. Meaningful information must be disclosed even if the clinician does not believe that the information will be beneficial.

Integrity: Maintaining integrity involves acting consistently with personal values and the values of the profession. In a healthcare system often burdened with constraints and self-serving groups and organizations, threats to integrity can be a serious pitfall for nurses.

Interdisciplinary healthcare team: The interdisciplinary healthcare team can be especially effective in outpatient services. Here, the physician or nurse practitioner sees the client, and consultations are put into practice as needed. The teams deal with client-related problems and help the patients progress through the clinic and hospital efficiently.

Interpersonal role conflict: Can occur when individuals are working together and the expectations are incompatible and can affect interdisciplinary collaboration.

Iowa Model of Evidence-Based Practice: Resembles a decision-making tree that identifies either problem-focused or knowledge-focused triggers that initiate the process in the organization.

Jenner, Edward: In Britain, Edward Jenner discovered an effective method of vaccination against the dreaded smallpox virus in 1798.

Journaling: The process by which one sits down quietly on a daily or regular basis to think and record one's thoughts and ideas in writing. Keeping a journal of clinical experiences that were meaningful or troubling to you is a recommended way to help enhance and develop reasoning skills.

Justice: The fair distribution of benefits and burdens. In regard to principlism, justice most often refers to the distribution of scarce healthcare resources.

Klebs, Edwin: Edwin Klebs (1834–1913) proved the germ theory, that is, that germs are the causes of infectious diseases. This discovery of the bacterial origin of diseases can be considered the greatest achievement of the 1800s.

Koch, Robert: Robert Koch (1843–1910), a physician known for his research in anthrax, is regarded as the father of microbiology. By identifying the organism that caused cholera, *Vibrio cholerae*, he also demonstrated its transmission by water, food, and clothing.

Leadership, *Nurse of the Future Nursing Core Competencies*: The Nurse of the Future will influence the behavior of individuals within their environment in a way that will facilitate the establishment and acquisition/achievement of shared goals.

Learning domains: Identification of the learning domain reflects the type of learning desired as a result of the patient education process. Learning occurs in three domains: the cognitive, the psychomotor, and the affective.

Learning style: A particular method of interacting with, taking in, and processing information that allows an individual to learn. Learning styles are generally categorized as visual, auditory, or tactile/kinesthetic.

Licensure: The granting of permission to perform professional actions that may not be legally performed by persons who do not have this permission.

Life management: Entails determining what is truly important to you and making positive choices about how, where, and with whom you spend your precious hours.

Lifelong learning: A professional and personal approach that embraces opportunities to increase one's understanding and skills throughout one's career and life.

Lister, Joseph: Joseph Lister (1827–1912) was a physician who set out to decrease the mortality resulting from infection after surgery. He used

Pasteur's research to eventually arrive at a chemical antiseptic solution of carbolic acid for use in surgery. Widely regarded as the father of modern surgery, he practiced his antiseptic surgery with great results, and the Listerian principles of asepsis changed the way physicians and nurses practice to this day.

Listservs: A form of group email that provides an opportunity for people with similar interests to share information.

Living will: A formal legal document that provides written directions concerning medical care that is to be provided in specific circumstances.

Lobbyist: Person who develops expertise on proposed legislation and presents to legislators that information clearly and concisely.

Malpractice: The failure of a professional to use such care as a reasonably prudent member of the profession would use under similar circumstances, which leads to harm.

Managed care: Managed care is a market approach based on managed competition as a major strategy to contain healthcare costs and is still the dominant approach today.

Manager: All nurses are managers. They direct the work of professionals and nonprofessionals to achieve expected outcomes of care.

Medical directive: A medical directive is not a formal legal document but provides specific written instructions concerning the type of care and treatments that individuals want to receive if they become incapacitated.

MEDLINE: The largest biomedical literature database that provides authoritative medical information on medicine, nursing, dentistry, veterinary medicine, the healthcare system, and preclinical sciences.

Mental health: A level of cognitive or emotional well-being. The definition of mental health is affected by cultural differences, subjective assessments, and competing professional theories. As professional nurses experience the stresses that come with today's healthcare environment, they are obliged to assess their own mental health needs.

Mentoring: A developmental, empowering, and nurturing relationship that extends over time and in which mutual sharing, learning, and growth occur in an atmosphere of respect, collegiality, and affirmation.

Metaparadigm: The most global perspective of a discipline; acts as an encapsulating unit, or framework, within which the more restricted structures develop.

Mind mapping: The technique of arranging ideas and their interconnections visually; a popular brainstorming technique. It is used to generate, visualize, structure, and classify ideas and is used as an aid in organization, problem solving, and decision making.

Mission statement: A clear, concise statement of who you are and what you are about in life. It can be a powerful tool for helping you find meaning and give direction to your life.

Models of patient care delivery: Nurses are leaders and managers within various models of patient care delivery. The methods might differ significantly from one organization to another. The purpose of a nursing care delivery system is to provide a framework for nurses to deliver care to a specific group of patients.

Moral reasoning: Pertains to making decisions about how humans ought to be and act.

Moral right: The right to perform certain activities (1) because they conform to the accepted standards or ideas of a community (or of a law, or of God, or of conscience); or (2) because they will not harm, coerce, restrain, or infringe on the interests of others; or (3) because there are good rational arguments in support of the value of such activities.

Moral suffering: Can be experienced when nurses attempt to sort out their emotions when they find themselves in situations that are morally unsatisfactory or when forces beyond their control prevent them from influencing or changing these perceived unsatisfactory moral situations. Suffering can occur because nurses believe that situations must be changed to bring well-being to themselves and others or to alleviate the suffering of themselves and others.

Morals: Specific beliefs, behaviors, and ways of being based on personal judgments derived from one's ethics. One's morals are judged to be good or bad through systematic ethical analysis.

Multiculturalism: There is diversity among the members of the nursing profession in race, age, and socioeconomic backgrounds. However, the presence of this multiculturalism force can lead to people feeling threatened, especially if the culture within the profession does not encourage mutual respect and acceptance.

National Guideline Clearinghouse: Includes structured summaries containing information about each guideline, including comparisons of guidelines covering similar topics that show areas of similarity and differences; full text or links to full text; ordering details for full guidelines; annotated bibliographies on guideline development, evaluation, implementation, and structure; weekly email updates; and guideline archives.

Negligence: Defined as the failure to act as a reasonably prudent person would have acted in a specific situation.

Networking: The process by which you get to know people within your organization and within your profession.

Nightingale, Florence: Nightingale was identified as a true "angel of mercy," having reformed military health care in the Crimean War and having used her political savvy to forever change the way society views the health of the vulnerable, the poor, and the forgotten. She is perhaps one of the most written about women in history.

Nonmaleficence: The injunction to "do no harm" is often paired with beneficence, but a difference exists between the two principles. Beneficence requires taking action to benefit others, whereas nonmaleficence involves refraining from action that might harm others.

Nonvoluntary euthanasia: Occurs when persons are not able to express their decision about death.

Novice: Benner's model identifies the stages of novice, advanced beginner, competent, proficient, and expert that are based on the nurse's experience in practice. The first stage, novice, is characterized by a lack of knowledge and experience. In this stage, the facts, rules, and guidelines for practice are the focus. Rules for practice are context free, and the student's task is to acquire the knowledge and skills.

Nurse-managed centers: Also called nursing clinics and nurse practice arrangements, these healthcare delivery options are meeting needs in communities across the country. Based on the philosophy of primary care and education, nurses are offering vital services at a lower cost.

Nursing: (1) Attention to the full range of human experiences and responses to health and illness without restriction to a problem-focused orientation; (2) integration of objective data with an understanding of the subjective experience of the patient; (3) application of scientific knowledge to the processes of diagnosis and treatment; (4) provision of a caring relationship that facilitates health and healing; and (5) one of the four concepts of the metaparadigm of nursing; the nursing actions themselves.

Nursing ethics: Sometimes viewed as a subcategory of the broader domain of bioethics, just as medical ethics is a subcategory of bioethics. However, controversy continues about whether nursing has unique moral problems in professional practice.

Nursing faculty shortage: This shortage is limiting student capacity in nursing programs across the nation.

Nursing informatics (NI): The synthesis of computer science, information science, and nursing science in the organization and comprehension of data that directs nursing practice.

Nursing process: The nursing process is the tool by which all nurses can become equally proficient at critical thinking. The nursing process contains the following criteria: (1) assessment, (2) diagnosis, (3) planning, (4) implementation, and (5) evaluation.

Nursing shortage: Because of the growing complexity of health care, limited educational opportunities for nursing students, the aging of the population, and the overall growth of the population, a shortage of registered nurses has occurred and will continue to worsen. The current nursing shortage began in the year 2000 when there was an estimated supply of 1.89 million nurses and a projected demand of 2 million, or a 6% shortfall.

Nursing's Agenda for Health Care Reform: A demand for healthcare reform in the late 1980s. The nursing profession heralded the way in healthcare reform with an unprecedented collaboration of more than 75 nursing associations, led by the American Nurses Association and the National League for Nursing, in the publication of *Nursing's Agenda for Health Care Reform*.

Objectives: Specific measures that you will take to achieve your goal. Objectives should be specific and measurable, serving as milestones that mark your progress.

Osborne, Mary D.: Supervisor of public health nursing for the state of Mississippi from 1921 to 1946, Osborne had a vision for a collaboration with community nurses and granny midwives, who delivered 80% of the African American babies in Mississippi.

Palliative care: Providing comfort rather than curative measures for terminally ill patients.

Paradigm: The lens through which you see the world. Paradigms are also philosophical foundations that support our approaches to research.

Passive euthanasia: Occurs when a person allows another person to die by not acting to stop death or prolong life. An example of this type of euthanasia is withholding treatment that is necessary to prevent death at a point in time.

Pasteur, Louis: A French chemist, Pasteur first became interested in pathogenic organisms through his studies of the diseases of wine. He discovered if wine was heated to a temperature of 55–60°C, the process killed the microorganisms that spoiled wine. This discovery was critical to the wine industry's success in France. This process of pasteurization led Pasteur to investigate many fields and save many lives from contaminated milk and food.

Paternalism: Nurses might decide to act in ways that they believe are for a patient's "own good" rather than allowing patients to exercise their autonomy. The deliberate overriding of a patient's autonomy in this way is called paternalism.

Patient-centered care, *Nurse of the Future Nursing Core Competencies*: The Nurse of the Future will provide holistic care that recognizes an individual's preferences, values, and needs and respects the patient or designee as a full partner in providing compassionate, coordinated, age and culturally appropriate, safe and effective care.

Patient education: Any set of planned, educational activities designed to improve patients' health behaviors, health status, or both.

Patient Self-Determination Act: Legislation designed to facilitate the knowledge and use of advance directives.

Patient teaching: Activities aimed at improving knowledge are known as patient teaching.

PDAs: Personal digital assistants (PDAs) are handheld devices that have wireless connectivity and can synchronize data and information between the PDA and a computer. Use of the PDA is becoming widely popular in health care and nursing.

Performance improvement: Collaboration and evidence-based practice are key elements of successful quality programs, or performance improvement programs.

Person: One of the four concepts of the metaparadigm of nursing; the person receiving the nursing.

Personal dignity: Often mistakenly equated with autonomy; judging others and describing behaviors as dignified or undignified are of an evaluative nature.

Philosophy: The discipline concerned with questions of how one should live; what sorts of things exist and what are their essential natures; what counts as genuine knowledge; and what are the correct principles of reasoning. Philosophies set forth the general meaning of nursing and nursing phenomena through reasoning and the logical presentation of ideas. Philosophies are broad and address general ideas about nursing. Because of its breadth, nursing philosophy contributes to the discipline by providing direction, clarifying values, and forming a foundation for theory development.

Physician-assisted suicide: According to Oregon's Death with Dignity Act, "lethal medications, expressly prescribed by a physician for that purpose."

PICO: An acronym that assists in the formatting of clinical questions: P = Patient, Population, or Problem; I = Intervention or Exposure or Topic of Interest; C = Comparison or Alternate Intervention (if appropriate); O = Outcome. Using this format helps the nurse to ask pertinent clinical questions, focus on asking the right questions, and choose relevant guidelines.

Practitioner, caregiver, advocate, educator, leader, manager, collaborator, and researcher: Several of the roles of nurses.

Primary nursing care: The primary nursing care model of delivery was developed in the 1960s after team nursing first became popular and was designed to put the nurse back at the bedside. Primary nursing allows the nurse to provide care to a small number of clients for their entire stay. The nurse provides and is accountable for care, communicates with clients and their families and other healthcare providers, and performs discharge planning. The actual care is given by the primary RN or associate nurses (other RNs).

Privacy: The right of a person to be free from unwanted intrusion into the person's personal affairs.

Professionalism, *Nurse of the Future Nursing Core Competencies:* The Nurse of the Future will demonstrate accountability for the delivery of standard-based nursing care that is consistent with moral, altruistic, legal, ethical, regulatory, and humanistic principles.

Professional values: Beliefs or ideals that guide interactions with patients, colleagues, other professionals, and the public.

Proficient: Benner's stage 4 refers to the professional who is able to grasp the situation contextually and as a whole. Such nurses have a solid grasp of the norms as well as solid experiences that shed light on the variations from the norm. Incorporated into practice is the ability to test knowledge against situations that might not fit and to solve problems with alternative approaches.

Propositions: Propositions are statements that describe relationships among events, situations, or actions.

PsycINFO: Contains nearly 2 million citations and summaries of journal articles, book chapters, books, dissertations, and technical reports, all in the field of psychology.

Public speaking: By being a spokesperson for the organization, a nurse can increase his or her visibility dramatically. This a daunting task for many nurses who are otherwise fearless in their other professional activities.

Pure autonomy standard: Decisions made on behalf of an incompetent person based on decisions that the formerly competent person made.

Quality improvement: QI focuses on systems, processes, satisfaction, and cost outcomes, usually within a specific organization.

Quality improvement, *Nurse of the Future Nursing Core Competencies:* The Nurse of the Future uses data to monitor the outcomes of care processes, and uses improvement methods to design and test changes to continuously improve the quality and safety of healthcare systems.

Rathbone, William: A wealthy ship owner and philanthropist, Rathbone is credited with the establishment of the first visiting nurse service, which eventually evolved into district nursing in the community. He was so impressed with the private duty nursing care that his sick wife had received at home that he set out to develop a "district nursing service" in Liverpool, England.

Rational suicide: Self-slaying that is categorized as voluntary active euthanasia.

Readiness to learn: Patient's readiness or evidence of motivation to receive information at that particular time.

Realism: Realism contains these assumptions: The world is static. Seeing is believing. The social world is a given. Reality is physical and independent. Logical thinking is superior.

Referral: The practice of sending a patient to another practitioner for consultation or service.

Reflective thinking: The process of analyzing, making judgments, and drawing conclusions to create an understanding through one's experiences and knowledge and exploring potential alternatives.

Reformation: Religious changes during the Renaissance were to influence nursing perhaps more than any other aspect of society. During the Reformation, the monasteries were abolished. The effects on nursing were drastic: Monastic-affiliated institutions, including hospitals and schools, were closed, and orders of nuns, including nurses, were dissolved.

Research utilization: Involves the critical analysis and evaluation of research findings and then determining how these findings fit into clinical practice.

Respondeat superior: The doctrine that indicates the employer may also be responsible if the nurse was functioning in the employee role at the time of the incident.

Robb, Isabel Hampton: In 1896, she founded the Nurses' Associated Alumnae, which in 1911 officially became known as the American Nurses Association (ANA).

Role transition: The transition from the role of nursing student to the role of registered nurse is sometimes described in terms of reality shock. The experience of moving from the known role of student to the role of practicing professional is known as role transition shock.

Roman era: The periods of Roman history in classical antiquity, lasting ca. 146 B.C. (the Roman conquest of Greece) or 31 B.C. (defeat of Mark Antony by Augustus at the Battle of Actium) to ca. A.D. 476 (fall of the Roman Empire). Roman civilization is often grouped into classical antiquity with ancient Greece, a civilization that inspired much of the culture of ancient Rome. The development of policy, law, and protection of the public's health was an important precursor to our modern public health systems.

Rule of double effect: Usually defined narrowly in health care as the use of high doses of pain medication to lessen the chronic and intractable pain of terminally ill patients even if doing so hastens death.

Safety, *Nurse of the Future Nursing Core Competencies*: The Nurse of the Future will minimize risk of harm to patients and providers through both system effectiveness and individual performance.

Saint Vincent de Paul: In 1633, Saint Vincent de Paul founded the Sisters of Charity in France, an order of nuns who traveled from home to home visiting the sick.

Sanger, Margaret: Margaret Sanger worked as a nurse on the Lower East Side of New York City in 1912 with immigrant families. She was astonished to find widespread ignorance among these families about conception, pregnancy, and childbirth. After a horrifying experience with the death of a woman from a failed self-induced abortion, Sanger devoted her life to teaching women about birth control. A staunch activist in the early family planning movement, Sanger is credited with founding Planned Parenthood of America.

Scales, Jessie Sleet: Scales is considered the first African American public health nurse. Scales provided district nursing care to New York City's African American families and is credited with paving the way for African American nurses in the practice of community health.

Search engines: Search engines assist in finding specific topics on the Web by compiling a database of Internet sites.

Self-care: Acknowledging and meeting your own physical, psychological, social, and spiritual needs. It means caring for yourself before you care for others, not after you have tended to everyone else.

Self-efficacy: A person believes that he or she is capable of performing a behavior.

Shattuck Report: Lemuel Shattuck, a Boston bookseller and publisher who had an interest in public health, organized the American Statistical Society in 1839 and issued a census of Boston in 1845. Shattuck's census revealed high infant mortality rates and high overall population mortality rates. In his *Report of the Massachusetts Sanitary Commission* in 1850, Shattuck not only outlined his findings on the unsanitary conditions but made recommendations for public health reform. He also called for services for well-child care, school-age children's health, immunizations, mental health, health education for all, and health planning. The report was revolutionary in its scope and vision for public health.

Snow, John: John Snow, a prominent physician, is credited with being the first epidemiologist by demonstrating in 1854 that cholera rates were linked with water pump use in London.

Social justice: A virtue that guides us in creating those organized human interactions we call institutions. In turn, social institutions, when justly organized, provide us with access to what is good for the person, both individually and in our associations with others. Social justice also imposes on each of us a personal responsibility to work with others to design and continually perfect our institutions as tools for personal and social development.

Social learning theory: If a person believes that he or she is capable of performing a behavior (self-efficacy) and also believes that the behavior will lead to a desirable outcome, the person will be more likely to perform the behavior.

Social media: Internet-based applications that enable people to communicate and share resources and information.

Socialization: Professional socialization involves a process by which a person acquires the knowledge, skills, and sense of identity that are characteristic of a profession.

Standard of substituted judgment: Used to guide medical decisions that involve formerly competent patients who no longer have any decision-making capacity.

Statutory law: Consists of ever-changing rules and regulations created by the U.S. Congress, state legislators, local governments, and constitutional law. The statutes are the rights, privileges, or immunities secured and protected for each citizen by the U.S. Constitution.

Stereotypes: A standardized mental picture that is held in common by members of a group and that represents an oversimplified opinion, prejudiced attitude, or uncritical judgment. For example, Nightingale defined nursing as "female work." Nurses need to face the stereotypes present in our society and erase the lines that define us.

Success: Success in life can be defined as doing what you want, where you want, and with the people you want to do it with. This implies balance within the various arenas of your life: professional, personal, social, and spiritual.

Systems-based practice, *Nurse of the Future Nursing Core Competencies*: The Nurse of the Future will demonstrate an awareness of and responsiveness to the larger context of the healthcare system, and will demonstrate the ability to effectively call on microsystem resources to provide care that is of optimal quality and value.

Team nursing: The team nursing model of care is used in the United States most frequently in hospitals and in long-term and extended-care facilities. This arrangement evolved after the functional nursing of the 1940s. With this approach, the nursing staff is divided into teams, and total patient care is provided to a group of patients.

Teamwork and collaboration, *Nurse of the Future Nursing Core Competencies*: The Nurse of the Future will function effectively within nursing and interdisciplinary teams, fostering open communication, mutual respect, shared decision making, team learning, and development.

Telehealth: Using electronic communication for transmitting healthcare information such as health promotion, disease prevention, professional or lay education, diagnosis, or actual treatments to people located at a different geographical location.

Terminal sedation (TS): When a suffering patient is sedated to unconsciousness, usually through the ongoing administration of barbiturates or benzodiazepines. The patient then dies of dehydration, starvation, or some other intervening complication, as all other life-sustaining interventions are withheld.

Theory: A theory is an organized, coherent, and systematic articulation of a set of statements related to significant questions in a discipline that are communicated in a meaningful whole.

Tort: Refers to acts that result in harm to another.

Total patient care: As early as the 1920s, the first model of patient care delivery was total patient care. In this model, the RN has the responsibility for all aspects of care of the patient(s). The RN works directly with the client, other nursing staff, and physician in implementing a plan of care. The objective of total patient care is to have one nurse provide all care to the same patient(s) for the entire shift. Currently, this model is practiced in areas such as critical care units or postanesthesia recovery units, where a high level of expertise is required.

Tyler, Elizabeth: Lillian Wald hired African American nurse Elizabeth Tyler in 1906 as evidence of her commitment to cultural diversity. Although unable to visit white clients, Tyler made her own way by "finding" African American families who needed her service.

Unavoidable trust: Zaner's contention that patients, in most cases, have no option but to trust nurses and other healthcare professionals when the patient is at the point of needing care.

Utilitarianism: Contrasted with deontology, the ethical approach of utilitarianism is to promote the greatest good that is possible in situations (i.e., the greatest good for the greatest number).

Values: Refer to a group's or individual's evaluative judgments about what is good or what makes something desirable. Values refer to what the normative standard should be, not necessarily to how things actually are. Values are the principles and ideals that give meaning and direction to our social, personal, and professional life. Professional values are integral to moral reasoning. Values in nursing encompass appreciating what is important for both the profession and nurses personally, as well as what is important for patients.

Values clarification: The process of values clarification can occur in a group or individually and helps us understand who we are and what is most important to us. The outcome of values clarification is positive because the outcome is growth.

Violence: The exertion of physical force so as to injure or abuse. Objectives toward the prevention of violence and abuse are included in *Healthy People 2010*.

Virtues: *Arête* in Greek; refer to excellences of intellect or character.

Voluntary euthanasia: Occurs when persons with a sound mind authorize another person to take their life or to assist them in achieving death. Also, this type can include the taking of one's own life.

Wald, Lillian: A wealthy young woman with a great social conscience, Wald graduated from the New York Hospital School of Nursing in 1891 and is credited with creating the title "public health nurse."

Wholeness of character: Pertains to knowing the values of the nursing profession and one's own authentic moral values, integrating these two belief systems, and expressing them appropriately. Integrity is an important feature of wholeness of character.

Index